Contested Illnesses

Contested Illnesses

Citizens, Science,
and Health Social Movements

———

Edited by

Phil Brown
Rachel Morello-Frosch
Stephen Zavestoski
and the Contested Illnesses
Research Group

UNIVERSITY OF CALIFORNIA PRESS
Berkeley   Los Angeles   London

University of California Press, one of the most distinguished university
presses in the United States, enriches lives around the world by advancing scholarship in the humanities, social sciences, and natural sciences. Its
activities are supported by the UC Press Foundation and by philanthropic
contributions from individuals and institutions. For more information,
visit www.ucpress.edu.

University of California Press
Berkeley and Los Angeles, California
University of California Press, Ltd.
London, England

Library of Congress Cataloging-in-Publication Data

Brown, Phil.
    Contested illnesses : citizens, science, and health social movements /
Phil Brown, Rachel Morello-Frosch, Stephen Zavestoski, and the
Contested Illnesses Research Group.
        p. ;   cm.
    Includes bibliographical references and index.
    ISBN 978-0-520-27020-6 (cloth : alk. paper) — ISBN 978-0-520-27021-3
(pbk. : alk. paper)
        1. Environmental health.   2. Social medicine.   I. Morello-Frosch,
Rachel.   II. Zavestoski, Stephen.   III. Contested Illnesses Research
Group.   IV. Title.
    [DNLM: 1. Environmental Health.   2. Consumer Organizations.
3. Environmental Illness.   4. Social Change. WA 30.5]
    RA565.B76   2012
    362.1—dc23   2011025412

Manufactured in the United States of America

21 20 19 18 17 16 15 14 13 12
10 9 8 7 6 5 4 3 2 1

In keeping with a commitment to support environmentally responsible
and sustainable printing practices, UC Press has printed this book on
50-pound Enterprise, a 30% post-consumer-waste, recycled, deinked fiber
that is processed chlorine-free. It is acid-free and meets all ANSI/NISO
(Z 39.48) requirements.

CONTENTS

For additional appendixes, see www.ucpress.edu/go/contestedillnesses

ILLUSTRATIONS

FIGURES

TABLES

ACKNOWLEDGMENTS

This volume would not have come to fruition without the critical support of colleagues, family members, students, foundations, and government funding institutions.

Many grants from government, foundations, and universities over the last several years have made possible the research described in this book. We are grateful for the following support: Robert Wood Johnson Foundation Investigator Awards in Health Policy Research Program (grant number 036273); the National Science Foundation Program in Science, Technology, and Society (SES-9975518, SES-0401869, SES-0350691, SES-0450837, SES-0822724, and SES-09242441); the National Institute of Environmental Health Sciences (1 R25 ES013258-01, P42 ES013660-01); National Institute of Allergies and Infectious Diseases (T15 A149650-01); National Heart, Blood, and Lung Institute (T15 HL069792); UC Berkeley Center for Environmental Public Health Tracking, Cooperative Agreement number U50/CCU922409 with the Centers for Disease Control and Prevention; the California Air Resources Board (Grant Agreement number 04-308); US EPA Regional Applied Research Effort (RARE) grant (Cooperative Agreement number X3-83338901-1); the California Environmental Protection Agency; the California Wellness Foundation; the California Endowment; the Ford Foundation; and the Brown University Salomon Faculty Research Award Program.

Current and former members of the Contested Illnesses Research Group (CIRG)—including ourselves, the coauthors—contributed to the work described here. They include Crystal Adams, Carrie Alexandrowicz, Rebecca Gasior Altman, Mara Averick, David Ciplet, Alison Cohen, Alissa Cordner, Sarah Fort, Margaret Frye, Leah Greenblum, Angela Hackel, Elizabeth Hoover, Tania Jenkins,

Ellie Leonardsmith, Meadow Linder, Theo Luebke, Mercedes Lyson, Joshua Man-delbaum, Brian Mayer, Sabrina McCormick, Heleneke Mulder, Bindu Pannikar, Laura Senier, Ruth Simpson, Allison Waters, and Pamela Webster. In addition, this volume benefited greatly from research assistance by students, some of whom are also members of CIRG: Aracely Alicea, Benjamin Bregman, Annie Gjelsvik, Nathaniel James, Ilissa Lazar, Bindu Pannikar, Michelle Rome, Ruth Simpson, and Valerie Tran.

We have been privileged to collaborate with many different organizations, including Alliance for a Healthy Tomorrow, Alternatives for Community and Environment, the Bay Area Environmental Health Collaborative, the Boston Environmental Hazards Center, the Boston School Department, the Boston Urban Asthma Coalition, the Collaborative Initiative for Research Ethics and Environmental Health, Commonweal, Communities for a Better Environment, the Environmental Justice League of Rhode Island, the Environmental Neigh-borhood Awareness Committee of Tiverton, the International Union of Paint-ers and Allied Trades District Council Number 35, the Massachusetts Committee on Occupational Safety and Health, the New Jersey Work Environment Council, Silent Spring Institute, the Southern California Environmental Justice Collabora-tive, the Toxic Use Reduction Institute, and West Harlem Environmental Action.

We thank Kim Boekelheide, Richard Clapp, Peter Conrad, Elizabeth Cooksey, David Eifler, Steve Epstein, Adriane Genette, Ann Grodzins Gold, David Hess, Maren Klawiter, Sheldon Krimsky, Jim Mahoney, Kelly Moore, Kelly Pennell, Susan Proctor, Dianne Quigley, Madeleine Kangsen Scammell, and Sally Zierler for helpful readings of various chapters.

We are indebted to our editors at the University of California Press, including Jenny Wapner and director Lynne Withey, who both encouraged us to develop our book idea into a reality. Hannah Love, our editor throughout, was an enthu-siastic supporter and critical reader. Jacqueline Volin was an outstanding produc-tion editor, along with Erika Büky, whose meticulous copy editing ensured that our facts were straight and arguments clear. Thérèse Shere's indexing work has made the book more accessible to readers. For the beautiful art that graces our book cover, we thank San Francisco Bay Area mural artist Marta Ayala, who gave us permission to use a photograph of one of her Richmond works.

Finally, our partners, David Eifler, Ronnie Littenberg, and Marion Christ, patiently provided encouragement, support, essential critiques, and feedback. This book is dedicated to them.

ABBREVIATIONS

ACE	Alternatives for Community and Environment (Boston)
AChEi	acetylcholinesterase inhibitor
API	Academic Performance Index
BCA	Breast Cancer Action (San Francisco)
BPA	bisphenol-A
BUAC	Boston Urban Asthma Coalition
BVHP	Bayview–Hunters Point
CAA	Clean Air Act
Cal-EPA	California Environmental Protection Agency
CBE	Communities for a Better Environment (Oakland, CA)
CBEDS	California Basic Educational Data System
CBOs	community-based organizations
CBPR	community-based participatory research
CDC	Centers for Disease Control and Prevention
CERCLA	Comprehensive Environmental Response, Compensation, and Liability Act
CFS	chronic fatigue syndrome
CHEJ	Center for Health, Environment, and Justice (Falls Church, VA)
CIRG	Contested Illnesses Research Group
CITI	Collaborative Institutional Training Initiative
COAL	Communities Organized against Asthma and Lead (Houston, TX)
COSH	Committee(s) on Occupational Safety, and Health
CSA	citizen-science alliance
DEET	N,N-diethyl-m-toluamide

DEP	dominant epidemiological paradigm
DoD	Department of Defense
DTSC	Department of Toxic Substances Control
EBCM	environmental breast cancer movement
ECHO	Environmentally Compromised Home Ownership program
EDCs	endocrine-disrupting compounds
EHM	embodied health movement
EJ	environmental justice
EJLRI	Environmental Justice League of Rhode Island
ENACT	Environmental Neighborhood Awareness Committee of Tiverton (RI)
EPA	Environmental Protection Agency
EPP	environmentally preferable products
EWG	Environmental Working Group (Washington, DC)
FACE	For a Cleaner Environment (Woburn, MA)
GAO	General Accounting Office
GASP	Groups against Smokers' Pollution
GWV	Gulf War Veteran(s)
HAP	hazardous air pollutant
HES	Household Exposure Study
HHS	US Department of Health and Human Services
HSM	health social movement
HUD	US Department of Housing and Urban Development
IOM	Institute of Medicine
IRB	institutional review board
LAUSD	Los Angeles Unified School District
LIBCSP	Long Island Breast Cancer Study Project
MassCOSH	Massachusetts Committee on Occupational Safety and Health
MBTA	Massachusetts Bay Transit Authority
MTA	Metropolitan Transit Authority (New York)
NBCC	National Breast Cancer Coalition (Washington, DC)
NCI	National Cancer Institute
NIEHS	National Institute of Environmental Health Sciences
NIH	National Institutes of Health
OHRP	Office for Human Research Protection
PAH	polycyclic aromatic hydrocarbon
PB	pyridostigmine bromide
PBDE	polybrominated diphenyl ether
PCB	polychlorinated biphenyl
PCE	perchlorethylene
PEJEF	Providence Environmental Justice Education Forum

PERC	perchlorate
PFOA	perfluorooctanoate
PhilaPOSH	Philadelphia Project for Occupational Safety and Health
PTSD	post-traumatic stress disorder
RAC	Research Advisory Committee on Gulf War Veterans' Illnesses
RaDAR	Research and Data Access Review
REEP	Roxbury Environmental Empowerment Project
RIDEM	Rhode Island Department of Environmental Management
RILS	Rhode Island Legal Services
SMO	social movement organization
SRP	Superfund Research Program
TCE	trichloroethylene
TRI	Toxic Release Inventory
TSCA	Toxics Substances Control Act
TURA	Toxic Use Reduction Act
TURI	Toxics Use Reduction Institute
TURN	Toxics Use Reduction Networking
US EPA	US Environmental Protection Agency
USPSTF	US Preventive Services Task Force
VA	Veterans Administration
WE ACT	West Harlem Environmental Action (NY)
WEC	Work Environment Council (Trenton, NJ)
WRWC	Woonasquatucket River Watershed Council (RI)

PART ONE

Setting the Stage

Introduction, Theory, Methods

Introduction

Environmental Justice and Contested Illnesses

Rachel Morello-Frosch, Phil Brown, and Stephen Zavestoski

Hazards are produced by business operations, to be sure, but they are defined and evaluated socially—in the mass media, in the experts' debate, in the jungle of interpretations and jurisdictions, in courts or with strategic-intellectual dodges, in a milieu of contexts.

—ULRICH BECK, *RISK SOCIETY*, 1992

As mirror and conscience of society, sociology must define, promote, and inform public debate about deepening class and racial inequalities, new gender regimes, environmental degradation, market fundamentalism, state and non-state violence. I believe that the world needs public sociology— a sociology that transcends the academy—more than ever. Our potential publics are multiple, ranging from media audiences to policy makers, from silenced minorities to social movements. They are local, global, and national.

—MICHAEL BURAWOY, "2004 PRESIDENTIAL ADDRESS: FOR PUBLIC SOCIOLOGY," 2005

During the summer of 2008, community members in Richmond, California, filed out of a packed and raucous city council meeting after being handed a major setback. Despite Herculean organizing efforts and passionate testimony by fence-line neighbors,[1] council members had voted to approve a conditional-use permit allowing the Chevron oil refinery to increase its production capacity by refining lower-grade crude oil with a higher sulfur content, resulting in increased emissions of harmful sulfur dioxide, sulfates, and metals (Jones 2008; Baker 2007). The Richmond Chevron refinery is one of the nation's largest, covering 2,900 acres, employing a thousand workers, and processing more than 240,000 barrels of crude oil daily into gasoline, jet fuel, diesel, and lubricants (Chevron Corporation 2009a, 2009b). At the meeting, community members presented scientific data from an

NIH-funded household exposure study conducted collaboratively by an independent research institute, two major universities, and a regional environmental justice organization. The data showed that refinery activities were adversely affecting indoor and outdoor air quality and that the refinery should reduce emissions, not increase them. After the meeting, one of the scientists spoke with a community organizer about whether science could play a productive role in localized, high-stakes policy decisions such as the one that had just unfolded. The organizer's assessment illuminates the potential, the limitations, and the contested role of science in struggles for environmental health and justice: "Science has its limitations, but it develops strong advocates—people can speak for themselves. The data generated supports the claims, experiences, and demands that the community members bring to the podium in policy settings. Community members can say, 'I know this because my home was tested and all these chemicals were found in my house!'"

As decisions about social policy and environmental regulation in the United States, are increasingly shaped by scientific and technocratic discourse, some communities and most industry stakeholders have used their own data and challenged scientific evidence to advance their interests. Yet the insistence on "better" science in decision making often reinforces dominant political and socioeconomic systems by slowing down policy making, precluding precautionary action, and ensuring regulatory paralysis through (over)analysis. Through this scientization of decision making, debates regarding the costs, benefits, and potential health and societal risks of new technologies and industrial production may be dominated by experts who work to ensure that battles over policy remain "objective" and divorced from their socioeconomic and political contexts. This outcome is achieved in three ways. First, questions are posed in scientific terms that may be impossible to answer scientifically, because of uncertainties in the data or the impracticality of carrying out a study. Second, political and moral questions are inappropriately framed in scientific terms, thereby limiting public participation (Weinberg 1972). Third, the scientization of decision making delegitimizes those questions that may not be amenable to scientific analysis. For example, racial, class, and transgenerational inequalities in environmental hazard exposures have been largely downplayed or ignored in the regulatory arena. All of these processes exclude the public from important policy debates and diminish public capacity to participate in the production of scientific knowledge itself.

Scientization is closely related to the perennial debate over what counts as science and what lies outside the scientific realm. This boundary is highly contested, because different actors struggle over the resources and authority associated with science. Scientists and nonscientists alike engage in what sociologists call *boundary work*, the active construction and contestation of the legitimacy, authority, and resources associated with the scientific enterprise (Gieryn 1983, 1999). From this boundary-work perspective, debates over scientific authority in policy making result from efforts by scientists to expand and legitimize their authority and by policy makers to use scientific authority to justify their regulatory decisions. These types of boundary work can exclude public voices from the decision-making process.

For nearly four decades, a class of social movements known as health social movements (HSMs) has challenged political power and scientific and professional authority. Examples include struggles to improve the quality of and access to health care (e.g., health insurance reform and advocacy of a single-payer health system); to eliminate persistent health inequalities based on race, ethnicity, gender, class, or sexuality (e.g., the women's health movement); and to push public health and medical institutions to address fundamental causes of disease and disability by reshaping scientific inquiry on etiology, diagnosis, treatment, and prevention (e.g., the HIV/AIDS and breast cancer movements). Historically, the emergence of HSMs focused on contested illnesses has involved scientific disputes and extensive public debates over the definition, causes, treatment, and prevention of disease. Among these, HIV/AIDS, breast cancer, and asthma HSMs have been central to promoting social and policy change; breaking new paths of scientific inquiry; and bringing attention to the politics of public health and prevention in the United States (Epstein 1996; Ferguson and Kasper 2000; Brown et al. 2004; Corburn 2005; Morello-Frosch et al. 2006). Indeed, HSMs have demonstrated that scientific knowledge is "coproduced" as government, industry, community advocates, and academic researchers all generate different forms of expert knowledge and scientific data that drive regulatory science and influence all parties (Jasanoff 2005). Furthermore, contested illness struggles highlight how regulatory science integrates scientific data and analysis with "large doses of social and political judgment" because the issues involve scientific uncertainty and contestation (Jasanoff 1990, 229; Jasanoff 1987). In short, health social movements shape and reshape science, and science in turn shapes and reshapes health social movements.

Despite the existence of a significant body of research on health social movements, the field of contested illnesses is still in its infancy. Methods for studying HSMs tend to be limited to deep ethnographic case studies of single movements or organizations. Only recently have scholars begun to examine more deeply the forces that give rise to HSMs and cross-movement coalitions focused on contested illnesses and policy goals. Moreover, little attention has been given to the collective influence that HSMs have had on scientific fact-making in public health, public policy, and regulation. This book addresses these gaps by discussing interdisciplinary research conducted by the Contested Illnesses Research Group (CIRG) on how contested illness struggles play out in three realms: the collective illness experience and movement building; scientific fact-making in public health and medical science; and policy making and regulation. We argue that the social movements emerging from contested illnesses have been catalyzed by three social forces: growing public awareness about the limited ability of medical science to solve persistent health problems that are socially and economically mediated, the rise of bioethical dilemmas in scientific knowledge production, and the collective drive to enhance democratic participation in the scientific enterprise. By using science to democratize knowledge production, contested illness struggles engage in effective policy advocacy, challenge aspects of the political economy, and transform traditional assumptions and scientific lines of inquiry regarding disease causation and prevention.

CONTESTED ILLNESSES IN CONTEXT

Recent contested illness struggles have moved into the realms of environmental and ecological health, as mounting scientific evidence has linked environmental and human well-being (Colborn, Dumanoski, and Myers 1996; Schettler et al. 1999). Disturbing trends in human health statistics, such as declining sperm counts, rising rates of fertility problems in young women, and increasing rates of breast, testicular, and prostate cancers suggest environmental causes (Schwartz and Woodruff 2008). The prevalence of asthma and certain neurological problems in children also appear to be on the rise (Beasley et al. 2000; Gurney et al. 2003; Newschaffer et al. 2005; Holguin 2008). Although environmental links to human disease remain hotly contested, scientific evidence strongly suggests that increasing and ubiquitous chemical exposure where we live, work, and play may partially explain these trends (Schettler et al. 1999; Landrigan et al. 2002; Grandjean and Landrigan 2006; Wilson and Schwarzman 2009). Since World War II, chemical production in the United States has increased more than twentyfold. "In 2006, more than 34 million metric tons of chemical substances were produced in, or imported into, the United States each day" (Schwarzman and Wilson 2009, 1065), and the number of chemicals registered for commercial use in the United States has increased by more than 30 percent since 1979 (Schwartz and Woodruff 2008). Many of these chemicals are showing up in our air, water, food, ecosystems, and body tissues (Morello-Frosch et al. 2009a).

For over a decade, the CIRG has focused on social movements dealing with environmental health. Its members represent the disciplines of environmental and medical sociology, science studies, environmental health science, epidemiology, and medical and environmental anthropology. (For details on the CIRG's history, see Senier et al. 2006.) With support from the National Science Foundation and the Robert Wood Johnson Foundation, the CIRG initially sought to address the lack of knowledge on health social movements related to contested illnesses and to improve understanding about the role of these struggles in reshaping scientific inquiry and pushing for policy change. Our first case studies entailed disease controversies with potential environmental links, including asthma, breast cancer, and Gulf War illness. Our work centered on understanding stakeholder struggles related to the underlying causes of these diseases—including, in the case of Gulf War syndrome, disputes over whether the veterans' physical and mental symptoms were real. Over time our analytical gaze has broadened to examine contested illnesses in domestic and global contexts and specific controversies related to medical and environmental health science, the politics of public health prevention, and regulatory decision making.

This shift has required us to expand the scope of the health social movements that we examine and rethink our ethnographic methods for studying these struggles. CIRG has moved beyond *studying* scientific controversies to *engaging directly* in the environmental health and science enterprise using community-based participatory research (CBPR). One key premise of CBPR is that involving the communities that experience hazardous exposures and diseases can promote new lines of inquiry and analytical techniques. Further, CBPR allows substantive community participation in the research process, including formulating research questions, collecting data, and disseminating results to diverse constituencies and the scientific community (Israel et al. 1998; Minkler and Wallerstein 2003). In pursuit of this objective, CIRG began to strengthen the links between its ethnographic and scientific work and the environmental policy and regulatory goals of its community collaborators.

TYING RESEARCH TO POLICY

By collaborating with organizations that contest traditional approaches to regulatory science and environmental health policy making, we positioned ourselves to explore scientific, ethical, and political challenges in three realms: doing science, interpreting science, and acting on science. *Doing* science involves assessing how scientists (and sometimes their community collaborators) choose research topics, conduct research, collect data, and manage their relations with funding institutions and support organizations. It also incorporates the study of how government and nongovernment organizations shape the funding and directions of scientific inquiry. *Interpreting* science involves examining the ways scientists make sense of data, assess how study results fit with existing bodies of knowledge, and develop qualitative and quantitative criteria for standards of proof. *Acting* on science relates to advocacy and organizing; it also encompasses the dissemination of new scientific results through peer review, the media, government agencies, and the general public in order to gain the support of scientific colleagues and decision makers to improve policy making. This triad model uncovers complex paradigm shifts in scientific and community knowledge production by integrating community and expert knowledge and qualitative and quantitative methods (Brown et al. 2006).

CIRG's decision to collaborate on scientific work and policy advocacy with some of the groups we were studying may seem unconventional. Yet this form of public engagement has deep roots in both public health (Gottlieb 2005; Corburn 2007) and sociology (ASA 2005). CIRG's transition from observer to participant-observer has enabled us to examine contested illnesses by assessing the effectiveness of different scientific methods for answering regulatory and policy questions (e.g., assessment and reduction of exposure to pollutants versus epidemiologic studies searching for definitive links between pollution and disease). We also moved from observer to participant status by engaging in the politics of regulatory science with diverse constituencies at multiple sites (e.g., sites of industrial production, sites of household product consumption, and sites of chemical persistence in environmental justice communities) (Altman 2008).

Our collaboration on a scientific project with community organizations was initially motivated by our study of the environmental breast cancer movements in Massachusetts and the San Francisco Bay Area and our long-term collaborative relationships with environmental justice advocates in California. This CBPR project entailed a partnership among three entities: CIRG; Silent Spring Institute, a research institute that examines links between women's health and the environment; and Communities for a Better Environment (CBE), an organization that combines science, litigation, policy advocacy, and community organizing to address environmental justice in California. With funding from the National Institute of Environmental Health Sciences (NIEHS) Environmental Justice Grants Program, our collaborative launched the Northern California Household Exposure Study in neighborhoods bordering an oil refinery and major transportation corridors in Richmond and in a comparison community, Bolinas, in rural Marin County. The project brought together the breast cancer advocacy and environmental justice communities by conducting a household exposure study that measured endocrine-disrupting compounds (EDCs) and other contaminants in household dust, indoor air, and outdoor air. The chemicals of interest to environmental justice advocates included urban air pollutants, industrial chemicals, and pesticides to which low-income minority populations are disproportionately exposed (Morello-Frosch and Shenassa 2006). Some of these compounds have also been linked to asthma, premature puberty, obesity, and cognitive development problems (Gold et al. 2005; Carpenter 2008; Holguin 2008). EDCs from sources ranging from consumer products to industrial processes are also a central concern for breast cancer activists, because many EDCs mimic the human hormone estrogen, a known risk factor for breast cancer (Brody et al. 2007b; Rudel et al. 2007). EDCs are also emerging as a health equity concern because of the disproportionately high breast cancer mortality among African American and poor women (still largely unexplained), as well as rising rates of breast cancer among some immigrant groups (Deapen et al. 2002; American Cancer Society 2007; Baquet et al. 2008).

Both breast cancer and environmental justice advocates have sought to reshape scientific approaches in ways that highlight potential causes of disease and suggest opportunities to reduce chemical exposures and safeguard community health. Our group chose to conduct an exposure study, because an epidemiologic breast cancer study within Richmond would not have been informative given the community's small size and the lack of data on relevant historical chemical exposures (Brody et al. 2009). An exposure study of potentially hazardous compounds can assess the extent of a pollution problem and inform action to reduce exposures. Moreover, exposure studies are not as resource-intensive and are more conducive to an academic and community partnership incorporating collaborative design of study protocols, data interpretation, and dissemination of results.

To decide how to collect data that would advance the shared goals of the three project partners, we conducted a year-long deliberative process. This entailed gathering information on community health concerns through community meetings; building on CBE's relationships with public officials in Richmond to gain support for our work; and convening an advisory council of neighborhood activists, breast cancer and biomonitoring activists, a state health official, an environmental justice advocate, and an outside academic researcher. Using the results of this input, we designed research to assess the cumulative exposures and specific sources of indoor pollution originating from outdoor industrial emissions, transportation sources, and consumer products. CBE staff were equipped and trained to conduct interviews and collect air and dust samples that were subsequently analyzed for industrial and traffic-related pollutants, such as particulates, metals, polycyclic aromatic hydrocarbons (PAHs), ammonia, and sulfates, and also for compounds found in consumer products, such as pesticides, flame retardants, phthalates, and phenols.

CIRG's experience with the Northern California Household Exposure Study demonstrates how joint community and academic production of environmental health science can enhance the rigor, relevance, and reach of scientific research projects. The scientific rigor of the study was ensured through collective discussion and negotiation of study design issues such as choosing study sites, recruiting study participants, finalizing the list of chemicals for analysis, and developing protocols for reporting study results. For example, CBE encouraged the study team to collect a subset of air and dust samples from a community that did not have significant outdoor industrial and transportation source emissions, so that these results could be compared to those from Richmond. As a result, we added Bolinas as a comparison site. Similarly, the relevance of the study was bolstered through the development of bilingual (Spanish and English) graphic displays to communicate aggregate and individual sampling results for dissemination to individuals and at community meetings. This effort helped to ensure that study results were transparent and scientifically valid, conveyed uncertainties, and elucidated strategies for exposure reduction. Finally, CBE's engagement in the study helped us to reach broader audiences and thus apply scientific results to making better decisions about land use. For example, scientists and CBE trained community residents to effectively present scientific data at community meetings and to testify before regulatory and policy forums.

Our experience with the Household Exposure Study and other CBPR projects has taught us that collaborative enterprises encourage all partners to consider the political and moral contexts that shape how we do, interpret, and act on science. As this book demonstrates, linking environmental health research with organizing and policy applications not only improves the scientific enterprise but also ensures that diverse groups can use good science to protect community health, push for innovation in scientific methods, and forge new paths of inquiry.

OVERVIEW OF CHAPTERS

This book is organized into three parts. Part 1 provides a theoretical framework and overview of CIRG's methods for examining contested illnesses. Part 2 presents several scientific and ethnographic case studies that represent the trajectory of CIRG's work. Part 3 explores policy applications of this work.

Chapter 2 revisits and updates some of CIRG's early theoretical work on embodied health movements (EHMs). EHMs are a relatively new subset of health social movements that challenge science and medicine on all aspects of contested illnesses. They introduce the biological body into social movements in compelling ways, using the embodied experience of illness to counter the authority of established institutional actors. In this way, EHMs elucidate the political economy of health and disease to shift intervention strategies upstream, beyond treatment and toward prevention. Very often, EHMs simultaneously challenge and collaborate with researchers and health professionals to pursue new paths of inquiry about the fundamental causes of disease, including social and environmental factors. These activities lead to a shift in what we term the dominant epidemiological paradigm (DEP) of disease causation.

Chapter 3 grounds our current work by examining qualitative methods used by various environmental health scholars. It further addresses issues of reflexivity: the researcher's impact on the field and the field's impact on the researcher. Chapter 3 demonstrates that qualitative methods are important instruments that allow community narratives to be constructed and shared. Furthermore, they provide social scientists with an opportunity to contribute to community activism and advocacy.

Chapter 4 proposes a new approach to the ethnography of contested illnesses that is multisited and focused on policy. Our field-analysis method situates social movements within social and institutional worlds that include diverse allies and coalition partners, some with conflicting perspectives. These may include government, academic, scientific, and civic organizations. What we call policy ethnography employs field analysis as one analytical tool. It explores the spaces and boundaries between science, policy, and civil society. Specifically, policy ethnography combines traditional interviews, content analysis (of government and organizational documents and media), and participant observation with historical analysis of movement trajectories, evaluation of current policy strategies, assessment of political contexts and opportunities, and the evaluation and use of scientific evidence. Most important, policy ethnography assumes a policy goal. In some cases, those carrying out policy ethnography are themselves actors in the policy realm.

In part 2, chapter 5 discusses a scientific analysis conducted by the Southern California Environmental Justice Collaborative. This community-based participatory research project, focusing on environmental health in Los Angeles schools, used secondary data analysis to answer scientific questions that informed policy advocacy and the organizing strategies of community partners. The chapter presents quantitative results from the analysis on environmental inequality in exposure to ambient-air toxics and associated health risks among schoolchildren. It examines the implications of this work for regional and state policy and the possibility of better application of the precautionary principle to issues of environmental justice.

Chapter 6 revisits and updates our analysis of the contested terrain of Gulf War illnesses. We examine the dramatic shifts in scientific and public controversies over myriad symptoms reported by veterans of the 1991 Gulf War. We begin by describing illness associated with the Gulf War, the sources of conflict, and the scientific complexity of its definition and etiology. We initially expected to find strong evidence for environmental links to this collection of debilitating symptoms and conditions but found a lack of scientific data supporting that perspective. Indeed, early theories of Gulf War illnesses centered on stress as the dominant cause. The dominant epidemiological paradigm now attributes the illness to contextual stress as well as chemical exposure. This paradigm shift culminated in a recent federal report concluding that "scientific evidence leaves no question that Gulf War Illness is a real condition with real causes and serious consequences for affected veterans" (RAC 2008, 5).

Chapter 7 updates our earlier examination of the politics and embodied health movement strategies of environmental justice advocates working on asthma issues: Alternatives for Community and Environment (ACE), based in the Roxbury area of Boston, and West Harlem Environmental Action (WE ACT), based in New York City. Here we demonstrate how asthma is transformed from a disease affecting an individual to a politicized collective illness experience. Community-based environmental justice organizations link asthma with the social determinants of their health, such as discrimination and social inequality.

Chapter 8 examines Cape Cod residents' discovery of and response to pollution exposures inside their homes and bodies. This chapter shifts the focus to embodied experiences other than the manifestation of potential disease and symptoms.

We demonstrate that science—not just the direct experience of environmental problems—shapes participants' embodied health experiences. Until recently, most work on environmental pollution has focused on measuring chemicals in air, water, and soil. However, advances in exposure assessment science have led to the analysis of more intimate spaces in people's homes and body tissues. This chapter highlights how science influences people's discovery and understanding of environmental health threats. It suggests future opportunities for social scientists to expand their examination of contested illnesses by characterizing how exposure experiences vary and are mediated by environmental science.

Chapter 9 revisits our earlier investigations of the environmental breast cancer movement (EBCM) in Massachusetts; Long Island, New York; and the San Francisco Bay Area. Our research began with an in-depth study of one organization dealing with environmental links to breast cancer: Silent Spring Institute in Massachusetts. However, it soon became apparent that there was a broader environmental breast cancer movement that was directly challenging the traditional medical focus on individual-level factors associated with disease (e.g., diet, physical activity, and genetics) and advancing a new epidemiological paradigm centered on environmental causes. We describe the framework, history, and strategies of the environmental breast cancer movement, demonstrating the importance of understanding the fluidity of social-movement actors and allowing us to develop the concept of a "boundary movement." Boundary movements straddle the scientific and nonscientific realms, blur distinctions between laypeople and experts, and connect activist groups with nonactivist reform agents like public health officials. These movement sometimes employ "boundary objects" that have different meanings for diverse parties: for example, an air-quality monitor may represent an official data-gathering device for a government agency but a triumph of organizing success for a community group.

In part 3, chapters 10 and 11 provide two case studies that investigate the potential and pitfalls of cross-movement coalitions between labor advocates and environmentalists. Scholars have written extensively about cases in which such "blue-green" coalitions have overcome class tensions that seemingly force workers to choose between job security and occupational or environmental health. Our first case study (in chapter 10) examines a successful coalition that worked to replace potentially hazardous cleaning products used in Boston public schools with safer alternatives. This coalition succeeded in part through the role of bridge builders who, through application of the precautionary principle, were able to unify community and environmental health advocates, labor activists, labor unionists, and school administrators to eliminate the use of toxic chemicals.

Chapter 11 examines another labor and environmental health coalition, the New Jersey Work Environment Council. Again, a strategic cross-movement frame emphasizing environmental health and human rights helped the coalition achieve its goal of establishing reporting requirements for industry chemical use. Its campaign culminated in the passage of the most sweeping right-to-know laws in the United States. However, this cross-movement coalition experienced significant political challenges when some members attempted to expand the discursive frame and policy goals from the right to know to the right to act.

Chapter 12 discusses a case study of the Brown University Superfund Research Program, in which academic researchers and state agency personnel collaborated with community activists in developing legislation to give temporary financial relief to residents of a contaminated neighborhood while they awaited cleanup. Relationships between stakeholders in cases involving contaminated sites are often contentious, in part because biomedical and engineering scientists are not trained to recognize and address the social problems that accompany the environmental hazards. By creating opportunities for cooperation, outreach efforts that make the research results more accessible can begin to repair trust among stakeholders and thus may pave the way for speedier site cleanup and reuse. This case study also shows how the inclusion of social scientists in a research translation and outreach program can contribute to a broader understanding of the social and political contexts that shape interactions between professionals and affected communities.

Chapter 13 explores the ethical and scientific challenges of communicating results to communities and study participants in biomonitoring studies, which measure the presence and concentrations of chemicals and their metabolites in human tissues. Technological advances have made biomonitoring studies more common, but often scientists are faced with dilemmas regarding whether and how to report results to participants when the health implications of chemical exposures are not well understood. We identify three frameworks for reporting such data: traditional clinical ethics; community-based participatory research; and citizen science "data judo." The first approach emphasizes reporting results only when the health significance of exposures is known, whereas the latter two represent new communication strategies in which study participants are engaged in interpreting, disseminating, and applying results to promote community health. We then suggest five critical considerations for planning future biomonitoring studies.

Chapter 14 delineates the challenges of obtaining institutional review board (IRB) coverage for community-based participatory research (CBPR) projects.[2] This discussion draws on our experiences guiding a multipartner CBPR project through university and state IRB deliberations as well as on other CBPR colleagues' accounts. In general, IRBs are unfamiliar with this approach to research, reluctant to take responsibility for the actions of community partner organizations, and resistant to interaction between researchers and participants. Their hesitation causes significant delays and may prevent effective research and dissemination of results. We suggest concrete ways in which IRBs and funders can develop clear review guidelines that respect the unique qualities of CBPR.

Chapter 15 discusses the implications of our work for further scholarship on health social movements. We draw conclusions about the need for future research, interdisciplinary training of undergraduate and graduate students, and funding opportunities to support community-based collaborative enterprises that reshape science and policy making. Finally, we direct readers to appendixes of supplementary material for research groups working in the fields of environmental health, CBPR, and health social movements. These appendixes, which are accessible online, include questionnaires and coding sheets to illustrate our approach to interviewing, along with meeting observations and literature and document reviews. We also provide a template for reporting exposure assessment results to diverse public audiences, incorporating both text and graphics. These materials can be used to address issues of results communication, research ethics, and scientific literacy in CBPR projects rooted in environmental health. An additional appendix discusses the logistical aspects of running our research group, whose faculty, postdoctoral fellows, and graduate and undergraduate students are from an array of disciplines and whose community partners are located in Massachusetts, Rhode Island, and California.

Throughout this book we provide extensive quotations from our many interviews and observations. All unreferenced quotations come from these sources.

This volume demonstrates that the realm of health social movements, and contested illness struggles in particular, is diverse and fluid, and there is no single ethnographic or scientific approach to engaging with this burgeoning field. The body of work discussed here suggests that just as health social movements can transform scientific knowledge production, science also shapes these social movements in unexpected ways. Indeed, communities that engage in scientific projects to advance policy change find that they must grapple with the same polemical issues and contradictions they had previously challenged. Nevertheless, we believe that contested illness struggles can be of critical importance in democratizing and reshaping science, social policy, and regulation. Ultimately, such changes can transform the structural conditions affecting social justice, racial equality, public health, and environmental sustainability in the United States and globally.

NOTES

1. The term *fence line* refers to people, homes, schools, and other places adjacent to polluting facilities or other hazards.

2. IRBs are legally mandated to protect human subjects in research.

2

Embodied Health Movements

Phil Brown, Rachel Morello-Frosch, Stephen Zavestoski,
Sabrina McCormick, Brian Mayer, Rebecca Gasior Altman,
Crystal Adams, Elizabeth Hoover, and Ruth Simpson

What we really need is a new women's health movement, one that's sharp
and skeptical enough to ask all the hard questions: What are the environ-
mental (and possibly lifestyle) causes of the breast cancer epidemic? Why
are existing treatments, such as chemotherapy, so toxic and heavy-handed?
And, if the old narrative of cancer's progression from "early" to "late" stages
no longer holds, what is the course of this disease (or diseases)?
* What we don't need, no matter how pretty and pink, is a lady's auxiliary*
to the cancer-industrial complex.

—BARBARA EHRENREICH, "WE NEED A NEW WOMEN'S HEALTH
MOVEMENT," 2009

When the US Preventive Services Task Force recommended in late 2009 that
women not start regular mammography until age fifty, it sparked an uproar in
the media, in policy circles, and among women's health advocates. Although this
new recommendation was based on a body of scientific studies demonstrating the
limits of mammography in reducing breast cancer mortality rates among women
under fifty, it threatened to undermine dominant medical and public health messages regarding mammography as a reliable strategy for disease "prevention" or
"early detection." Drawing from her personal experience with breast cancer, Barbara Ehrenreich boldly advocates prevention and treatment through a more politically and institutionally transformative women's health agenda. Ehrenreich's call
epitomizes the characteristics that make embodied health movements (EHMs) an
important area of analysis for scholars of social movements, medical sociology,
and environmental sociology.

The United States has seen more than a century of social activism to improve
health and health care, beginning in the Industrial Revolution with concerns
about occupational health and continuing through to more recent fights for

15

disability rights, mental health rights, women's health, and national health care. Embodied health movements are a subset of a relatively recent and understudied type of social movement that we term "health social movements" (HSMs). These are social movements centered on health that challenge medical policy and politics, belief systems, research, and practice.

Some HSMs, which we term access health movements, focus on improving access to health care services: these include Physicians for a National Health Plan, local movements that try to prevent hospital closings, and movements seeking the legitimation of complementary and alternative medicine. Other HSMs target health inequalities. These, known as constituency health movements, focus on group membership based on race, ethnicity, gender, class, disability status, or sexuality. For example, the women's movement has advocated successfully for improved treatment of breast cancer and other illnesses, changed medical research practices, expanded funding and services in many areas important to women, and broadened reproductive rights (Ruzek 1978; Ruzek, Olesen, and Clarke, 1997; Morgen 2002). The HIV/AIDS movement expanded funding for AIDS research, fought the stigmatization of AIDS patients, gained medical recognition of alternative treatment approaches, and effected major shifts in how clinical trials are conducted (Epstein 1996). Indeed, constituency always matters, even if it is not the central orientation of an entire HSM or a single HSM organization. Interaction between individuals affected by a particular disease or condition can lead to the development of a politicized collective illness experience and constituency.

EHMs, as a subset of HSMs, tend to emphasize the embodied experience of illness—that is, people's everyday lived experience. Indeed, EHMs identify the collective experience of health and illness as their core—a source of solidarity, motivation, and urgency. At the same time, EHMs link the personal experience of illness with the collective experience and with the institutional and political-economy structures that can cause disease as well as treat it.

Figure 2.1 demonstrates the diverse ways that HSMs interact with one another by emphasizing their different components. The central component for the environmental breast cancer movement is embodiment. This EHM intersects with the mainstream breast cancer movement, which seeks to improve access to care and alter research funding streams, and with the women's health movement, which represents a broader constituency.

Although we focus on EHMs in this chapter, health advocacy typically involves much crossover between different types of HSMs. For example, constituency-based groups seeking to improve working conditions for farmworkers in agricultural areas have historically taken up the embodied illness experiences of those affected by pesticide exposure and other occupational hazards (Pulido 1996). Like other social movements, HSMs include formal and informal organizations, supporters, networks of cooperation, and media. In pursuit of their objectives, HSMs

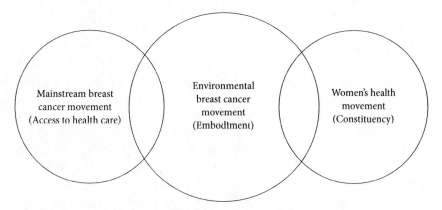

FIGURE 2.1. Intersection of three types of health social movement, with embodiment at the center

may challenge political power, professional authority, and existing definitions of personal and collective identity.

In part, the emergence of HSMs is a response to the increase in industrial and technological risks in modern society (Beck 1992). Such risks are thought by many to have introduced new types of illness. As concerns have been raised about possible connections between industrial hazards and disease, HSMs have been formed to investigate and publicize those links. This trend both reflects and contributes to the "scientization" of society: battles over policy making are expected to involve experts and to be scientific and "objective," and they have the potential to discredit lay perspectives and the lived experience of illness. In this scientized, risk-filled, HSMs use medical science and public health to marshal resources, conduct research, and produce their own scientific knowledge. Thus they simultaneously embrace the principles of science—the systematic use of theory, method, and evidence—and use them to challenge the authority of scientific institutions in public debates about health.

The past decade has seen increasing scholarly attention to health social movements.[1] We see the study of HSMs in general, and EHMs in particular, as drawing on multiple perspectives. Earlier studies of health-related activism typically did not adopt social-movement perspectives, and scholars of social movements have paid little attention to health-related movements. EHMs are the quintessential example of HSMs. They have theoretical relevance for social-movement theory, the sociology of medicine, environmental sociology, policy studies, and related fields. By studying EHMs, and by applying policy ethnography to our investigations (see chapter 4), we hope to bridge the gap between the insights of individual experience with illness and the implementation of effective policy for a community.

CATEGORIZING EMBODIED HEALTH MOVEMENTS

Embodied health movements have as their primary motivating force the individual experience of a physical disease process and the related, shared experience of treatment. EHMs address illness experience by challenging science and medicine. Many EHMs focus on "contested illnesses"—conditions whose causes are either unexplained by current medical knowledge or whose purported environmental explanations are in dispute—and organize to achieve medical recognition, treatment, and research. Other movements advocate improved medical care for conditions that are better understood. Some established EHMs may include constituents who are not ill but who perceive themselves as vulnerable to a disease. Many activists concerned with the environmental causes of breast cancer, for example, have not personally experienced breast cancer but have joined the movement out of a sense of shared collective risk.

EHMs are defined by three characteristics. First, they insert the biological body into social movements, particularly through the embodied experience of people who have the disease. Second, they challenge the ways medicine and science define these experiences (as do other movements, such as the environmental and antinuclear movements—though, as we discuss below, EHMs are unusual in the nature of their challenge to science). Third, EHMs collaborate with scientists and health professionals in pursuing treatment, prevention, research, and expanded funding.

The Embodied Experience of Illness

In EHMs, the bodily experience of disease is a unifying and mobilizing force. The progression of identity from aggrieved sufferer to a participant in collective action results from the disease process happening inside the individual's body and the ways that others perceive and react to the disease. This identity represents the intersection of social constructions of illness and the personal experience of disease. Our focus on embodied health movements meshes with recent social movements scholarship stressing the importance of emotion and lived experience in the development of social movements and social movement activists (Goodwin, Jasper, and Polletta 2001; Morgen 2002). As Morgen writes, we cannot "understand the agency of political actors without recognizing that politics is lived, believed, felt, and acted all at once" (2002, 230).

The body is often also implicated in other social movements, especially identity-based movements, but these are typically movements that emerge because a particular ascribed identity causes a group of people to experience their bodies through the lens of social stigma and discrimination. Such is the case with the women's and lesbian and gay rights movements, for example. With EHMs, on the other hand, the disease process results in the development of a particular disease identity, which may or may not be stigmatized.

Illness sufferers can work either with or against the system that produces and applies scientific and medical knowledge. Though some seek alternative or complementary therapies, many others need or seek immediate care and are forced to pursue solutions within the system they may perceive as failing their health needs.[2] Most important, illness sufferers uniquely experience not only the direct effects of the disease process but also its effects on other aspects of their physical and mental existence, effects on their personal relationships, and broader social ramifications. These personal experiences give people with the disease or condition a lived perspective that is unavailable to others. They also lend moral credibility to the mobilized group in the public sphere and scientific world.

Challenges to Medical and Scientific Knowledge

As science and technocratic decision making have become increasingly dominant in social policy and regulation in the United States, social movements have encountered new sources of authority against which they must contend and a need to mobilize new types of resources. The scientization of decision making privileges those questions or decisions that can be asked of science and marginalizes those questions that may not be amenable to scientific analysis. Framing political and moral questions in exclusively scientific terms limits public participation in the decision-making process (Weinberg 1972) and can prevent outside scrutiny, which in turn can reduce the quality of the science produced. These outcomes of scientization have spurred existing social movements to challenge science's monopoly on the production of respected or legitimate knowledge and to develop new forms of scientific expertise.

EHM activists often judge science on the basis of their own intimate, firsthand knowledge of their bodies and illness. Many EHMs develop a strong critique of medicine that points out how ideological and structural factors shape medical research and treatment. Some EHMs work outside science altogether. In these embodied movements, adherents have a strong critique of the dominant science, but rather than work to produce alternative science (with or without professional allies), they reject scientific explanations. For example, some participants in the "psychiatric survivors" movement resist traditional psychiatry, eschew all approaches to reform, and oppose the very idea that they have, or have had, a mental illness.

Activist Engagement with Science

Unlike many other movements that confront scientific knowledge and practice, EHMs must simultaneously challenge and collaborate with the scientific enterprise. Environmental groups, for example, quite often confront scientific justifications for risk-management strategies or resource use by drawing on their own scientific evidence for alternative courses of action. However, some environmental groups can circumvent scientific arguments, for example by appealing instead to the public's desire to protect open spaces for psychological or spiritual reasons or to preserve resources for enjoyment by future generations.

Such alternative organizing strategies are not available to EHMs, as treatment within the biomedical model requires a scientific understanding of disease. Although these groups may make nonscientific appeals to people's sense of justice or shared values, participants nevertheless remain heavily dependent on scientific understanding and continued innovation if they hope to receive effective treatment.[3] Disease groups depend on medical and scientific allies to raise funds for research and for support groups and to get health insurance coverage. The more persuasively scientists can testify to those needs, the stronger are the claims of patients and advocates. Indeed, an EHM's success is measured in part through any medical and scientific advances. EHMs are thus inextricably linked with science.

This dependence on science is particularly apparent for EHMs focused on contested illnesses. When little was known about AIDS, activists had to prod the medical establishment and the government to act quickly and with adequate knowledge (Epstein 1996). However, even EHMs that focus on already-understood and treatable diseases typically must point to scientific evidence of causation in order to demand public policies for prevention.

What sets EHMs apart from other movements is less the fact that they challenge science than how they go about doing it. EHMs often engage in citizen-science alliances (CSAs) in which activists collaborate with scientists and health professionals in pursuing treatment, prevention, research, and expanded funding. CSAs represent the willingness of citizens and scientists to go beyond an "us versus them" paradigm to develop innovative organizational forms that can address the social determinants of health. Citizens bring insights from their personal illness experiences, and scientists contribute their technical skills and knowledge. These alliances contribute to new knowledge, and they also challenge—and sometimes change—scientific norms by valuing the experience and knowledge of illness sufferers. CSAs may be initiated by citizens or professionals or created through a joint-affinity model in which lay and researcher interests are aligned.

There are numerous examples of CSAs in EHMs. AIDS activists have sought a place at the scientific table so that their personal illness experiences can help shape research design (Epstein 1996). Breast cancer activists have been involved in federal and state review panels, as well as in decisions about foundation funding (Brown et al. 2006). Asthma activists have cooperated with scientists in projects linking air pollution to respiratory illnesses in urban neighborhoods that house bus depots and transit hubs (Shepard et al. 2002). CSAs have also been important in the environmental breast cancer, environmental justice, and environmental health movements, which are concerned with the effect of exposure to industrial pollutants, such as those used in the petrochemical and plastic industries, on human health. Participants in these movements have become involved in a new form of activism.

Community-based participatory research (CBPR) programs are the most far-reaching example of citizen-science alliances. In CBPR, members of an affected community engage in the research process alongside scientists, social scientists, medical professionals, and other researchers. They participate in the definition of research questions and design, assist in carrying out the study, help disseminate findings to the community, and help shape any resulting policies. CBPR thus includes all affected parties and all potential end users of the research, including community-based organizations, public health practitioners, and local health and social services agencies (Shepard et al. 2002; Israel et al. 1998; Minkler and Wallerstein 2003; Minkler et al. 2008). More comprehensive citizen involvement in research often occurs as the social problem becomes more public and the social movement gains strength and momentum.

At first glance, some HSMs may not appear to fit the three characteristics of EHMs. For example, the tobacco-control movement may appear vastly different from the environmental breast cancer movement in terms of personal experience of illness, challenges to science, and collaboration with science. But this movement started with health testimony from smokers who developed lung cancer and respiratory diseases, and their families and friends. It was also rooted in non-smokers' grievances about the health effects of secondhand smoke. For example, a loosely organized group of organizations, GASP (Groups against Smokers' Pollution), pushed for clean-air policies at the state and national levels (Wolfson 2001). Further, this movement challenged science for failing to pursue its findings on the health hazards of tobacco or to take on secondary-smoke hazards in a timely fashion. Even before the movement had a strong scientific foundation, its activists had made a logical extrapolation from primary to secondary exposure, and they pressured researchers to examine this issue more closely. Indeed, one of the common features of EHMs is that they often initiate proposals for scientific research in advance of medical science. The tobacco-control movement also blurs several boundaries, as reflected in Wolfson's concept of state-movement interpenetration, in that it comprises single-issue groups, health voluntaries, state agencies, health care professionals, and health care organizations.

A NEW THEORY FOR A NEW BREED OF SOCIAL MOVEMENT

The study of new social movements explicitly focused on health requires a new approach. Possibly because so much health activism has taken place within the framework and objectives of other forms of activism, research has occurred across a range of disciplinary perspectives, with no general conceptual framework for studying health social movements per se. Most of this research has not made use of social-movement theory, and the social-movement literature itself has paid little attention to health-related movements of any sort, let alone EHMs.

Drawing on social movement theory and the unique characteristics of embodied health movements, we develop a three-point theoretical approach. First, we use the concept of politicized collective illness identity to explain how individual disease sufferers become mobilized for action. Second, we use the model of the dominant epidemiological paradigm to describe the context in which EHMs develop targets and identify the goals of their activism. Third, drawing on the concepts of boundary work and boundary objects from science studies, we conceptualize EHMs as boundary movements offering a new way to understand what constitutes a movement and who movement actors are while also allowing us to observe the hybridity and fluidity of EHMs.

THE POLITICIZATION OF COLLECTIVE ILLNESS IDENTITY

The centrality of the biological body in EHMs suggests a basic mechanism of mobilization: collective identity. We draw on the substantial body of work on collective identity (Polletta and Jasper 2001) and oppositional consciousness (Groch 1994; Mansbridge and Morris 2001) to arrive at what we term "politicized collective illness identity." Polletta and Jasper define collective identity as "an individual's cognitive, moral, and emotional connection with a broader community. It is a perception of a shared status or relation, which may be imagined rather than experienced directly, and it is distinct from personal identities, although it may form part of a personal identity" (Polletta and Jasper 2001, 285). Illness identity, on the other hand, is the sense of self shaped by the physical constraints of illness and by others' social reactions to that illness (Charmaz 1991). Collective illness identity is the cognitive, moral, and emotional connection an individual has with a broader community of illness sufferers and their allies. A collective illness identity requires the perception of a shared status or relation, rooted in some aspect of the illness experience that is distinct from, though it may form a part of, the personal illness identity.

A collective illness identity may be sufficient to motivate individuals to form a support group or a self-help group. But for a *politicized* collective illness identity to form, the collective illness identity must be linked to a broader social critique that views structural inequalities and the uneven distribution of social power as responsible for the causes or triggers of the disease. Oppositional consciousness reflects a "state of mind" that binds members of a group against dominant ways of thinking (in this case, the dominant epidemiological paradigm) by attributing problems to structural factors (Groch 1994; Mansbridge and Morris 2001). When the lived experience is subordinate to dominant groups or ideas, an oppositional consciousness often develops among laypeople who recognize that group-based inequalities are structural and unjust. These actors turn to collective action as a means to address perceived injustices (Mansbridge and Morris 2001). The development of an oppositional consciousness enables aggrieved people to politicize their collective illness identity.

The structural critique triggered by an oppositional consciousness and embedded in the politicized collective illness identity also places responsibility on social institutions, instead of individuals, for treating and preventing the disease (e.g., government may be held responsible for harms caused by chemical pollutants because of failures to regulate industry and reduce population exposures). In short, a politicized collective illness identity begins the process of transforming a personal trouble into a social problem. At this stage, people with the disease focus primarily not on treatment access, support groups, or expanded research, but on seeking political-economic and institutional explanations and the requisite structural changes. In this latter development, people without the disease can be part of the collective identity, either because they are friends or relatives of someone with the disease or because they have reason to fear they will get the disease in the future. This latter stage clearly offers the potential of creating a critical mass of sufferers who will identify with and join EHMs.

Part of what causes individuals with illness to begin experiencing a politicized collective illness identity is their common experience of dealing with the government, medical, and scientific institutions that create the dominant epidemiological paradigm. The institutional beliefs and practices that shape the discovery and understanding of a disease also partly shape the illness experience for the affected population. As individuals experiencing illness enter formal health care systems, these institutions shape their perceptions of the disease. When disease groups experience their conditions in ways that contradict scientific and medical explanations, and these contradictions are identified as a source of contention, a politicized collective illness identity may emerge.

In some cases, social movement spillover (Meyer and Whittier 1994) enables disease groups to make connections between their collective illness experience and some form of perceived inequality. For example, environmental justice activists have influenced asthma activists to view asthma as related to race-related inequities in exposure to air pollution and toxic substances. As Meyer and Whittier explain, "Taken together, one movement can influence subsequent movements both from outside and from within: by altering the political and cultural conditions it confronts in the external environment, and by changing the individuals, groups, and norms within the movement itself" (1994. 281–82). Further, the notion of spillover captures the variety of outcomes movements can have, and it moves beyond the notion that a social movement's successes are measured simply by influence on the state. Such a conceptualization is ideally suited to EHMs, which are hybrid movements in which the collective identities, tactics, styles of leadership, and organizational structures of movements intersect with a disease's powerful effect on the body and which therefore transcend traditional conceptions of social movements and their attendant organizations. Observing the spillover that EHMs experience invokes the notion of EHMs as boundary movements.

EMBODIED HEALTH MOVEMENTS AS CHALLENGES TO THE DOMINANT EPIDEMIOLOGICAL PARADIGM

When challenging science, social movements confront a powerful set of institutions and belief structures. This dominant epidemiological paradigm (DEP) is the codification of beliefs about a disease and its causation that are held by science, government, and the private sector. It incorporates the views of institutions entrusted with the care of disease sufferers as well as professional journals, the popular media, universities, medical philanthropic organizations, and government officials. Many structures and institutions may contribute to a generally accepted view of disease without their role being visible. Actors can challenge the dominant epidemiological paradigm, attempt to reshape it at different locations, and take action on one or more of its components.

The dominant epidemiological paradigm is involves a complex set of interactions (figure 2.2). Social actors such as government, industry, academics, nonprofit organizations, health voluntaries, and the media draw on public understanding, scientific knowledge, and policy frameworks to identify and define disease as well as determine its etiology, proper treatment, and acceptable health outcomes. This process shapes future awareness and policy in ways that influence the illness experience of a disease sufferer.

A disease sufferer who is dissatisfied with what science tells her about her disease may be motivated to challenge the DEP. A movement may mount an organized challenge to a DEP's approach to disease etiology because the movement opposes the notion of holding individuals responsible for their health status. Embodied health movements point to population data that demonstrate the importance of social structures and environmental factors in determining health and disease in populations. They challenge the emphasis on lifestyle risk factors, implicit or explicit in the DEP, that singles out apparent choices (such as smoking, diet, and alcohol use). EHMs argue that the lifestyle approach fails to recognize that personal behaviors are largely shaped by social structures, much as C. Wright Mills (1959) argued that we often miscast "social problems" as "personal troubles." In short, the process of challenging a DEP is often an attempt to move away from the idea that illness is a personal problem for which the individual is responsible and over which she or he has control, and toward the idea that illness is a

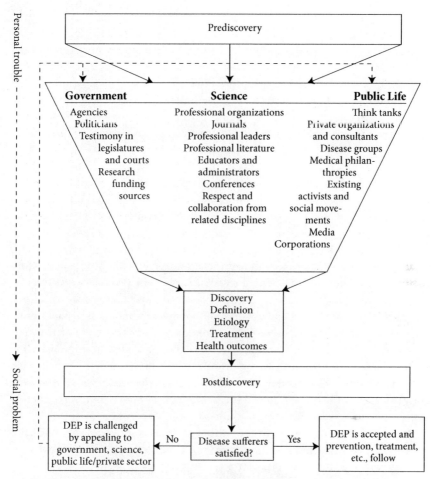

FIGURE 2.2. The dominant epidemiological paradigm (DEP). Government, industry, academics, nonprofit organizations, health voluntaries, the media, and other relevant actors draw on public understanding, scientific knowledge, and policy frameworks to identify and define disease and determine treatment and acceptable health outcomes. These in turn influence the illness experience. The bottom of the figure illustrates how a disease sufferer may opt to challenge the DEP when dissatisfied with the resulting definition of the disease, beliefs about its etiology, norms for treatment, or accepted outcomes. The left side of the figure captures what we see as a pattern in health social movement organizing: an organized challenge to the DEP's bias toward individualistic approaches to disease.

social problem that must be dealt with systematically at higher levels of social organization.

Science and medicine, like other institutions, have increasingly come under scrutiny by social movements, but because they differ from other institutions commonly targeted, they are subject to a different set of strategies. Rapid changes in scientific innovation, investment in new areas of research, and the lack of a strongly held consensus on a scientific issue may create windows of opportunity for protest and action. Medicine and science are in a nearly constant state of flux. In addition to creating new knowledge that may be contested by social movement actors, scientific progress may destabilize the rules and relationships that govern institutions. When an organization receives a large influx of research dollars or experiences rapid growth in membership or staffing, or when the expansion of the knowledge base triggers a paradigm shift, this may destabilize the organization, opening up opportunities for social-movement actors to challenge the institutions. In such circumstances, the institution may present opportunities for challenges by EHMs. As Moore notes, a scientific field undergoing rapid change presents "multiple locations of challenge and access for protesters and dissenting scientists" (1999, 113). Moore argues that social movement actors (including sympathetic scientists and the general lay public) can alter institutional practices when they take advantage of these windows of opportunity. For example, the rapid expansion of breast cancer research funding under the administration of President Clinton opened up opportunities for different kinds of challenges, such as calls for improved detection devices and better treatment (Casamayou 2001), and, from the environmental breast cancer movement, for a very different approach to prevention (McCormick, Brown, and Zavestoski 2003).

Second, the heterogeneous field of actors involved in creating and maintaining the DEP presents multiple points of leverage for social movement activists. Medical and scientific institutions are not unanimous in their views of disease causation or analytical approaches to research. Although the DEP is dominated by an emphasis on individual and behavioral risk factors for disease, rather than environmental or social factors, it is not monolithic: some elements may be more receptive to environmental hypotheses of causation (Zavestoski et al. 2005). With respect to breast cancer, for example, some scientific institutions have embraced the endocrine-disruptor hypothesis (Krimsky 2000), and some institutes within the National Institutes of Health (especially the National Institute of Environmental Health Sciences, NIEHS) have funded extensive research on environmental causation of disease (McCormick et al. 2004). The existence of sympathetic elites in the science policy arena and a lack of consensus among the scientific actors involved in creating or maintaining the DEP may allow social-movement actors to gain entry into an institution of authority.

Third, science policy is enacted at multiple levels, and activists can target local, statewide, or federal agencies. Locally based research institutions may be responsive to the interests of local advocates. Silent Spring Institute is one such organization. It was founded by the Massachusetts Breast Cancer Coalition to conduct research on women's health and the environment, with a strong component of citizen involvement. At the national level, research initiatives like those within NIEHS have facilitated federal initiatives to foster collaborations between academic researchers and community organizations that have a social justice component (Felix 2007).

Medical institutions that attempt to resolve illnesses similarly operate on various scales. While local practitioners may relate observed disease phenomena to community concerns, higher-level health care foundations and philanthropic institutions transcend the concerns of a single community and draw national attention to the issue, such as the panoply of breast cancer foundations like Komen for the Cure and the Breast Cancer Research Foundation (McCormick and Baralt 2006).

Finally, many scientific and medical institutions are connected to the state through funding and regulatory channels, which create additional targets for social-movement action. Activists can mount challenges to scientific research by questioning funding decisions or demanding additional government funding for certain projects. For example, passing legislation mandating the Long Island Breast Cancer Study Project in 1993 was a part of breast cancer activists' establishment of a new agenda focused on elucidating environmental links to breast cancer and thus potential keys to disease prevention, rather than treatment and cure. This important milestone was preceded by activism highlighting environmental links to breast cancer on Long Island and across the country.

EMBODIED HEALTH MOVEMENTS
AS BOUNDARY MOVEMENTS

Blurring the boundaries between social movements is just one example of how EHMs represent what we call boundary movements. In the sociology of science, the term *boundary work* describes the efforts of scientists, policy makers, and laypeople to distinguish good science from bad (Gieryn 1983).This demarcation effort is based not on a positivistic notion of truth but on different kinds of proof and certainty that vary with the issue at hand. Star and Greisemer (1989) also focus on boundaries, examining how actors use them to define "boundary objects" that overlap different social worlds and are malleable enough to be used and contested by different parties. For example, a mammography machine may represent a major diagnostic technology for medicine, while environmental breast cancer activists may view it as an obstacle to preventive approaches when it is touted as a form of disease prevention.

Because EHMs so often depend on challenging medical and scientific knowledge and practice, they constantly engage in boundary work and use boundary objects. Consequently, they can be thought of as boundary movements in four different ways. First, they attempt to reconstruct the lines that distinguish science from nonscience and good science from bad science. For example, environmental health activists have criticized the science of chemical risk assessment for failing to adequately consider the health impacts of cumulative exposures to toxic contaminants, and they have opposed the widespread notion that early-detection strategies (such as mammography) are viable approaches to disease prevention. By pushing science in new directions, and by bringing previously unaddressed issues and concerns to the attention of clinical and bench scientists, EHMs push the boundaries of science. EHMs can also use boundary objects in ways that blur the lines between science and nonscience. For example, a particular scientific tool, like an inexpensive air sampler, may serve as a boundary object that an EHM can employ both to produce scientific data to help scientists and to empower movement followers to push for regulatory action.

Second, EHMs blur the boundary between experts and laypeople. Some EHM activists become experts by using the Internet and other resources to gain medical and scientific knowledge that can empower them in discussions with their medical care providers. Others gain a more readily acknowledged form of expertise by working with scientists and medical experts to better understand their disease. Through this process, movements gain power and authority by erasing the boundary between expert and layperson. In some cases, rather than just blur the boundary, activists redefine or even eliminate it, as with the National Breast Cancer Coalition's Project LEAD, which helps activists become versed in the policy and scientific literature so that they can serve on peer review panels for allocating research funding (Dickersin et al. 2001). Some EHM organizations have evolved beyond lay organizations because they deal so much with science and contend with the world of science. They become hybrids through this process of breaking down longstanding boundaries.

Third, EHMs cross the boundaries of government and philanthropic institutions: for example, tobacco-control activists have allied in varying combinations with health voluntary organizations and government agencies (Wolfson 2001). Hence, rather than distinct entities, EHMs are savvy social actors moving between social worlds. This approach redefines activists, just as scientists who can move easily between the lay and expert worlds of knowledge often take on the role of "advocacy scientists" (Krimsky 2000).

Finally, EHMs take advantage of the malleability of boundary objects to acquire political resources to raise funds, recruit new members, and generate legitimacy.

For example, the Boston environmental justice organization Alternatives for Community and Environment (ACE) pressured state and federal environmental agencies to install an air monitor on its roof. The monitor is a boundary object that crosses several social worlds. It is a symbol of ACE's political effectiveness; it is a device that facilitates teaching and community organizing; and it is a tool for research by ACE and public health researchers. Using the monitor, ACE was able to gather data to press the regional transit agency to adopt low-emissions buses.

For the environmental breast cancer movement, boundary objects include mammography machines, genetic testing for breast cancer, patents on the BRCA-1 and BRCA-2 breast cancer gene sequences, pharmaceuticals, and events such as Breast Cancer Awareness Month and Avon's Breast Cancer Walk. The mammography machine is a mainstay of hospitals and their breast cancer centers as well as a point of contention for activists who have criticized its overuse and the lack of attention to mammography's harmful consequences (exposure to radiation, false positive test results, and consequent unnecessary surgery), especially for younger women. This controversy was highlighted in November 2009, when the US Preventive Services Task Force (USPSTF) issued new screening recommendations for women who are asymptomatic and who are not at elevated risk of breast cancer. The task force called for an end to routine mammography screening for women age 40–49 and encouraged screenings every two years rather than annually for postmenopausal women. This recommendation has redirected public attention toward a question that has long troubled breast cancer activists, sufferers, clinicians, and policy makers: does the technology do harm? That is, does it produce false positives and hence lead to unnecessary interventions, and does it unnecessarily expose people to radiation, itself a cause of breast cancer? The mammogram represents more than an imaging technology.

The BRCA sequences are medical diagnostic tools that detect high levels of genetic risk for breast cancer; they are also an example of the dangers of allowing private firms to patent gene sequences. Myriad Genetics, Inc., uses that patent to prevent laboratories from conducting very inexpensive screening, thus limiting many people's access to knowledge about whether they have mutations. Likewise, National Breast Cancer Awareness Month calls attention to breast cancer, but it emphasizes treatment over prevention. And because the event is copyrighted by the nonprofit healthcare foundation of the pharmaceutical giant AstraZeneca, breast cancer activists are limited in their involvement and the messages they can communicate to the public.

CONCLUSION

Health has emerged as a powerful frame for many grievances. Health movements have changed the landscape of state and scientific institutions and have helped promote social equality and change. Because health is a vital human and social issue, many social movements not explicitly concerned with health have nonetheless come to champion health-related causes. Following the work of Rachel Carson in identifying environmental pollutants in the 1960s and the public outcry over the toxic waste disaster in Love Canal, New York, in the late 1970s, the environmental movement expanded beyond its initial concerns with wildlife conservation and habitat preservation to consider the environment's effects on human health. Civil rights activists cited the notorious Tuskegee syphilis experiment (in which effective treatment was withheld from black men with syphilis) to demonstrate how the health care system itself promoted racism. Environmental justice activists built their movement on this civil rights framework. Housing activists demonstrated that poor housing conditions contribute to poor health, especially asthma. Repeatedly, social movements with disparate objectives have gravitated toward health issues.

Health social movements feed off the growing public awareness of and involvement in health issues. As a result, they have taken up struggles against targets that were previously seen as untouchable, such as the tobacco industry. In the United States, there is growing opposition to an expensive health care system, consuming 16 percent of the country's gross domestic product, that still fails to serve our needs. A huge uninsured population, the lack of treatments for new and mysterious chronic diseases, and dissatisfaction with the increasingly impersonal nature of managed care have led to a widening distrust of the health care system and provided grounds for engaging in social movement activity, or at least for supporting others who do so.

EHMs, and the theoretical insights they afford us, have implications for various fields, including social movement theory and the related fields of environmental sociology and medical sociology. For example, in social movement theory, the "political opportunity" approach argues that as political networks change, social movements may find allies among sympathetic political parties and government agencies where previously none existed (Tilly 1978; McAdam 1982; McAdam, Tarrow, and Tilly 2001). In a number of cases, EHMs have taken advantage of such circumstances. For example, to a certain extent, greater opportunities for gay rights activism made AIDS activism feasible. Similarly, veterans struggled for years to get government acknowledgment of chemical and biological weapons use during the Gulf War (see chapter 6). The eventual uncovering of evidence that thousands of soldiers had been exposed to such hazards enabled Gulf War veterans to appeal for funding for research into and compensation for their health problems.

While EHMs demonstrate the importance of political opportunities for social movements, they also encourage us, as theorists, to avoid attributing too much power and significance to external factors. EHMs are strongly rooted in the illness experience. Those experiencing serious illness cannot, and do not, wait for advantageous political circumstances before mobilizing. Although their efforts are likely to be more successful when such opportunities exist, they often organize in the face of political constraints.

While some EHMs struggle against state action or inaction, others focus on nonstate targets, for example by challenging AstraZeneca on its direct advertising of the drug tamoxifen for the prevention of breast cancer. Many activists believe that the prophylactic use of tamoxifen is not as effective as the manufacturer claims, and there are concerns that long-term use may increase breast cancer risk in people without the disease. EHMs also show that social movements can have complex and seemingly paradoxical relationships with the state, allying with some components of the state to challenge others. For example, some asthma activists have worked with the EPA to persuade the federal government to enact stronger air-quality regulations.

Like many social movements, EHMs engage in "frame alignment," setting their agendas in ways that resonate with the personal experiences, values, and expectations of potential constituents (Snow et al. 1986; Benford and Snow 2000). This process aligns the illness experience of potential constituents and the illness experience defined by the movement, thereby transforming individuals' experiences from personal troubles into a social problem. EHMs may also align the collective illness experience with the policies of medicine, science, and government actors, as those sectors offer the potential for legitimation and resources.

Class remains a salient feature of many, though not all, health movements, and any effort to understand these movements must consider class and other social structures. For example, our research on asthma activism shows that it is often led by poor, inner-city communities of color, and they integrate their organizing with efforts to address class-based discrimination in housing, transportation access, and economic development (Brown et al. 2003).

Our approach represents a unique way of looking at certain types of movements, such as those concerned with aspects of scientific knowledge. The concerns of such movements include natural resources, energy, genetically modified organisms, and hydroelectric dams. In all these cases, activists cross scientific boundaries. They are compelled to learn science in order to advance their causes, and they eventually seek and may obtain seats at the table where science-based decisions are made. David Hess (2002) addresses this trend in his notion of "technology-oriented social movements," including those concerned with organic foods, nutritional therapeutics, renewable energy, recycling, and human-centered transportation. Kelly Moore (2008) looks at challenges to the military uses of science, and Scott Frickel and Neil Gross (2005) examine "science and intellectual movements."

EHMs encourage medical sociologists to scrutinize the intersection of health inequalities and environmental justice. Academic study of health inequalities has not usually taken that interest to an applied or activist level; nor has the field grasped the connections with environmental justice. Some environmental justice scholars view health inequalities as central to environmental justice concerns, but even they tend to rely more on justice and legal scholarship than on medical sociology to make sense of environmental justice struggles.

Apart from medical sociology, environmental sociology is the field that most closely examines health social movements. Environmental sociologists have addressed the problem of contaminated communities by explaining how conflicts emerge between ecological realities (e.g., contamination), and a community's interpretation of contamination (Kroll-Smith and Couch 1991; Couch and Kroll-Smith 1994). Moving beyond a conflict between reality and symbolism, our framework for understanding EHMs views community contamination as a more fundamental conflict between biological bodies and the social meaning of illness.

The following chapters present accounts of EHMs that we have studied and collaborated with. Most of those, although not all, have been engaged in CBPR. As affected members of a community, whether linked geographically or by a disease, they draw on their own experiences to help define research objectives and methods, to conduct the studies, to disseminate information to the community, and to apply their work to influence social policy. Our characterization and analysis of these movements are based on our direct involvement with them, and this involvement also shapes our theoretical thinking and methodological approaches.

NOTES

1. Examples include special streams at the 2001 and 2003 conferences of the Society for the Social Study of Science; a workshop at the American Sociological Association's Collective Behavior and Social Movements Section conference in 2002; a symposium on medical social movements in Sweden in 2003, which led to a special issue of the journal *Social Science and Medicine* on patient-based social movements in 2006; a special issue, "Health and the Environment," of *Annals of the American Academy of Political and Social Science* (2002; edited by Phil Brown); the *Sociology of Health and Illness* 2004 annual monograph on health social movements (later published as a book edited by Phil Brown and Stephen Zavestoski); a 2005 conference at the University of Victoria, British Columbia, titled "Illness and the Contours of Contestation: Diagnosis; Experience; Policy," which led to the publication of *Contesting Illness: Processes and Practices* in 2007; a conference on social movements and health institutions at the University of Michigan in 2007, from which a volume was published (Zald et al. 2009); and a workshop at the 2008 US-UK Medical Sociology conference.

2. Reflecting the contested nature of the illnesses that EHMs address, any term we might choose is inevitably problematic from some perspective. Not all EHM actors identify as illness "sufferers" (antipsychiatry advocates, for example, do not), and many prefer more empowered terms, such as *survivor*.

3. This claim should be qualified because, as previously acknowledged, some illness sufferers exit the system of Western medical care by seeking alternative and complementary therapies or abandoning treatment altogether. As this group of individuals represents a small minority of the ill who are seeking to restore their health, we focus on the dependence on science that characterizes those who turn to mainstream medical care providers.

3

Qualitative Approaches in Environmental Health Research

Phil Brown

Health researchers are increasingly turning to qualitative methods, used either on their own or in combination with quantitative methods (Bourgeault, DeVries, and Dingwall 2010). Qualitative methods give a voice to individuals and community organizations and provide fuller, more complex descriptions of the affected community. For this reason, these approaches often support laypeople's discovery of, and action on, hazards and disease. Quantitative data are helpful for demonstrating the existence of environmental exposures and health effects but offer only a partial picture. Only through qualitative data can we understand how people and communities experience and act on these problems.

There is growing acceptance of qualitative methods among federal agencies, but in some cases they are still very subsidiary to traditional quantitative approaches (Office of Behavioral and Social Sciences Research 1999). Program officers at the National Institute of Environmental Health Sciences and the Centers for Disease Control have extended environmental health research and intervention into an array of diseases and conditions, including obesity and diabetes, that stem from the combined environmental assault of fast food and high-fructose corn syrup, lack of safe and healthy walking areas and green space, and dangerous housing conditions (Srinivasan et al. 2003; Jackson 2007). In-depth qualitative studies of contaminated communities are undertaken mainly by sociologists but also by geographers, psychologists, public health scholars, and political scientists. Researchers typically enter a community to study how laypeople have discovered environmental problems and acted on this knowledge. Such ethnographic research usually follows a crisis or discovery that has placed the "contaminated community" in the public eye

(Edelstein 2004). Sometimes social scientists enter the research setting as part of an epidemiological research team.

While this chapter focuses on in-depth ethnographic studies of contaminated communities, other forms of qualitative methods are also used in environmental health research. These include structured interviewing (O'Connell 2003), focus groups (Scammell et al. 2009), policy analysis (Raffensperger and Tickner 1999; Weisman 2000), media analysis (Anderson 1997; Foskett, Karran, and LaFia 2000; Brown et al. 2001a), content analysis of documents (Markowitz and Rosner 2002), and cultural critique (Miller 2000; O'Neal 2000). Qualitative methods can play important roles in environmental epidemiology and environmental justice (EJ) research. For example, qualitative approaches to community mapping, often a part of environmental justice organizations' work, are now frequently being integrated with quantitative GIS techniques (Corburn 2005). As hybrid qualitative-quantitative approaches gain acceptance, methods may evolve to a point where there is no distinction between health-effects research and community ethnography: any project examining environmental health would combine epidemiological approaches with social science analysis rooted in community collaboration.

Robert Bullard's *Confronting Environmental Racism: Voices from the Grass-roots* (1993), a collection of accounts of the environmental justice movement, many written by activists themselves, demonstrates how environmental racism leads to health inequalities by excluding certain ethnic and socioeconomic groups from environmental decision making. Studies of environmental justice organizing efforts weave community voices extensively into their scholarship. Sze's profiles of four community struggles include fliers, posters, and photos of rallies to describe the EJ campaigns more richly. This approach helps situate the effect of EJ organizing throughout a city. Similarly, work by Roberts and Toffolon-Weiss (2001), presenting four case studies of EJ campaigns, provides a sense of EJ organizing throughout Louisiana, allowing us to see that state as a crucible for such efforts.

Virtually all cases of contaminated communities are detected by residents, largely because they are more sensitive to environmental problems than are scientists and government agencies doing routine surveillance. Furthermore, problems detected by such surveillance are rarely reported to directly to the community: for example, a state cancer registry may be mandated to publish annual reports of cancer excesses by town and city but not required to notify residents of areas where such excesses are observed. Even when pressed by communities to investigate environmental health concerns, many agencies or health departments require extensive data before taking action. The role of laypeople as the typical discoverers of environmental health crises can be fully understood only through qualitative research. When neighborhood residents are trying to figure out what is happening to them, they often face a long and complicated route to get anything done about it. They have a multitude of stories of learning about hazards, sharing their

problems, organizing politically, challenging scientific and government authority, dealing with resistance within the community, and becoming scientifically
capable. To convey the richness of these narratives, I begin with a review of several
ethnographic studies of contaminated communities. I then discuss personal and
scholarly insights on qualitative research from my study of the Woburn childhood leukemia cluster, and from other community studies.

THE HISTORY AND LEGACY
OF QUALITATIVE RESEARCH

In 1972, at a coal mine near Buffalo Creek, West Virginia, a poorly constructed
and inadequately maintained dam broke, allowing a torrent of coal-mining sludge
to sweep down the hollow. The Buffalo Creek flood destroyed whole villages with
hundreds of homes, uprooted miles of railroad tracks, killed 125 people, injured
many others, and left immense psychological scars on the residents (Erikson
1976). Attorneys for the residents suing the coal company asked the sociologist
Kai Erikson to report on the damage done to the poor Appalachian community.

Erikson's *Everything in Its Path: Destruction of Community in the Buffalo Creek
Flood* was the first book-length study of the effects of a human-caused environmental disaster on individuals and community. Using the residents' own eloquent
descriptions, Erikson fashioned an emotionally powerful, sociologically astute
account that connected the shock of individual trauma with the effects on the
community and assessed both mental health and physical health outcomes. He
situated the disaster in the cultural, social, and historical context of the community and sought to improve the situation of the affected people.

This legacy continued with Adeline Levine's *Love Canal: Science, Politics, and
People* (1982), which recounted the story of a buried-waste site in a small suburb
of Niagara Falls, NY, and the environmental disaster it caused. The story begins
with the routine dumping of hazardous chemicals in the 1940s and ends with the
insidious poisoning of children and families, some of whom were forced into a
fight with local and national authorities. For several years, Levine and her students
conducted interviews with residents and local organizations and attended public
meetings and events.

Michael Edelstein's *Contaminated Communities: The Social and Psychological
Impacts of Residential Toxic Exposure* (2004) examined the social and psycho-
logical effects of a water contamination episode in Legler, NJ. Steve Kroll-Smith
and Stephen R. Couch's *The Real Disaster is Above Ground: A Mine Fire and
Social Conflict* (1990) studied social conflicts between affected groups dealing
with an underground mine fire in Centralia, PA. Michael Reich's *Toxic Politics:
Responding to Chemical Disasters* (1991) compared a dioxin explosion in Seveso,
Italy, polybrominated biphenyl cattle-feed contamination in Michigan, and PCB

contamination of cooking oil in Japan. Lee Clarke's *Acceptable Risk: Making Decisions in a Toxic Environment* (1989) detailed hazard perception following a fire at the state government office in Binghamton, NY. Martha Balshem's *Cancer in the Community: Class and Medical Authority* (1993) looked at the hazard perception of people in a Philadelphia working-class neighborhood; and Steven Picou published *Social Disruption and Psychological Stress in an Alaskan Fishing Community: The Impact of the* Exxon Valdez *Oil Spill* (1990). These studies recounted stories not told in the mainstream scientific literature on these disasters, creating a rich texture of personal experiences and community effects. They emphasized the democratic rights of individuals and communities to learn about the hazards and disasters befalling them and to obtain remediation, compensation, and justice.

In *No Safe Place: Toxic Waste, Leukemia, and Community Action* (Brown and Mikkelsen, 1997 [1990]), I developed the concept of popular epidemiology to describe lay involvement in community health studies and to demonstrate an approach for using ethnographic data alongside clinical, epidemiological, and natural science findings. The approach emphasizes concerns of access, trust, confidentiality, sharing of data, reflexivity effects, and benefits to the people and community being studied. Families in Woburn, MA, pressured state and federal agencies to investigate the cluster of leukemia cases in their community (mostly in children) and sued W. R. Grace and Beatrice Foods for contaminating municipal water wells with organic compounds known to be animal carcinogens, especially trichloroethylene (TCE) and perchlorethylene (PCE). The residents, without prior activist experience or health knowledge, educated and organized themselves in a highly effective way. They worked with biostatisticians to conduct 5,010 interviews, covering 57 percent of Woburn residences that had telephones, and the results showed clear correlations between contaminated water and the incidence of leukemia and other negative health outcomes. Their efforts made national headlines, putting the Woburn case alongside Love Canal as an example of community research into and action against hazardous toxic-waste disposal practices.

COMPONENTS OF QUALITATIVE
RESEARCH METHODS
Access and Trust

Researcher access to activists is important in qualitative methods to enable personal and emotional contact. It must be negotiated, and it often results from preexisting connections, sometimes with lawyers as an intermediary. Kai Erikson was brought in by lawyers to assess the impact of the Buffalo Creek flood; his idea to write a book came later. My *No Safe Place* coauthor, Ed Mikkelsen, interviewed the Woburn families to prepare psychiatric data for the lawsuit they filed, and they trusted him as a confidant who had helped them examine their emotional reactions to illness, suffering, and death. When I became involved, Ed Mikkelsen initially accompanied me on interviews; later I continued interviews and observations alone. I had additional access to the families through the attorney Jan Schlictmann, whom they trusted as the person who was bringing their story to light and helping hold W. R. Grace and Beatrice accountable. Jan called each family personally to encourage them to cooperate with me. Access and trust are inseparable.

Access can also derive from the deep interest of a sympathetic researcher. At Love Canal, Adeline Levine presented herself as a trustworthy scholar who could help tell the residents' story to the world. A key organizer may help provide access to a community, as Lee Clarke found with his study of the toxic contamination in Binghamton after the state office building fire.

Connections do not guarantee that residents will share their experiences. The researcher still has to generate personal trust and confidence, as well as a belief that the research will be helpful to people and the community. Earning trust requires sincerity. Community groups can tell which outsiders are sincere, having already had opportunities to test the sincerity of public health and environmental officials. Sincerity, however is not enough; researchers must also be well informed about the events and the situation in order to signal their interest, their competence, and their respect for the residents' time.

Trust means that the people you are researching have faith in your rationale for doing the study and your support for their point of view. Once you have earned that trust, they will include you in gatherings, help connect you to other people, and give you broad access to information about themselves and to other relevant materials.

Study Design

The qualitative researcher must decide how to frame the study and thus how to tell the story. In truth, it is sometimes not clear until well into the project where the emphasis should be placed. Often research will change directions and take new tacks in the midst of the work as a result of the researcher's own realizations about the material and ongoing interaction with people.

Framing the study also entails deciding how much historical and cultural context to include. Kai Erikson's Buffalo Creek research was saturated with the social history of the Appalachian region, going back to the nineteenth century, in order to show both the isolation and the resiliency of the people. Kroll-Smith and Steve Couch's research on the underground mine fire in Centralia and Steve Picou's work on the Exxon *Valdez* oil spill are other studies that incorporate intense local background. Louise Kaplan's 1997 work on lay efforts to uncover the Hanford historical documents, which recorded accidental and deliberate radiation releases at the nuclear weapons facility in Hanford, WA, required a review of the salience of a pronuclear culture in a community that primarily wanted to avoid conflict. Not all researchers go into such depth. In *No Safe Place*, preferring to focus on the contamination crisis, I provided a very small amount of such background, primarily the town's history of tanning and chemical production.

The researcher must decide how much attention to place on conflicts within the community. Again, the specific constellation of community, industry, and government actors determines the focus. Kroll-Smith and Couch's *The Real Disaster is Above Ground* details the events in the following the discovery of the rapidly spreading coal fire underneath the town. Residents differed on how to respond, and there were conflicts over threats to jobs and property values. The authors later expanded their concern to a generalized idea of "corrosive communities," as related events in other areas provoked similar conflict among residents. Levine's Love Canal research mentioned such conflicts but did not make them central. My choice in Woburn was to mention but not dwell on internal conflicts, largely because they did not seem a major part of the situation or appear to affect the outcomes.

How closely grained should the research process be? Kroll-Smith and Couch decided that one of them should actually move into the community to ensure access to residents and community meetings. For eight months Kroll-Smith became part of the contaminated community and was able to "observe and experience daily life in a hazardous area" (Kroll-Smith and Couch 1990). He was also subject to the divisions within the community. This close relationship with the community forced Kroll-Smith and Couch to face a "complex moral and methodological quandary" over the objectivity of their work (1990, 175): they felt that the line between social science research and advocacy was blurred. Their joint efforts provided enough objectivity, however, to produce a balanced interpretation of the events in Centralia. Kai Erikson lived and breathed the aftermath of the Buffalo Creek flood during prolonged stays in the area. I came to Woburn too late to be present at the many meetings that fashioned that struggle, but I tried to attend any subsequent meetings to observe the continuing organizing.

Most scholars working in this area use open-ended interviewing as their primary data source, along with observation and documentary materials such as activist newsletters and leaflets, newspaper articles, legal documents, government reports and documents, and medical and scientific reports. For my work in Woburn, I focused on the families who were parties to the lawsuit, who were by extension the main activists, but I also interviewed other activists whose health was not affected and who were thus not part of the lawsuit. I interviewed relevant state and federal officials involved in the case as well as health professionals who conducted health studies with and for the residents. I attended community meetings as well as academic presentations by activists.

Deciding on the nature of the study involves choosing what theoretical frameworks to employ and what themes, concepts, and issues to analyze. It is important to have a theoretical foundation before beginning, as it shapes the way the research is framed and conducted. I drew on several frameworks—Edelstein's (2004) notion of "inversion of the home," Krimsky and Plough's (1988) work on lay versus professional disputes in environmental hazards, scholarship on citizen participation by Nelkin (1984), and a variety of critiques of value-neutral science and the political economy of environmental hazards.

Themes, concepts, and issues for analysis are decided in several ways (and need not be all in hand before starting). First, they may be known from prior research by other scholars. Such sources are especially useful, since shared concepts facilitate well-grounded research instruments and contribute to a standard body of knowledge. Second, they may emerge from pilot interviews, initial examination of observations and interviews, and expanded analysis of the observations and interviews. Recurring themes can be determined by word counts, concept counts, and skilled multiple readings of transcribed material.

The above elements of flexible study design are congruent with our discussion of multisited ethnography in chapter 4. Individual research sites, while amenable to rich description and analysis, do not reveal larger trends. Our multisited approach describes the original research on disputes over environmental causes of asthma, breast cancer, and Gulf War illnesses.

Empathy, Bias, and Personal Shifts in the Researcher's Worldview

Policy ethnography can introduce a strong value component to a project, which in turn may introduce a serious reflexive element, through researchers' development of sympathetic relationships with the people and settings they study. My empathy for the Woburn families' plight was visible to them and helped enhance access and trust. I let my interest and concern show and tried to avoid the voyeurism of a few journalists who had sought catchy quotes (some had even asked parents to stage reenactments of their children getting in the car to go to the hospital). My sadness in talking to people who had lost a child colored my approach to the book: I wanted readers to sense these families' loss and understand how it was amplified by the corporations' mean-spirited responses and by the problems in the state and federal agencies' research processes. Deep empathy is necessary in order to study contaminated communities. It opens the way for engaged policy application, better access to participants, and deeper and more complex responses.

Carrying out research in this way can dramatically affect the researcher. The quintessential example of a researcher transformed by the research process is

Martha Balshem, a health researcher for the Fox Chase Cancer Center. Hired as a medical anthropologist by a Philadelphia cancer prevention project in the Tannerstown neighborhood, she began to distrust the cancer center's medicalized approach, which focused on individual risk factors, especially smoking, drinking, and diet. Balshem observed that this approach clashed with belief system of the predominantly white, working-class residents of the neighborhood. Tannerstown residents countered this worldview with their belief that the local chemical plant and other sources of contamination were responsible for elevated cancer rates in the area. The professionals approached the working-class community as a monolithic group. They identified many unhealthy behaviors and nonscientific attitudes that they referred to as working-class "fatalism," which they actually termed a "disease." Balshem, however, came to view residents' health behaviors as a reasonable response to financial insecurity in the face of Philadelphia's declining industrial economy. The health educators focused on people's failure to comply with cancer prevention experts' recommendations. Yet, from a community standpoint, mainstream lifestyle change approaches to prevention amount to what Balshem notes is "to adapt to life in the 'cancer zone.'" (1993, 57). When Balshem shifted from attributing the area's cancer rates to individual behaviors to believing that there were broader, structural explanations, she could no longer tolerate her job, and left it.

Regardless of how access is achieved, the emotional and political context of such endeavors puts researchers into close contact, and often friendships, with the people they are studying. Critics of such reflexive research argue that this closeness introduces bias. I would argue that some bias—if that is really the appropriate term—is inherent in our choice of research topic: we study these situations because we sympathize with the affected citizens. Indeed, all research has some implicit values, despite claims to the contrary. In conducting a research project with Edwin Mikkelsen, the Woburn plaintiffs' psychiatric expert, I recognized the potential for siding with the residents. But sympathy does not mean that a researcher accepts uncritically all the beliefs and perspectives of informants. Rather, the goal is to understand the social-scientific nature of community discovery and action, both to make our society healthier and to increase our knowledge of how people, organizations, and communities perceive and act on important matters. Many sympathetic researchers have had to acknowledge, after careful investigation, that community claims of environmental health effects could not be confirmed and to adjust their conclusions as a result (see Ozoneff and Boden 1987).

Are environmental sociologists and other environmental researchers already biased toward community groups in general? All environmental sociology is tinged with a procommunity ethos. Social scientists often perceive community contamination episodes as insults brought about by corporate malfeasance and amplified by government inattention or failure to act. If they believe that affected populations lack the resources to learn about and act on environmental crises, they may feel a responsibility to balance the resource inequity by offering their own expertise in support of the affected people. From the researcher's point of view, such alliances yield higher-quality data, as residents have a strong motivation to cooperate with data collection.

Researchers have the tools to examine their own biases. Becker (1967) argues that conducting research uninfluenced by personal and political sympathies is impossible for social scientists. He proposes instead that we ask ourselves whose side we are on. By confronting that question directly, we can examine possible sources of bias. Only by not allowing sympathy to rule our work and by recognizing and reporting the limitations of our studies will we move in the direction of eliminating bias from our work (Becker 1967). A "symmetrical analysis," purporting to equally represent competing sides of a dispute, is an illusion, and researchers who fail to acknowledge it as such perpetuate the illusion of symmetry (Scott, Richards, and Brian 1990).

More generally, the initial choice of topics, research sites, and specific organizations is itself full of value commitments. Qualitative researchers, typically well versed in critiques of positivism, usually believe that all research is based on some sort of commitment, implicit or explicit. When fieldworkers end up actually intervening in the process they are studying, some scholars argue that the intervention is justified, because deciding not to intervene is just as much a value choice as is the choice to intervene. Research cannot be value-neutral, despite claims to be so (Scott, Richards, and Brian 1990; Martin 1996). Opposing such an interventionist stance, Collins (1996) holds that rather than choosing one side in a debate, it is the role of researchers to demonstrate the asymmetrical nature of scientific controversies.

Roles, Reflexivity, and Member Validation

Positivism seeks to use natural science as a model for social science, attempting to apply universal laws and employ neutral language. Positivist approaches try to quantify data as much as possible and to use measures that appear universally valid. By contrast, many researchers seek to take an approach that claims to study the world in its "natural" state, undisturbed by the researcher. They try to describe phenomenologically the community or group they are studying without being involved in it. But in truth, this approach is similar to positivism in that it assumes a "natural" world that all observers would view similarly: it seeks to identify a positive fact or phenomenon. The seemingly opposite poles of positivism and naturalism in epistemology and research methodology both maintain a sharp distinction between social scientists and the group or community being studied.

Qualitative researchers seek to repair that distinction by acknowledging that the people we study, and our interactions with them, also shape the data. Our conversations and observations with people at our research sites lead them to make their own analyses, which may then influence their perceptions and experiences. By entering the field, we have changed it: when people know what we are interested in, they may change their thoughts, conversations, and actions to reflect our interests.

Such influence raises concerns about the role we are taking in our research site. Do we seek as neutral as possible a stance, hoping that it will avoid such co-construction of data, or do we move toward that level of co-construction of data while simultaneously making all efforts to identify and grapple with it? It is not always possible to make this choice ahead of time, because roles change as a project evolves. My collaboration with Ed Mikkelsen in Woburn put me into the role of an interested party who was attached to the case. But I also sought an independent role as a scholar with knowledge about other environmental struggles and as a political activist. Both these roles gave me an understanding of the Woburn situation beyond the bounds of the legal case. It would not have been wise, or even possible, to take a markedly detached and disinterested stance, because residents might lose trust and limit my access to people and their stories.

Acknowledging reflexivity helps avoid the problems associated with both positivist and naturalist attempts to remove the effects of the researcher on the data. As Hammersley and Atkinson point out, "We are part of the social world we study" (1995, 18). Awareness of reflexivity also forces us to acknowledge that another researcher, even one with similar personal values and views, would likely experience and analyze the case differently, and hence we must analyze the reasons why we do it a particular way. For example, my published work on the Woburn case presented a public account of the situation that in some sense represents the residents and their organized efforts. Therefore it was important for me to get it right, using member validation techniques (Bloor 1988). These involve sharing parts of the research process and its products with the people being studied.

Member validation can correct factual errors, but, more important, it can point to areas for current and future research. As participants learn what you have said about them, they can reassess their initial interview responses or come up with new material, thus enriching the whole data set. This process changes the field and alters subsequent narrative content. Member validation and data sharing communicate narratives that might otherwise have been kept private. Social scientists draw from a perspective different from that of participants, precisely because participants are embedded in the situation and their purpose is direct action rather than social research and publication. Member validation may provide new concepts or language from which community members may draw when constructing subsequent narratives, and thus it is highly congruent with the community-based participatory research that characterizes this volume.

Member validation also fulfills an ethical responsibility to involve community members in the research. I shared my completed book manuscript with three leaders of the Woburn citizens' group (FACE), one epidemiologist involved in the case, and the plaintiffs' lead attorney. Their reviews helped to uncover some factual inaccuracies.

Michael Bloor notes of his own work: "While my accounts were recognizable to members, they were not isomorphic with their common-sense knowledge of their work practices" (1988, 165). Indeed, they should not be isomorphic. Woburn residents did not employ the concept of popular epidemiology. From their perspective, they were simply doing what they and members of other contaminated communities had to do: investigate the environmental health crisis in which they were enmeshed. Qualitative researchers can feed back not just facts but also analytic concepts, thus helping residents shape the social-scientist research literature on their community and similar places. Residents might later come to accept such an analytic concept, but it is not part of their initial framework.

Kai Erikson's approach to member validation in his study of an underground petroleum leak in East Swallow, CO, is unique. He asked twenty-one residents to read copies of his court testimony and to record comments on a tape recorder. He did so "to bring the people I was writing about into the composing of their own story" (Erikson 1994, 102). He also wanted them to come up with material that could be useful in cross-examination of the residents by the defendant's lawyers. Erikson's book *A New Species of Trouble* includes the text of the entire report, with almost half the space devoted to footnotes in which he provided the residents' tape-recorded responses. This interactive approach gives rich voice to the people being studied.

Lay participation in science forces professional scientists to step outside their traditional training and to consider the importance of firsthand knowledge possessed by the community. This concern brings us back to concepts such as the role of "advocacy scientists" who extend their personal responsibility and commitment to their professional work. While investigating the emergence of the environmental endocrine-disruptor hypothesis, Krimsky witnessed several scientists become visible activists for the hypothesis despite gaps in their knowledge and the risks for their image and careers. Advocacy scientists, Krimsky tells us, "view their role as bifurcated between advancing the scientific knowledge base and communicating to the public, the media, and policymakers" (Krimsky 2000, 151).

Discussion of reflexivity also gives weight to considerations about "citizen-science alliances," as one form of advocacy science. Collaboration between community groups and scientists educates both parties. While researchers clearly benefit from the input of community members, the collaboration also educates the community about the strengths and limitations of the scientific process. Citizen groups often have unrealistic expectations about science. Collaboration between citizens and scientists also eases mutual apprehensions: community members may feel exploited by outside researchers, and researchers can feel intimidated by activist groups. Overall, the citizen-science alliance benefits both parties by introducing laypeople's concerns into the research project and by allowing the researcher an insider's view of the community. Ethnographies of contaminated communities help to uncover data that might not otherwise surface. This is a notable contribution, but to what extent does it benefit the community? Another way to increase community control is to share data freely. Researchers who study contaminated communities and other environmental health and justice issues have often presented their work at activist conferences so that community groups can engage with the data publicly; indeed, they have an ethical obligation to do so, given the history of problems with many forms of research on communities. Sharing data also taps a growing scientific interest in open access to research and publications. A leading environmental justice group, West Harlem Environmental Action, has consistently provided excellent vehicles for sharing information through conferences that highlight activist concerns but also include academic researchers and government agencies. Topics have included race and genetics, climate justice, and children's environmental health.

CONCLUSION

Qualitative methods are important in enabling community narratives to be constructed and shared. They also provide social scientists with an opportunity to contribute to community activism and advocacy. Research efforts over the past two decades have laid a foundation for qualitative methods, used either alone or in tandem with quantitative epidemiological studies.

Not all environmental social-science researchers practice this form of advocacy, but many do. Their work helps create, modify, and present to the world the community narratives of grassroots environmental health research and advocacy that might otherwise remain unknown. Gareth Williams writes about "narrative reconstruction," the ways that people reconstruct how they believe they developed diseases (1984). People often employ broader viewpoints than does the biomedical model: some infer a political and economic causality; others locate the etiology in a nest of social relationships and in their own psychological makeup; others may supply a mystical explanation. Their goal is to produce a coherent self-analysis for their own narrative, thus providing a way to repair the rupture that disease causes in their relationship with the world. That repair can empower them in their efforts, and the researchers' account can convince relevant parties of the nature of the problem.

Environmental health research can make valuable contributions through its connections to two primary audiences: professional organizations in social science

and life science, and the affected communities. To maintain these links, researchers need to obtain support from sympathetic government agencies and programs,
from private foundations, and from scientists and their organizations. They also
need to cement alliances with community groups, which can exert influence on
the funding organizations. Finally, researchers must carefully document their
methods, especially those that improve academic and community partnerships.

NOTE

Originally published as Phil Brown, "Qualitative Methods in Environmental Health Research," *Environmental Health Perspectives* 111 (2003): 1789–98. Reproduced with permission from *Environmental
Health Perspectives*.

4

Getting Into the Field

New Approaches to Research Methods

Phil Brown, Rachel Morello-Frosch, and Stephen Zavestoski

Chapter 2 discussed the theoretical foundation underlying our work, which addresses the lack of suitable frameworks on health movements involving contested illnesses and their resistance to scientization. Research on contested illnesses also requires methodological innovations. This chapter presents three such innovations: analytical methods we term *field analysis* and *policy ethnography,* and our adaptation of community-based participatory research. Field analysis situates social movements within social and institutional worlds that include diverse strategic allies and coalition partners, some of them with conflicting perspectives. These may include government, academic, scientific, and civic organizations. Policy ethnography, which employs field analysis as an analytical tool, studies social movements by including organizational and policy analysis alongside ethnographic observations and interviews, and it operates with a policy goal in mind. Some of those carrying out policy ethnography are themselves actors in the policy realm. These methods move beyond traditional divisions between researcher and subject and acknowledge the effects that researchers themselves may have on policy. Our approach is centered on the belief that science, activism, and policy are all part of the same phenomenon and need to be examined holistically.

This chapter also presents our adaptation of an existing research method, community-based participatory research (CBPR). We simultaneously engage in and study CBPR projects. These often entail citizen-science alliances in which environmental health movement organizations challenge and also engage directly in the scientific enterprise, with the aim of changing policy and regulation or transforming dominant theories of disease causation.

Our innovations on existing methods were driven by the need for better tools to understand our research sites and questions. For example, our research studying environmental factors in breast cancer initially focused on one organization, Silent Spring Institute, that was established by an activist organization, the Massachusetts Breast Cancer Coalition. It soon became clear, however, that advocacy efforts to highlight environmental links to breast cancer were emerging in other sites as well and that these local and regional movements were networking with each other. As a result, we expanded our ethnographic work to include organizations on Long Island that had successfully advocated for the National Institutes of Health to launch the Long Island Breast Cancer Study Project (a multistudy investigation of environmental links to breast cancer), and advocacy groups in the San Francisco Bay Area engaged in related activities, such as Breast Cancer Action and the Breast Cancer Fund (see chapter 9). Field analysis that situated Silent Spring Institute within a larger network of research and activism was necessary to track and understand the evolution and heterogeneity of this emerging movement.

The environmental breast cancer movement was using scientific research to influence policy, primarily in the arena of chemical regulation. Both Silent Spring Institute and the Massachusetts Breast Cancer Coalition played pivotal roles in the Precautionary Principle Project (later the Alliance for a Healthy Tomorrow), which was a key actor in developing and articulating precautionary approaches to decisions about policy and regulations governing chemical use. The advocacy efforts of this diverse coalition resulted in the rapid rise in understanding of the precautionary principle among the public, environmental activists, the scientific community, and some decision makers in the United States, as evidenced by the enactment of municipal purchasing programs to promote toxics-use reduction in San Francisco and Mendocino County, California.

To elucidate the policy orientation of this broad-based movement required a change in our methodological approach, which ultimately made local and national policy outcomes a core subject for our ethnographic work. This issue became even more significant as our work with Silent Spring broadened into a research collaboration with Communities for a Better Environment (CBE), an environmental justice advocacy organization in California. We jointly conducted a household exposure study in Richmond and Bolinas, CA, that had significant implications for local and statewide regulation of consumer products and outdoor sources of pollution. Policy ethnography enabled us to study and respond to these emerging regulatory issues.

Our work on contested illnesses evolved from studying CBPR projects to participating in them. In our work with Silent Spring Institute in the later stages of its Cape Cod Household Exposure Study, we examined the ethical and policy implications of reporting personal exposure assessment and biomonitoring data to individual study participants (Brody et al. 2007a; Altman 2008; Morello-Frosch et al. 2009a). Similarly, our work with Silent Spring and CBE on the Northern California Household Exposure study entailed CBPR strategies such as coproduction of study protocols and dissemination of results to diverse audiences. We collaboratively conducted air and dust sampling, reported results to community members, disseminated the study results to the public and the media, and assessed the effects of our scientific work on policy. CBE, however, focused its organizing and advocacy efforts on challenging the expansion of a major oil refinery near the fence line of our Richmond study site.

For each research method discussed in this chapter, we examine what it is, how we do it, and why it is important. All these methods respond to some of the issues arising from our theoretical framework. For example, field analysis offers a way to examine theoretical concerns such as movement fields and interpenetration of movements. Policy ethnography serves our theoretical interest in how activists challenge authority structures. CBPR helps us address our theoretical concerns with power imbalances in science and knowledge. Indeed, CBPR provides a framework for both studying and acting on power imbalances in collaborations between community and academia.

FIELD ANALYSIS

What It Is

Field analysis stems in part from Raka Ray's "fields of action" (1999), Maren Klawiter's "cultures of action" (1999), David Meyer and Nancy Whittier's "social movement spillover" (1994), and Adele Clarke's "social worlds" (2005). It considers both the antecedents of health social movements and concurrent movements. Field analysis helps researchers situate a movement within a complex historical, socioeconomic, political, and institutional web. For example, we can better understand the ways environmental breast cancer movement (EBCM) activists challenge science by looking at what they learned from AIDS activists, who a decade earlier demanded greater participation in research decisions about the design of clinical trials (McCormick, Brown, and Zavestoski 2003). Sources of information on this historical legacy include the print and electronic newsletters of organizations like Breast Cancer Action and the Breast Cancer Fund and interviews with movement leaders.

This plotting of the history and the ways it shapes contemporary connections between social movements helps to elucidate a movement's own awareness of its origins and the context in which it functions, both of which significantly influence its strategies and tactics. Groups and actors look at the experience of antecedents to learn how similar issues were framed, allies sought, and strategies and tactics devised. Field analysis also examines conflicts and incongruencies between movement constituents, which may arise from differing assumptions, experiences, motivations, and knowledge. It highlights how movements develop and evolve, as the organizations' own hindsight may not always provide adequate data.

Our approach to field analysis draws on field theory, which has been used in the social sciences to explain how relationships shape the behavior of social movement organizations and actors (Martin 2003). In this tradition, the analysis of fields maps the dynamic relationships between actors in a particular social space. This approach is perhaps best developed in the work of Pierre Bourdieu (1984), who uses the concept to understand how actors struggle within a shared space to appropriate power and capital to monopolize authority, as well as how actors cooperate in shaping the field. This analytic approach also highlights the rules that govern relationships among various organizations and the institutional norms they create (DiMaggio and Powell 1983; Scott and Meyer 1992). Social scientists have used this approach in studying epistemic communities (Haas 1992; Knorr-Cetina 1999) and transnational issue networks (Keck and Sikkink 1998).

Sometimes, the communities we study are not place-based. The children's environmental health community, for example, encompasses a broad range of actors and organizations addressing specific issues of concern to children's health, such as lead poisoning and various developmental toxins. Communities may begin as place-based and then evolve into broader networks: the environmental breast cancer movement emerged separately in several locales (Massachusetts, Long Island, and the San Francisco Bay Area). And researchers' focus may shift over time: concern over compounds like perfluorooctanoates (PFOAs), for example, began with an examination of production workers, then extended to local communities whose drinking water was contaminated by local chemical production, and then, in light of evidence indicating ubiquitous exposures in the US population, to the nation as a whole (CDC 2010).

How We Do It

The set of groups, individual actors, and organizations involved in a movement constitute a *movement field*. Because movement growth and generation are continual, researchers may need to remap the movement field periodically. Mapping offers the opportunity to examine historical connections that might not otherwise be apparent; diagramming a particular antecedent might, for example, reveal connections to other antecedents, some indirect. Figure 4.1 illustrates the application of field analysis to understand the origins and networks of a social movement field, in this case for the environmental breast cancer movement.

We originally posited the existence of this movement as a result of our early interviews with activists in Long Island, the San Francisco Bay Area, and the Boston–Cape Cod area. We then located breast cancer activist groups nationwide that focused on environmental factors. Although some of these groups were in contact, they had only a rudimentary awareness that their advocacy efforts were

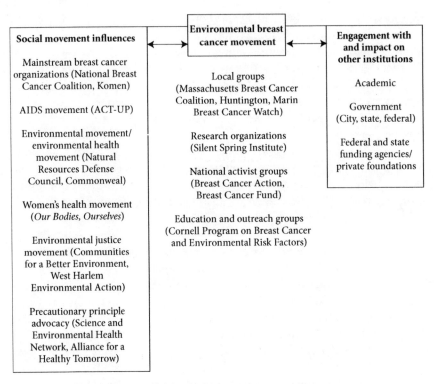

FIGURE 4.1. Field analysis model for the breast cancer movement

converging to address environmental links to breast cancer and that this work was evolving into a new movement. As we interviewed the groups' leaders and members, observed group activities, and read their newsletters and other publications, It became apparent that a new form of the breast cancer movement, with a strong focus on environmental concerns, was emerging. A movement can exist even if people are not aware that it is a movement. Members may still see themselves as part of the original, broader breast cancer movement, even though their theoretical, political, and strategic differences define them as part of a new movement.

The next step was to query these organizations more deeply about their interactions with each other and finally to suggest to them the idea that their work constituted a fundamental shift in breast cancer advocacy and the emergence of a distinct environmental breast cancer movement. We also analyzed the approach of mainstream breast cancer activists to environmental factors, both to counterpose the environmental focus and to identify nascent and potential shifts toward environmental causation within the mainstream breast cancer movement. Such research tracks changes in published statements and in funding priorities as well as interaction between mainstream and environmental groups. In this case, remapping the field meant observing the growing contact of breast cancer groups with other environmental health organizations as part of their efforts to mobilize constituencies by increasing public awareness about the failures of chemical regulation and policy in the United States.

For example, the collaboration of the Breast Cancer Fund with the Environmental Working Group in its milestone Body Burden Study (Environmental Working Group 2003a), recruited nine volunteers, most of whom were prominent breast cancer and environmental advocates, to have their blood and urine tested for the presence of 210 chemicals commonly found in consumer products and industrial pollution streams. An average of 91 industrial compounds, pollutants, and other chemicals were found in the blood or urine of the study participants, with a total of 167 chemicals found in the entire group. Results from this study were published in the peer-reviewed literature and released as an online report that presented a thumbnail photo of each participant and a list of the contaminants in that person's body. Release of the Body Burden Study came a few years after the first report by the Centers for Disease Control on biomonitoring of a representative sample of the US population, which showed ubiquitous exposures to a wide array of chemicals from diverse sources, including consumer products (CDC 1999).

We used interviews and observations with other relevant movements to validate our findings. For example, analysis of the precautionary principle movement (Mayer, Brown, and Linder 2002) provided a form of triangulation to show the connection between the EBCM and environmental justice movements. Direct engagement with some environmental justice groups involved in breast cancer issues helped show the connection between the environmental justice and EBCMs. Discussions and collaborations with academic leaders gave a basis for that connection.

Field analysis is connected to the dominant epidemiological paradigm (see figure 2.2), because new movements, such as the environmental breast cancer movement, often seek to transform or overturn a dominant paradigm of disease causation. Indeed, the EBCM challenges academic research, foundation and government funding sources, industry production and public relations practices, and government regulatory policy, which traditionally have downplayed environmental links to breast cancer. To promote environmental factors research, the movement even nourishes its own fundraising mechanisms, for example through the Breast Cancer Fund. It also pushes scientific journals and conferences to focus more attention on how chemicals function as endocrine disruptors. As scientific evidence mounts to validate the endocrine-disruptor hypothesis, the legitimacy of movement claims regarding environmental links to disease is enhanced. Movement critiques of corporate "pink ribbon" campaigns that encourage consumerism (e.g., Shop for the Cure) reveal how industry practices contribute to environmental contamination and human exposures that may be linked to the rising incidence of breast cancer. The EBCM also challenges the prevalent public messages of health voluntary organizations, such as the American Cancer Society, that often downplay environmental links to disease. In addition, it conducts sophisticated media advocacy to educate audiences about environmental links to disease by writing op-ed pieces, engaging with journalists, and writing articles for popular environmental magazines.

Why It's Important

Field analysis enables us to identify the actors, organizations, and influences that make up a social movement. As with our identification of the environmental breast cancer movement, it provides social movement researchers with tools to see movements in formation. Field analysis provides a method for studying the practices of fields of action while also being engaged in those fields. The more fully researchers understand groups they are studying, the better prepared they are for future collaborations. But field analysis does not require collaboration; it can be used without researchers' being directly involved with the groups under study.

Field analysis can also help social movement organizations see how they fit into the socioeconomic and political landscape, gain a better sense of their origins, and understand their role within a broader social movement. Their limited resources often leave groups with little time to reflect on their origins and their changing relations with other organizations. A group's field of activism may be politically or geographically limited, so that even if its work fits with the work of groups elsewhere, it may not immediately grasp those connections. Sharing field analysis data through CBPR collaborations can help inform these groups' efforts. In the Northern California Household Exposure Study, we interviewed community partner groups, with all partners present, to explore connections and means of mutual support.

Field analysis can also seed new collaborations as organizations discover new connections to other movement actors. Such relationships can lead to the development of new proposal ideas that elicit discussion of organizations' strengths and new developments. Many funding mechanisms require that proposals discuss the benefits of a group's work to community partners, and this requirement prompts such field-analysis discussions when proposals are prepared. Through this sharing, researchers can affect the movement field; our work with Silent Spring Institute and CBE helped them see common interests and work together, which they might not otherwise have done. In another example, we received a grant in 2009 to study the data reporting process in four biomonitoring projects across the country. In developing that grant, we expanded our connections to environmental health and environmental justice groups doing biomonitoring. In the process, these organizations, which included the Is It In Us? national network, the Little Hocking, Ohio, activists dealing with PFOA contamination, and the Commonweal Biomonitoring Resources Center (an environmental health education and research group), became more aware of each other's work and were able to see each other as part of the same movement field.

Field analysis can also help groups gain a deeper understanding of their history. Some social movement organizations have a presentation of self and an institutionalized account of their history that may not completely reflect their complex origins. A group's current political stance, constituency, and activities may have evolved considerably after its founding. For instance, a group that is very grassroots-oriented, with leaders and a constituency largely composed of people of color, may have been founded at least in part by white professionals. Understanding this kind of historical evolution can help situate and trace changes in organizations' concerns and advocacy strategies. Analyzing "fields of action" (Ray 1999) can also reveal potential for new political opportunities and strategic partnerships: these may include coalitions or short-term collaborations, such as one-time cosponsorship of a rally or press conference. Such analysis can help scholars to understand the development of new movements and the evolution of existing ones.

POLICY ETHNOGRAPHY

What It Is

Policy ethnography is a form of extended, multisited ethnography that studies social movements by supplementing organizational and policy analysis with ethnographic observations and interviews. *Policy* includes institutional policy, science policy, and government policy, as shown in table 4.1. Often policy is not developed or applied solely in one sector, and hence policy ethnography must straddle these sectors. For instance, in the Northern California Household Exposure Study, our approach to reporting biomonitoring and household exposure results to participants is governed by science and medical policy (peer review of our analytical results at conferences and peer-reviewed journals), academic policy (institutional review board permission to report data to study participants), and government policy (provision of funding to support such work).

Policy ethnography combines ethnographic interview and observation material; organizational history; current and historical policy analysis; evaluation of the scientific basis for policy making and regulation; and, in some cases, engagement in policy advocacy. Our approach acknowledges and responds to important developments in social movement theory and research showing that social movements confront not singular authority structures but rather the multiple, interconnected authorities of policy structures and science (Myers and Cress 2004; Zavestoski et al. 2004). We conduct analysis at the micro level (personal experiences and interactions), meso level (organizational and institutional factors), and macro level

TABLE 4.1 Examples of policy types in our analysis and practice

Government (local, state, national, or international)	Academic	Scientific and medical
Legislation	University institutional review board (IRB) practices	Peer review of publications and grants
Regulation	University support of community-based participatory research	Practices of scientific organizations
Funding mechanisms	Internal funding sources	Clinical practice

(government structures and political and economic forces). Throughout, we focus on the spaces and boundaries *between* science, policy, and civil society, because health problems and solutions are defined and debated through interactions and exchanges at these boundaries rather than within any one sector. Policy ethnography applies the concepts of boundary work, in which hybrid movements blur the boundaries between lay and expert forms of knowledge and between activists and the state (Star and Greisemer 1989; Gieryn 1999; Brown et al. 2004).

Traditional ethnography may be inadequate for studying health social movements because they are so tightly interwoven with the government, medical, and scientific realms they challenge (Frickel and Gross 2005). To address this deficiency, we devised policy ethnography at a time when other, similar ethnographic methods were being developed to situate groups under study in extralocal and historical contexts (Burawoy 2000; Gille and O'Riain 2002). Multisited ethnography, Rapp notes, "break[s] the connection of space, place, and culture," because there are no clear boundaries to the research sites and their participants (1999, 12). We sought to identify interconnected locales that make up environmental and health social movements without being tied together in a formal organizational form. This strategy has enabled us to tie ethnography more explicitly to policy study and practice.

Ethnographic work on illness experience has been valuable in uncovering the ways people recognize and cope with various components of disease and illness. But we found that environmentally induced diseases entail a larger concern: the collective illness experience, and ultimately the politicized collective illness experience (Brown et al. 2004). Because this realization led to a push for policy change, we found it necessary to incorporate policy into what might be considered a basic illness ethnography. This approach should also be broadly applicable to many other illnesses that are not environmentally induced, because politicization and economic control are widely involved in illness experiences. For example, the study of reproductive rights, silicone breast implants, or childhood obesity requires a thorough policy assessment. Hence, for a substantial number of medical concerns, policy ethnography may in fact be a logical extension of basic ethnography. Many researchers have made significant transformations of ethnographic methods. However, to our knowledge, no one has systematized this method for the study of social movement organizations or analysis of movement fields.

How We Do It

Policy ethnographies engage multiple perspectives, multiple sectors, multiple sites, and multiple phases of mobilization. They are thus both "multi-sited ethnography" (Marcus 1995), and "multi-sighted" (Altman 2008), considering the perspectives of multiple social groups and stakeholders in an ever-changing socioeconomic and political milieu. Our approach differs from earlier forms of multisited ethnography in that we tie each of these foci to policy concerns.

Multiple Perspectives.   Multiple groups may hold diverse views of illness, treatment, and prevention. The environmental breast cancer movement has a perspective on breast cancer etiology and prevention that diverges from commonly held biomedical establishment views, which attribute the disease to genetics or lifestyle factors. Activists in the EBCM press for more research into the association between environmental exposures and disease incidence. Our multisighted approach works to document these diverse perspectives and to locate them within broader discursive and political trends in policy and science. Because of the contested nature of illness, movement groups often have dissimilar positions, even if they share concerns. For example, during deliberations over how to frame California's biomonitoring legislation, environmental health and some environmental breast cancer organizations disagreed over the value of breast-milk monitoring for contaminants, compared to monitoring other biological samples, like blood serum. Breast Cancer Action (BCA) argued that breast milk biomonitoring had critical ethical implications and that any state program needed to clarify how it would report such information in ways that would not just make breastfeeding mothers worry but would help them turn their concerns into effective action. BCA pointed out the importance of helping people interpret their results in ways that would not discourage breastfeeding, especially in communities of color, where rates of breastfeeding are low (Brenner 2003).

When illness, its etiology, or treatment is not contested, policy debates involve less conflict, because there is greater consensus on how to resolve a given problem (Brown et al. 2002). This pattern follows from our understanding of the dominant epidemiological paradigm, which health social movements challenge in order to overturn or transform established theories of disease causation.

Multiple Sectors.   With the increasing involvement of science and social movements in policy making on health issues, researchers must examine multiple sectors: government, science, academia, industry, public opinion, and social movement organizations. They observe as much activity in policy chambers as in scientific laboratories or conferences; they also pay attention to street-corner protests where social movements and constituents call for, challenge, and deliberate proposed policy solutions. Policy ethnography thus engages the articulation between science, policy, and the public. In our study of the breast cancer movement, we observed how policy makers allocated money for etiological research; we visited the labs of breast cancer scientists; we entered surgical suites as patients underwent mastectomies; and we marched at public rallies alongside cancer survivors and women living with breast cancer.

Researchers studying health social movements must not only move between disparate sectors but also investigate the interesting new hybrid spaces where the work of science, policy making, and social change take place. Science is increasingly being conducted outside laboratories, and policy is being formulated outside policy chambers; as a consequence, social movement groups often cross sector boundaries (as scholars of boundary work and interpenetration have shown). For example, when studying how community activists conduct and apply biomonitoring science in order to change policy and seek redress in the courts, Altman (2008) found herself in many such boundary spaces. She observed a social movement organization's press conference on chemical body burden and its public call to ban brominated flame retardants at the Maine State House, watched community organizers pack glass specimen-collection jars in the offices of an Alaskan environmental health and justice organization, and attended science-intensive discussions about contaminated drinking water held in a rural Appalachian high school auditorium.

Multiple Sites.   Studying issues across multiple sites allows us to tease out the influence of different contextual factors, such as social movement fields, lineages, and political-economic relations, on social movement behavior. Cases can vary by issue, by context, and by the stage or phase of movement or policy formation.

Multiple sites were helpful to us in examining how a variety of environmental breast cancer movement groups differed, networked, and converged. In the aggregate, those groups held a common position, differing from mainstream breast cancer groups on the issue of environmental causation; but within the environmental breast cancer movement, organizations differed considerably in the ways they worked with local, state, and federal agencies, in their strategy and style of work, and in their choices of allies. Thus the multisited approach helped us understand the broader social movement in which different groups operated (McCormick 2009). Multiple sites can be selected for their contextual differences. Our multiple locations for examining the EBCM differed according to demeanor and degree of activism, extent of collaboration with government, and connections to other social movements.

Multiple Phases of Mobilization. Policy ethnography can examine disease contestation and health social movements at different stages of mobilization or movement formation. In studying movement organizations that conduct research and in partnering with scientists, we found that our ethnographic involvement often led to research-based collaborations with the groups we studied. For example, one of our early field sites, Silent Spring Institute, asked us to collaborate on a research project to demonstrate a long legacy of community involvement in health research, which would justify the continuation and strengthening of community participation in research on environmental factors in breast cancer. This was part of a chain of events that led us to partner with Silent Spring Institute and Communities for a Better Environment in a four-year household exposure study that linked the scientific and policy goals of breast cancer advocacy and environmental justice activism.

Researchers may begin with one form of policy orientation and find it shifting in midstream. In our household exposure study, we tested air and dust in homes in Richmond, CA, next to a large oil refinery. We initially believed that our findings would be useful both as part of a national effort to introduce a more precautionary approach to policy on chemical regulation and as part of the neighborhood's efforts to reduce this refinery's emissions.

While our project was under way, the refinery sought a conditional-use permit that would allow it to refine lower-grade crude oil, resulting in increased emissions of harmful sulfur dioxide and sulfates (Baker 2007; Jones 2008). The Richmond Planning Commission and Richmond City Council hearings on the conditional-use permit issue were occurring while we were sharing aggregated study results with community members. The residents, seeing the results as valuable to their efforts to fight the conditional-use permit, moved the discussion of the data in that direction. As a result, one of our team members (see Morello-Frosch 2008 and online appendix) prepared a report to the planning commission that helped reopen what initially seemed like a final decision in favor of the refinery. Ultimately, however, the city council granted the permit to the refinery, forcing community members to file a lawsuit, in which they won an injunction. Some of the scientific results from the household exposure study were entered into evidence.

Our research was useful in support of another policy goal: regulation of flame retardants. In Richmond, our study of chemical exposures found the highest dust and blood levels of brominated flame retardants in the United States, a likely consequence of California's strict standards for the flammability of household furniture (Zota et al. 2008). This work may support academic and environmental activist efforts to ban the use of brominated and related flame retardants in the state (Blum 2007). Furthermore, this study adds to the body of work that may influence national and international flame-retardant standards. An alliance of scientists and citizens continues to try to overturn California's harmful flame-retardant standards on furniture and to prevent expansion of those standards to bed coverings, such as comforters, mattress pads, and pillows.

Why It's Important

Policy analysis is necessary because policy issues such as official diagnostic recognition, treatment, reimbursement, research appropriations, and legislation are contested. For example, asthma research and activism by many environmental justice groups are intimately tied to demands for stricter air particulate regulation, and environmental breast cancer organizing is tied to demands for tighter regulation or banning of various chemicals. Further, because the notion of interpenetration tells us that policy makers are part of some health social movements, examining those movements requires studying those actors (Wolfson 2001).

Although valuable research on HSMs can take place without such alliances, researchers need to examine whether their work serves particular ideologies or interest groups. Those who are engaged or collaborating with activists must allow space and time for reflexive analysis. They also need to be able to step outside the partnership in order to reflect on the causes and consequences of the actions of the HSMs they study. HSM organizations often seek counsel and guidance from movement allies, such as academic scientists and policy and regulatory agency staff, to assess the implications and impact of their work. This consultation often occurs when collaborators participate in project advisory committees and when collaborative partnerships involve community-engaged research methods, such as CBPR.

COMMUNITY-BASED PARTICIPATORY RESEARCH

What It Is

CBPR is a framework in which the community being studied partners with academics to design the research questions, protocols, and methods of data dissemination, with an eye toward applying the results to improve community life (Minkler and Wallerstein 2003). From a research perspective, community involvement in the process is essential (Israel et al. 1998), as outside researchers often fail to see or understand all of the factors that affect residents' health (Seifer and Sisco 2006). CBPR has been used mainly by public health researchers and practitioners; only recently has it been adopted by social scientists. From an environmental justice perspective, it is necessary for communities to participate in the policy and regulatory decisions that affect their lives (First National People of Color Environmental Leadership Summit 1991). CBPR seeks to balance scientific research goals with policy advocacy and organizing objectives (Minkler 2000), making it a natural fit for our work, which has an environmental justice orientation and a policy focus.

How We Do It

The fact that our research group is made up of environmental health scientists and epidemiologists, as well as sociologists, enables us to both study and participate in the CBPR enterprise. Our interdisciplinary skills (e.g., environmental health science, epidemiologic and statistical methods, qualitative data analysis, and ethnographic methods) have allowed us to collaborate with community partners seeking to conduct environmental health research while also evaluating its effect on policy, the regulatory environment, and social movements. Demand for such interdisciplinary work will likely increase as collaborations are sought and encouraged by patient advocacy groups, funding agencies, and movement organizations that want to assess the policy and regulatory consequences of scientific research. Conversely, the more fully activists and their social science allies understand the need to use data and scientific research to advance policy goals, the more likely they are to seek out joint efforts with scientists.

Interdisciplinary work entails far more than a set of professionals from different disciplines teaming up. It requires a version of CBPR in which team members work across disciplinary boundaries. Thus social scientists may engage directly in the scientific enterprise by helping to design research methods, analyze data, disseminate results, and report to participants; and scientists may study how social movement organizing reshapes scientific thinking about disease causation. Further, all research team members need to become conversant with each other's areas of expertise and be able to present the work in public venues; and all are involved in community outreach.

For example, in our California household exposure study, organizers at Communities for a Better Environment (CBE) went door to door in Richmond to solicit residents' participation in the study, and they organized community meetings with scientist partners to educate residents about the study and its possible effects. Sociologists led the design of questionnaires to assess community expectations about benefits of the household exposure study. Public health scientists, sociologists, and community members collected additional qualitative data on participants' attitudes to learning about the presence of chemicals in their homes. The sociologists on the team analyzed these data, and the entire research collaborative participated in discussions regarding interpretation of results and contributed to the writing of articles on the theme of community response to personal exposure data.

Meanwhile, environmental health scientists and toxicologists developed criteria for deciding which chemicals and pollutant compounds would be sampled in the study. They worked in close consultation with the community organizers, who wanted sampling of specific pollutants that they believed to be coming from industrial sources such as the nearby oil refinery. Similarly, scientists adapted air-sampling equipment and protocols to make them easier to use and taught community organizers how to collect samples to for laboratory analysis. This form of collaboration was facilitated both by the interdisciplinary nature of our research group and by CBE's strong technical experience, as science has long been a core part of its mission. Indeed, CBE is well known for pioneering the "bucket brigades" of volunteers conducting low-cost air sampling, used widely in California and Louisiana and now globally in fence-line communities living near large industrial facilities with hazardous emissions (Lerner 2005). In the San Francisco Bay Area and Los Angeles, CBE has a long history of tracking and analyzing flaring activity and emissions from large oil refineries; this scientific work led to the promulgation of a ground-breaking flare-control rule that became a front-page story in the *New York Times* (Marshall 2005). Training in new forms of air and dust monitoring enhanced CBE's in-house scientific capacity and ensured its co-ownership of the research process. This process also enabled CBE to demystify the science for its community constituents. For example, as CBE interviewers went through the preliminary exposure questionnaire and set up sampling equipment in residents' homes, the experience encouraged community members to think more deeply about sources of chemical exposure, such as industry, transportation corridors, and consumer products.

Decisions about how to report exposure data to individual participants and the community were made collectively. The goals were to facilitate understanding of the data, its significance for health, and its scientific uncertainties; and, where possible, to link results to individual or collective action for reducing exposures. Reports to participants included an individualized, one-page summary of compounds found in the home, along with more detailed data on the groups of compounds that were sampled. Graphs displayed the compounds found in homes and outdoors and compared the levels found to those for all other study participants. (See online appendix for an example.) Pollutant levels were also compared with regulatory benchmarks, where available. Information on the uses and sources of chemical compounds was included. All collaborators shared the task of writing summary letters, which were double-checked for scientific accuracy and clarity. CBE staff members were trained by scientists to meet with participants to go over these materials and to help them think through individual and collective strategies for reducing exposures.

All the collaborators worked together in planning community meetings in which aggregate results were shared and new collective-action strategies for reducing exposures were discussed and developed. The participatory approach of this research enterprise seeks to collaboratively do science, interpret it, and act on it. The production of knowledge is not linear, but rather cyclical and iterative (Brown et al. 2006). We believe such a unified approach improves the quality of scientific work, increases democratic participation in science, and enhances the effectiveness of science in supporting education, organizing, hazard reduction, litigation, and policy advocacy.

CBE's engagement in the household exposure study brought important benefits to its scientific partners by improving the project's rigor, relevance and reach. The scientific rigor of the study was ensured through discussion and negotiation of study design issues such as choosing study sites, recruiting participants, finalizing the list of chemicals for analysis, and developing protocols for reporting results. For example, CBE encouraged the study team to collect a second set of air and dust samples from another community (Bolinas) that did not have significant outdoor industrial and transportation source emissions, for comparison with results from in Richmond. Similarly, the relevance of the study was bolstered through the collective development of bilingual (Spanish and English) graphic displays for communicating results to residents. Finally, CBE's engagement helped extend the team's capacity to reach broad audiences and use the study results to improve regulation and land-use decision making. For example, scientists and CBE trained community partners to present the data effectively on their own at community meetings and in testifying before regulatory and policy forums (see the example of testimony in the online appendix).

In our household exposure study, academic scientists and Silent Spring Institute scientists trained postdoctoral fellows, graduate students, and undergraduates in CBPR methods. Silent Spring Institute used the Richmond part of the Household Exposure Study to strengthen its linkages with communities of color working on environmental health and justice issues. Similarly, through local fundraising, public education, participation on state and federal advisory committees, and involvement with national breast cancer organizations, the collaboration enabled the organization to encourage the broader breast-cancer community to embrace an environmental justice perspective.

To evaluate the effectiveness of the household exposure study in addressing the interests and objectives of each team member, partners interviewed each other about the benefits and challenges of the project. Setting aside time for such reflective evaluation is essential in assessing whether and how CBPR projects enhance the organizational capacities and the goals of each partner. By engaging in regular mutual evaluation, partners can adjust protocols, methods, and resource allocation as necessary. Moreover, lessons learned from such evaluation can help shape new projects.

Why It's Important

Reflection on the benefits of collaboration may enable partners to achieve more and broader objectives. For example, project partners in the household exposure study sought a social scientist for the research team to help document the project's effect on advocacy and social change. One such goal was to transform human-subjects protection into "participant inclusion." The project's decision to emphasize the reporting of results to individuals led to a challenge to the policies of the Brown University Institutional Review Board (IRB) and also influenced a broader audience about new community-level protections (see chapter 13).

CONCLUSION

Studying the many facets of health social movements and health social movement organizations requires methods that can simultaneously address science, activism, and policy, often across multiple sites and from multiple perspectives. Our field analysis approach readily leads to policy ethnography by identifying the universe of actors and activities we need to examine. We find it useful to emphasize overall social movements rather than case studies of individual social movement organizations. Ultimately, the strongest contribution of field analysis is that it can examine broad movements: it is especially useful for tracing the lineage, evolution, and trajectories of developing movements.

Our work has both scholarly and policy outcomes. For social movement scholarship, field analysis can contribute to three levels of attention. At the macro level it can show how social movements evolve through their interaction with the socioeconomic and political environment. At the meso (organizational) level, field analysis helps us study the diversity of strategies and tactics within a movement. For example, the environmental breast cancer movement works on toxics reduction and chemical regulation while also challenging researchers and funding organizations to pay attention to environmental causation. At the micro level, field analysis helps us understand how movements give capacity and legitimacy to individual experiences that might otherwise be invisible to the individuals themselves. Micro-level analysis can also show how and why individuals participate in the creation of a collective illness experience and move toward transformative political action.

In looking at policy outcomes, policy ethnography helps us understand how HSMs and HSMOs select allies and make strategic choices. Taking a multisited approach can explain a diverse range of such choices among participants in the environmental breast cancer movement; this perspective complements the meso-level understanding of collective action. Local groups on Long Island were more likely to link up with status quo allies, including Republican lawmakers, while more radical groups like Breast Cancer Action on the West Coast took direct action, such as demonstrations and challenges to mainstream breast cancer organizations (Brown et al. 2006). A multisited approach to biomonitoring can show diverse strategy approaches, ranging from anticorporate litigation in the mid-Ohio Valley to conflict in Alaska (where activists contested the state health department) to legislation in Maine that was developed by a strong alliance of activists and legislators (Altman 2008).

CBPR offers a way to both participate in and analyze the scholarly and policy concerns raised by field analysis and policy ethnography. The democratizing directions of health social movements call for a complementary democratizing impulse on the part of researchers, which is fulfilled by CBPR. One facet of this impulse is internal evaluation and reflection about the project. CBPR also produces better science, precisely because it values and integrates lay and scientific knowledge, understands local communities, and uses interdisciplinary and participant perspectives to improve research techniques.

Other scholars have analyzed social movements in ways that mirror our field analysis and policy ethnography approaches, but we have sought to integrate these methods with community-engaged research strategies such as CBPR. Though these methodological tools stem from our experience with health social movements, we believe that they are also applicable to the study of and engagement with other social movements.

5

Environmental Justice and the Precautionary Principle

Air Toxics Exposures and Health Risks among Schoolchildren in Los Angeles

Rachel Morello-Frosch, Manuel Pastor, and James Sadd

The emergence over the past three decades of the concepts of environmental justice and the precautionary principle have transformed environmental policy making, research, and community organizing. Yet despite the burgeoning literature on both of these frameworks and the fact that they share some important tenets, they have not been well integrated at either the theoretical or the policy level. In this chapter we examine their foundations and propose ways in which they can be better integrated to reshape policy making to protect public health, particularly for vulnerable populations, such as the poor and communities of color.

This chapter presents quantitative data from our community-based participatory research on environmental inequality in ambient-air toxics exposures and associated health risks among schoolchildren in Southern California and evaluates the study's effects on regional and state policy. We demonstrate how quantitative methods based on risk assessment can be used to advance policy goals in tandem with the qualitative work discussed in the rest of the book. We conclude by suggesting future paths of inquiry that link the precautionary principle with environmental justice concerns.

ENVIRONMENTAL JUSTICE AND THE FRAMEWORK FOR PRECAUTION

Environmental justice advocates contend that despite seemingly neutral and uniform regulations, legislation, and performance standards, the formal and informal dynamics affecting regulatory activities produce and perpetuate discriminatory outcomes. Activists have pushed environmental health researchers and regulatory authorities to move beyond assessments focused on single chemicals or facilities and toward a cumulative-exposure approach that takes into account where affected populations live, work, and play in order to elucidate how race and class discrimination increase community susceptibility to environmental pollutants (Morello-Frosch, Pastor, and Sadd 2001). Nevertheless, establishing that environmental pollution causes adverse health effects is an ongoing challenge, particularly where populations are chronically exposed to complex chemical mixtures (Institute of Medicine 1999). Environmental organizations and environmental justice activists have persuasively argued that in the quest for better data and unequivocal proof of cause and effect, some researchers and regulators have lost sight of a basic public health principle: the importance of disease prevention (Bullard 1994; Lee 2002). The quest for scientific certainty can paralyze environmental and health policy making. Consequently, some academics and regulators have integrated the precautionary principle into their work (Brown and Mikkelsen 1997). According to this principle, in the face of uncertain but suggestive evidence of adverse environmental or human health effects, regulatory action should be taken to prevent future harm.

Recently, children's health advocates have recommended implementing the precautionary principle to protect children from exposure to environmental hazards (Schettler et al. 1999; Tickner and Hoppin 2000). Evidence indicates that children are more susceptible than adults to the effects of environmental pollution because of fundamental differences in their physiology, metabolism, and absorption and exposure patterns (Guzelian Henry, and Olin 1992; NRC 1993; Crom 1994; Parkinson 1996; Schettler et al. 1999; Kaplan and Morris 2000). Increasing rates of exposures to myriad pollutants could also be aggravating chronic health problems such as asthma and affecting cognitive development (Landrigan and Goldman 2011). Anecdotal, epidemiologic, and exposure studies suggest potential short- and long-term health effects among children from outdoor and indoor air pollutants (Van Vliet et al. 1997; Jedrychowski and Flak 1998; Gilliland et al. 1999; Guo et al. 1999; Schettler et al. 2001; Ritz et al. 2002), potentially hazardous facilities (Ginns and Gatrell 1996; Gomzi and Saric 1997), and pesticides (Landrigan et al. 1999; US General Accounting Office 1999b; Northwest Coalition for Alternatives to Pesticides 2000). Partly because of this research, a 1997 executive order directs federal agencies to consider the particular vulnerability of children to environmental health risks (Executive Order 13045 1997). Despite mounting evidence that children of color and the poor bear a disproportionate burden of exposure to environmental hazards and their potentially adverse health effects (Schwartz et al. 1990; Gold et al. 1993; Clark et al. 1999; Sexton and Adgate 1999), little research has explicitly examined the environmental justice implications of inequalities in environmental hazard exposures or the unique vulnerabilities of children of color (Kraft and Scheberle 1995; Friedrich 2000).

THE SOUTHERN CALIFORNIA ENVIRONMENTAL
JUSTICE COLLABORATIVE

The Southern California Environmental Justice Collaborative (the Collaborative) is a regional partnership among Communities for a Better Environment (CBE), the Liberty Hill Foundation, and researchers from the University of Southern California, Occidental College, and the University of California, Berkeley. As an environmental justice organization with a strong community organizing base, CBE implements the "triangle strategy" in its work: this involves the balanced integration of grassroots organizing, science-based advocacy, and legal intervention to promote effective policy change (Communities for a Better Environment, n.d.). Despite CBE's awareness of the pitfalls of overreliance on litigation and science-based advocacy, it has expanded its capacity in these areas to supplement its primary emphasis on community organizing.

The Liberty Hill Foundation was founded in 1976 as a community foundation that promotes progressive social change in Los Angeles. Within the Collaborative, Liberty Hill plays a critical role in building regional environmental-justice organizing capacity through two mechanisms: providing seed funding to small neighborhood organizations working on environmental justice campaigns and offering training through its Environmental Justice (EJ) Institute. Grant recipients are trained by experts from a variety of disciplines (e.g., law, public health, computer science, environmental health science, organizational development, media advocacy, fundraising, and nonprofit management).

The university-based multidisciplinary research team includes three experts from environmental health and epidemiology, economics and urban planning, and environmental science. All three researchers came to the Collaborative with extensive community-based research experience and have focused their academic endeavors on supporting community economic development and improving environmental policy making (Sadd et al. 1999; Pastor et al. 2000; Pastor 2001; Morello-Frosch 2002a, 2002b).

Throughout Southern California, a very active environmental health and justice grassroots and nonprofit community has been working to demonstrate that disproportionately high rates of negative health impacts are linked to poor air quality, toxic chemicals in consumer products, and the pollution generated from traffic, power plants, and other industrial sites. Residents in heavily affected neighborhoods had organized to challenge such environmental health problems, but they lacked an effective regional voice. Their efforts were also weakened by a lack of scientific research documenting environmental inequality in Southern California. The Collaborative sought to redress these deficiencies by emphasizing regional organizing to create public awareness, voice, and political pressure; legal and policy work to promote change; and scientific research on environmental health and demographics to help environmental justice groups more effectively engage in "data judo" with regulators and policy makers. Data judo is a process in which communities marshal their own scientific expertise to conduct research and use the data in support of policy and regulatory change.

At the outset, Collaborative partners decided to make secondary data analysis the core of their research activities. Although primary data collection is generally considered the gold standard in research, it has some major drawbacks. First, it requires significant financial resources and organizational capacity. Second, primary data collection conducted in collaboration with community-based organizations that have a clear stake in study outcomes is vulnerable to criticisms of systematic bias and lack of objectivity from the mainstream scientific community and policy makers (Anderton 1996; Foreman 1998). The Collaborative decided instead to analyze data collected by government environmental regulatory authorities such as the US Environmental Protection Agency (US EPA), the California Environmental Protection Agency (Cal-EPA), and the California Air Resources Board. CBE and the researchers believed that analyzing the government's own data would be a powerful way to draw regulatory attention to environmental justice issues.

In 2000 the Los Angeles Unified School District (LAUSD) announced that it was temporarily suspending the construction of a state-of-the-art high school, known as the Belmont Learning Complex, following revelations that the $180 million construction project had been built over an abandoned oilfield without adequate cleanup of pockets of potentially explosive methane gas and other toxic contaminants (Anderson 2000). Community reaction to this announcement was mixed. Some residents believed that the controversy symbolized a systemic problem of environmental inequality, while others believed that the environmental problems were minor and that halting construction was a major setback to meeting the educational needs of this mostly low-income, immigrant Latino community. CBE believed that this incident pointed to the need for the Collaborative research team to evaluate whether there were systemic and broad-based patterns of environmental inequalities throughout the school district. As a result, CBE suggested that the research team conduct an EJ air-quality analysis for all LAUSD schoolchildren.

The LAUSD is the second largest school district in the country, spanning 704 square miles and enrolling more than 700,000 students. The project began with a districtwide preliminary analysis of estimated outdoor-air toxics exposures and associated health risks (Morello-Frosch, Pastor, and Sadd 2002). Because of evidence suggesting a link between childhood respiratory problems associated with air pollution and diminished academic performance (Fowler, Davenport, and Garg 1992; Bener et al. 1994; Perera et al. 1999; Diette et al. 2000), the study also assessed the relationship between estimated respiratory risks and overall school academic performance (Pastor, Sadd, and Morello-Frosch 2002a, 2002b).

Methodology and Data Sources

All school locations were geocoded to census tracts (often used as a proxy for neighborhoods) and linked to a set of environmental hazard indicators, including tract-level estimates of lifetime individual cancer risk and a respiratory hazard index, both of which are associated with ambient exposures to airborne toxics. Estimated cancer risk and respiratory hazard indices were derived by combining modeled estimates of ambient-air toxics concentrations with corresponding toxicity data information from the US EPA and Cal-EPA. The methodologies for calculating these risk estimates are discussed extensively elsewhere (Caldwell et al. 1998; Morello-Frosch et al. 2000; Morello-Frosch, Pastor, and Sadd 2001). Exposure data were derived from a modeling analysis undertaken by the US EPA's Cumulative Exposure Project and National Air Toxics Assessment that estimated long-term average concentrations for 148 airborne toxic substances for every census tract in the contiguous United States (US Environmental Protection Agency 1998). Emissions data used in the model take into account large, stationary sources (such as refineries or chemical plants), small area service industries and fabricators (such as dry cleaners, auto body paint shops, and furniture manufacturers), and mobile sources (such as cars, trucks, and aircraft). The modeling algorithm takes into account meteorological data and simulation of atmospheric processes (Rosenbaum, Ligocki, and Wei 1999; Rosenbaum et al. 1999).

Information about school enrollments came from the October 1999 California Basic Educational Data System (CBEDS), a program administered by the California Department of Education Demographic Research Unit that includes basic information about each school as well as data on annual enrollment and ethnic makeup of the student population. Indicators of students' school performance were derived from California's Academic Performance Index (API), an assessment program mandated by the state of California under the Public Schools Accountability Act of 1999, which provides a summary score of school performance based on the Stanford 9 achievement test. In order to contextualize measures of school performance, both the CBEDS and the API include a limited set of school-level variables, including student demography, a proxy for poverty, and a measure of teacher quality. (See Pastor, Sadd, and Morello-Frosch 2002a, 2000b for further discussion of data and methods.)

Results

Estimated lifetime cancer risks associated with outdoor air toxics exposures were found to be high throughout the Los Angeles Area, often exceeding the Clean Air Act goal of one in a million by a factor of between ten and one thousand (Morello-Frosch, Pastor, and Sadd 2001).[1] Respiratory hazards, although not as high, also exceeded health benchmarks in many locations (Morello-Frosch et al.

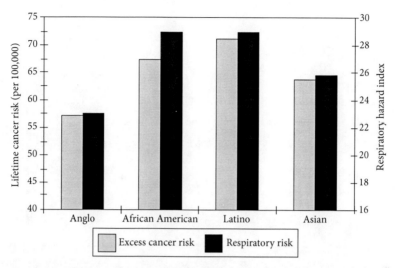

FIGURE 5.1. Cancer and respiratory risks for schoolchildren by race or ethnicity in the Los Angeles Unified School District

2000). Most of the estimated health risks originated from pollutants generated by mobile and small area sources rather than large point sources (Morello-Frosch, Pastor, and Sadd 2001).

Figure 5.1 shows the average lifetime cancer risk and the average chronic respiratory hazard index for schoolchildren of different racial and ethnic groups. The graph indicates that Latino and African American students bear the greatest burden of lifetime cancer risks associated with ambient-air toxics, but Asian schoolchildren also face higher risks than white students. A similar pattern emerges for estimates of respiratory hazard. Multivariate regression analysis demonstrated that after controlling for key covariates, the proportion of students of color at a school site continues to be a statistically significant factor for increased estimated cancer and respiratory risks associated with ambient-air toxics exposures (Pastor, Sadd, and Morello-Frosch 2002a, 200b).

To assess whether environmental hazards and estimated respiratory risks affect student school performance, we examined the relationship between school educational outcomes and estimated respiratory risk. This analysis does not use measures of individual student performance but rather an aggregate score for the entire school, by which it is ranked against other schools.[2] Such school-level studies are increasingly common because of the trend for school districts to focus on schools as the unit of accountability (Fowler and Walberg 1991).

Figure 5.2 shows the average academic performance index (API) score (a measure of schools' performance on standardized tests), ranked by three categories of

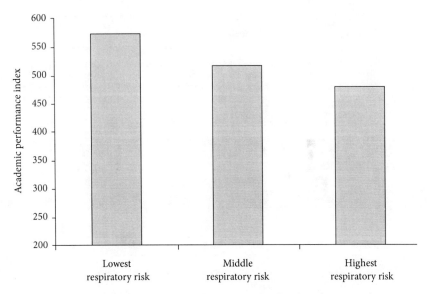

FIGURE 5.2. Public school academic performance index (API) and estimated cumulative respiratory risk from exposure to ambient-air toxics in the Los Angeles Unified School District

respiratory hazard. The differences are substantial: schools with the highest esti-mated respiratory hazard have APIs about 20 percent lower than schools with the lowest hazard level. This difference roughly matches the average academic per-formance difference between the bottom third and middle third of schools. Mul-tivariate modeling confirmed that increased respiratory risks have a statistically significant negative effect on overall school API performance, even when analy-sis controls for other factors that could explain variances in academic achieve-ment. These included the percentage of children receiving free school lunches (see Orfield 1997; Krueger 1999), the percentage of teachers with emergency cre-dentials (an indicator of teacher quality), average class and school size, whether schools were on year-round or semester schedules, the percentage of students who were just learning English,[3] a measure of student mobility (the number of students who are new to a school that year), and parents' educational attainment level. Moreover, the model indicated that reducing respiratory hazards from the highest level to the lowest would increase API scores by approximately 10 per-cent. Additionally, of the roughly 20 percent mean difference between white and African American academic performance in the API sample, about one-tenth can be attributed to disparities in the mean respiratory hazard levels experienced by these respective demographic groups at their schools. (See Pastor, Sadd, and Morello-Frosch 2002b for specific results.)

Thus this cross-sectional study demonstrated that minority students, particularly African Americans and Latinos, are more likely to bear the burden of attending school in locations where estimated cancer and respiratory risks from air toxics tend to be highest. Moreover, after controlling for demographic covariates, it appears that indicators of respiratory risk associated with air toxics are associated with diminished school performance.

POLICY IMPLICATIONS OF STUDY RESULTS

Preliminary results from our analysis indicated that there may be legitimate environmental-justice concerns for minority students attending Los Angeles public schools. Although all Los Angeles schoolchildren face exposure to outdoor air toxics and associated health risks, minority (especially African American and Latino) youth seem to bear the largest share of the burden. Moreover, the estimated respiratory hazards associated with air toxics appear to negatively affect school performance. Although the causal chain and biological mechanisms are not clearly specified, the association, even after controlling for other important covariates, is problematic, given the academic underperformance of predominantly minority and poor schools.

Although our results cannot be generalized beyond Los Angeles, our study offers some useful policy lessons and has implications for future research on the intersection of environmental justice and children's health. First, it reinforces the need for a holistic approach to environmental health and justice research. As more comprehensive data become available, future studies need to move from locational and pollutant-by-pollutant analysis toward a cumulative-exposure approach (Morello-Frosch and Shenassa 2006). Lacking comprehensive epidemiological data, we are often left with risk-assessment tools that, even within an equity-analysis framework, remain controversial among the public and policy makers (Latin 1988; Kuehn 1996). However, we sought to use risk assessment as a comparative tool. Although our analysis focused on one means of exposure, air pollution, it characterized potential health risks from cumulative exposures to multiple chemicals from multiple sources. Results here show that in the absence of good epidemiological data, risk assessment can still provide crucial information for communities grappling with high-stakes environmental equity issues related to school siting decisions.

As student enrollment rises and pressure mounts to ease severe overcrowding in schools, the LAUSD is faced with the Herculean task of building many more new schools over the next decade. Urban districts across the country face similar challenges in accommodating more students and balancing the need to enhance educational opportunities for students of color with the need to address environmental health concerns about siting new facilities. The Belmont Learning Complex controversy brought the difficulties of resolving this conflict to light.

As in the Belmont case, some might argue that building schools in dense urban areas will require the use of brownfields (land previously used for industrial or commercial purposes that contains low concentrations of hazardous waste or pollution), and that failing to quickly identify sites and slowing construction will reduce educational opportunities for minority schoolchildren (Hernandez 1999; Metropolitan Forum Project 1999; Blume 2000). Yet our study should encourage caution on the part of critics who argue against strict and potentially costly environmental standards for new schools. Indeed, both environmental justice concerns and the precautionary principle advocate that construction plans should seek to reduce environmental hazard exposure risks among minority schoolchildren, particularly given the overall poorer health of these populations (US Environmental Protection Agency 1992). Relevant policy decisions include zoning, siting decisions, and general school-based intervention strategies aimed at improving the health status and educational opportunities of minority students. At minimum, environmental inequity should not be further aggravated by expansion plans.

One lesson from the Belmont controversy is that environmental health concerns must inform decisions on where to site new school facilities. Standards for acquiring and cleaning up brownfields for school construction should be clarified and should take into account the particular vulnerability of children to environmental hazards. One result of the Belmont controversy is a new requirement that proposed school sites in California pass an environmental review by the state Department of Toxic Substances Control (DTSC). Although this is a step in the right direction, it raises a polemical social-justice issue for urban districts that are challenged to find suitable sites and also pressured to expedite the siting process to ensure adequate and timely state funding.

Until recently, state funds to support massive construction initiatives were awarded on a first-come, first-served basis. This seemingly neutral policy had the unintended consequence of placing urban school districts with few or no greenfield sites at a severe financial disadvantage and created a strong disincentive to integrating the precautionary principle and environmental justice concerns into siting decisions. California's school funding system is currently being overhauled to accommodate urban districts facing challenges in acquiring suitable property and redeveloping industrial land. Further efforts to address the overwhelming challenges faced by the LAUSD in accommodating its rapidly expanding student body will require leadership and collaboration between affected communities, the school district, city and state officials, and even the private sector to ensure that the environmental health and educational needs of children of color are addressed.

USING RESEARCH TO PROMOTE
REGULATORY CHANGE

Our study provides the preliminary data to justify new policy strategies that uphold both environmental justice and the precautionary principle. Creating a process to assess the environmental hazards of new educational construction sites and changing the California school-bond funding system to address the needs of urban districts serving predominantly minority students demonstrate how these two principles can be effectively integrated in the policy-making arena. The Collaborative's strategy of linking research, organizing, and advocacy to promote regulatory reforms and policy change has contributed to impressive victories at the regional and state levels. First, CBE used results from this study as well as a larger body of scientific work on environmental inequalities from the Environmental Justice Collaborative to advocate, along with other EJ organizations throughout the state, that Cal-EPA adopt a cumulative-exposure approach in its programs and regulatory enforcement activities. One result of this effort has been the integration of cumulative impacts into Cal-EPA's Environmental Justice Work Plan (Cal-EPA 2004).

Moreover, our study results were used by CBE to persuade the LAUSD to take a more precautionary approach in identifying and remediating school construction sites and to validate arguments for more equitable distribution of state monies for school construction between suburban and urban school districts (Morello-Frosch, Pastor, and Sadd 2002). Similarly, the California Air Resources Board issued its *Land Use Handbook,* which provides guidance for evaluating and reducing air-pollution effects in new projects that go through the land-use decision-making process (CARB 2005). The handbook specifies minimum distances for sensitive land uses, particularly schools, from sites where air pollution is likely to be a concern. (Although this recommendation addresses concerns about new school construction, the handbook does not address air-pollution concerns at existing sites.) In addition, environmental justice advocates helped shape LAUSD's integrated pest management policy to decrease pesticide use in the schools. This achievement further demonstrates how community organizing at a regional level can lead to significant local policy shifts that protect children, particularly children of color (Prussel et al. 2001).

Perhaps the most significant outcome has been the way in which the Collaborative effectively supported CBE's work with other environmental justice organizations statewide through their participation on Cal-EPA's Environmental Justice Advisory Committee, which is charged with developing recommendations on how the agency should address environmental justice. CBE presented the Collaborative's data and study results to industry and government stakeholders to argue for more stringent measures to address environmental health disparities.

This presentation resulted in the committee's consensus recommendations to Cal-EPA that emphasized developing resources and programs that enhance public participation in regulatory decision making related to environmental health; devising new regulatory and scientific approaches to assess the cumulative health impacts of pollution from multiple emission sources on neighborhoods and on vulnerable populations, such as children; and systematic integration of the precautionary principle in environmental regulation and enforcement activities (Cal-EPA Advisory Committee on Environmental Justice 2003). The latter two recommendations are now being implemented by the California Office of Environmental Health Hazard Assessment through a three-year initiative known as the Cumulative Impacts and Precautionary Approaches Project. This initiative is developing scientifically valid and transparent analytical methods to identify disparities in environmental hazard exposures and health status for key population groups (by race or ethnicity, socioeconomic status, and other vulnerability indicators) (OEHHA 2009).

THE PROMISE OF PRECAUTION AND ENVIRONMENTAL JUSTICE

Children's environmental health has been identified as a quintessential example of reasons to support environmental justice and the precautionary principle in environmental regulation and policy making (Bullard 1994; Tickner et al. 2000). As the tragic problem of childhood lead poisoning has shown, it is critical to integrate both of these frameworks to protect children's environmental health. Because of historical failures to exercise caution and act decisively to eliminate lead from paint and gasoline, one million U.S. children continue to exceed the recommended limit for blood levels of lead (Schettler et al. 2001). This failure has had a disproportionate effect on urban children of color, who have the highest average blood levels of lead and suffer the attendant neurological and developmental effects.

Integrating environmental justice and the precautionary principle is essential to protect vulnerable populations and eliminate persistent racial and class-based disparities in environmental hazard exposures and health outcomes. Environmental justice and the precautionary principle, although historically separate, have important overlapping goals. These include the following:

1. Public health and disease prevention: for advocates of environmental justice, this goal entails protecting communities of color and the poor from the environmental health effects of institutional and social discrimination. For advocates of the precautionary principle, this goal implies a commitment to

   preventing harm to human health or ecosystems in the face of inadequate scientific tools and incomplete but suggestive data.

2. Shifting the burden of proof: environmental justice advocates reject the
   notion that claims of environmental inequality must demonstrate a pattern of
   discriminatory intent and disparate impact, a requirement that creates formidable barriers to communities seeking remedies. Similarly, the precautionary
   principle proposes that chemicals should not be considered harmless until
   proven otherwise, but rather that supporters of a proposed new product or
   activity must bear responsibility for demonstrating that it is safe.

3. Procedural justice and democratic decision making: here adherents of
   environmental justice and the precautionary principle offer divergent yet
   complementary objectives for ensuring public participation in decisions that
   affect community environmental health. Environmental justice proposes a
   "political economy" perspective that advocates enhancing community capacity to shape policy making and regulation, and to advocate for regional and
   economic development activities that do not harm residents. The precautionary principle emphasizes procedural justice by promoting alternatives assessment, which entails a democratic and transparent examination of alternatives
   to potentially harmful activities. For example, this process can be applied
   to government through requirements of the National Environmental Protection Act, which requires an environmental impact statement describing
   adverse and beneficial consequences of federally funded projects and their
   alternatives. Alternatives assessment is also the key element of the Massachusetts Toxic Use Reduction Act (TURA), which requires industries using a
   threshold quantity of certain chemicals to periodically identify alternatives to
   reduce chemical use.

The integration of environmental justice and the precautionary principle offers
possibilities for new and innovative approaches to addressing issues of environmental health. The Southern California Environmental Justice Collaborative's
work in Los Angeles schools demonstrates that community participation is key
for developing long-term regulatory, enforcement, and land-use initiatives that
are sustainable and protect vulnerable communities. Moreover, decision making
about regulatory action in the face of limited scientific tools and uncertain data
must be transparent and democratic. Polemical questions of whether and how to
regulate hazards often transcend the realm of science and become political, economic, and moral judgment calls. In environmental policy making, the distinction between the scientific and sociopolitical realms is often unclear. Integrating
environmental justice and the precautionary principle offers a new framework for
creating policy tools that promote public health.

NOTES

Originally published as Rachel Morello-Frosch, Manuel Pastor Jr., and James Sadd, "Integrating Environmental Justice and Precautionary Principle in Research and Policy Making: Air Toxics and Health Risks among School Children in Los Angeles," *Annals of the American Academy of Political and Social Science* 584 (2002): 47–68.

1. In 1990 Congress established a health-based goal for the Clean Air Act: to reduce lifetime cancer risks from major sources of hazardous air pollutants to one in one million. The act required that over time, US Environmental Protection Agency regulations for major sources should "provide an ample margin of safety to protect public health" (Clean Air Act Amendments of 1990, § 112(f), Standard to Protect Health and the Environment).

2. For a general review of the quality of such educational indicators, see Koretz 1997.

3. English proficiency affects the overall Academic Performance Index scores, which are not adjusted for this variable. The exams used to calculate the API are administered in English only, in conformity with the 1998 California initiative that limits bilingual instruction and testing.

PART TWO

Working in the Environmental Health Field

Ethnographic Studies

6

A Narrowing Gulf of Difference?

Disputes and Discoveries in the Study of Gulf War–Related Illnesses

Phil Brown, Stephen Zavestoski, Alissa Cordner, Sabrina McCormick, Joshua Mandelbaum, Theo Luebke, and Meadow Linder

The contestations over symptoms reported by veterans of the 1991 Gulf War offer seemingly endless opportunities for investigating social disputes. According to our definition of contested environmental illnesses as diseases and conditions that engender scientific disputes and public debates over environmental causes, Gulf War–related illnesses represent contested illness par excellence.[1] In this chapter, we revisit our study "A Gulf of Difference: Disputes over Gulf War–Related Illnesses" (Brown et al. 2001b) in light of our more recent work on contested illnesses. Given the conclusion of a recent report that "scientific evidence leaves no question that Gulf War illness is a real condition with real causes and serious consequences for affected veterans" (RAC 2008), returning to our earlier study offers an opportunity to demonstrate how a dominant epidemiological paradigm evolves. Our analysis of the changing conflicts over and responses to Gulf War–related illness demonstrates how a dominant epidemiological paradigm—as both a structure and a process that is historically contingent—can be reexamined by social scientists.

HISTORICAL BACKGROUND

Roughly 700,000 U.S. military personnel served in the 1990–91 Persian Gulf War to end Iraq's occupation of Kuwait. The Gulf War was a quick and successful military campaign: a cease-fire was established only three days after the entry of ground troops into Kuwait, and fewer than 150 soldiers were killed in combat. Yet roughly one-quarter of those who served began reporting health problems in the ensuing years (RAC 2008). Symptoms of what has come to be known as

Gulf War–related illness include nausea, loss of concentration, blurred vision, fatigue, lack of muscle control and coordination, irritable bowels, headaches, respiratory problems, rashes, and other ailments that the affected individuals had not experienced prior to service in the Gulf.

Obtaining an appropriate diagnosis, treatment, and related benefits for Gulf War–related illnesses, however, has been a struggle for veterans. Initially, those experiencing symptoms suffered in isolation. A visit to a Veterans Administration (VA) hospital usually ended with suggestions to find ways to reduce stress in order to recover from the trauma of combat. Without a diagnosis linking the ailment to service in the conflict, the VA denied most veterans' requests for service-related disability compensation. The VA often claimed either that the symptoms were undiagnosable as a recognized medical condition, and therefore did not qualify for compensation, or that they were diagnosable but not caused by military service. Angered by the VA denials, many veterans began to speak out about their conditions and the perceived origins of their illnesses, and others began to realize that they and their fellow veterans might be likewise afflicted.

Mobilization has resulted in a number of breakthroughs for ailing veterans. Early organizing helped secure legislation in 1994 requiring the VA to award compensation benefits to chronically disabled Gulf War veterans with undiagnosed illnesses. As a result, today 33 percent of Gulf War veterans receive assistance for some type of service-connected disability, though only 5 percent receive disability for a service-connected "undiagnosed illness." Whereas 87 percent of diagnosed claims have been accepted, only 26 percent of undiagnosed illness claims have been approved as service-connected (RAC 2008).

To respond to the growing number of claims of service-related illness, the VA, along with the Department of Defense (DoD) and Department of Health and Human Services (HHS), began to fund research investigating the possible causes of veterans' illnesses.[2] Suspected chemical compounds included sarin gas, mustard gas, smoke from oil-well fires, pyridostigmine bromide (a prophylactic agent against nerve gas), depleted uranium, pesticides, the insect repellent DEET (N,N-diethyl-m-toluamide), anthrax vaccines, and other prophylactic medications. Plagued by poor data, disputes over how to study Gulf War health effects, and a long list of possible chemical substances that could be to blame, research through 2001 had resulted in no effective treatments of symptoms and no clear understanding of their causes.

By 1998, federal expenditure on research into Gulf War–related illnesses had grown from $7.1 million in 1994 to $37.9 million. A total of 121 research projects were funded between 1994 and 1998 at a total cost of $115 million. Between 1998 and 2003, this level of support more or less continued: an additional 119 research projects were funded by VA, DoD, and HHS at a cost of $132 million. Eighty percent of these studies were completed by 2003 (US General Accounting Office

2004). Much of this early research focused on stress and psychological conditions and examined behavioral or psychological treatments, rather than looking for markers of multisymptom or undiagnosed illnesses. Similarly, some researchers examined rates of diagnosed illness, hospitalization, or mortality, trends that would be unlikely to pick up the chronic symptoms most often experienced by Gulf War Veterans.

Government-funded research on Gulf War–related illnesses slowed down substantially after 2004. The DoD, which funded 70 percent of all government-sponsored Gulf War research through 2003, reasoned that its primary responsibility was to active-duty soldiers and that the number of Gulf War veterans still serving was too small by 2004 to justify extensive further research. The focus shifted to the potential long-term health effects of other deployments. The DoD currently funds Gulf War research through a significantly smaller Gulf War Illness Research Program under the Congressionally Directed Medical Research Program.

What did scientists, doctors, and government officials learn from all of this research, and how did their conclusions change over time? Early government-funded studies concluded that there was no environmentally caused Gulf War–related illness. A 1994 report of the Defense Science Board Task Force on Persian Gulf War Health Effects reported:

> There is no persuasive evidence that any of the proposed etiologies caused chronic illness on a significant scale in the absence of acute injury at initial exposure. . . . The epidemiological evidence is insufficient at this time to support the concept of any coherent "syndrome." We do recognize that veterans numbering in the hundreds have complained of a range of symptoms not yet explained by any clear-cut diagnosis—a number of cases in many respects resemble the "Chronic Fatigue Syndrome." . . . This is not to deny the possibility of service-connectedness, as severe stress, infection and trauma may well be precipitating causes of "CFS." (Defense Science Board Task Force on Persian Gulf War Health Effects 1994, 2)

These findings would shape the focus of veterans' struggles for the next fourteen years. As veterans organized, they found themselves fighting to have their symptoms acknowledged and the causes identified, and they struggled to counter the common explanation from VA and military doctors that their conditions were caused by stress.

Similarly, a 1996 report by the Presidential Advisory Committee on Gulf War Veterans' Illnesses explicitly linked Gulf War–related illnesses to stress and denied any environmental causes.

> Current scientific evidence does not support a causal link between the symptoms and illnesses reported today by Gulf War veterans and exposures while in the Gulf region to the following environmental risk factors assessed by the Committee: pesticides, chemical warfare agents, biological warfare agents, vaccines, pyridostigmine

bromide, infectious diseases, depleted uranium, oil-well fires and smoke, and petroleum products. . . .

Stress is known to affect the brain, immune system, cardiovascular system, and
various hormonal responses. Stress manifests in diverse ways, and is likely to be an
important contributing factor to the broad range of physical and psychological illnesses currently being reported by Gulf War veterans. (Presidential Advisory Committee on Gulf War Veterans' Illnesses 1996, 1)

Both these reports attribute Gulf War–related illnesses to postcombat stress and
expressly deny any environmental or toxic causality.

In sharp contrast to these early findings, and despite a precipitous decline
in federal research funding, in 2008 the Research Advisory Committee (RAC)
on Gulf War Veterans' Illnesses highlighted the following findings based on its
review of fourteen years of Gulf War research:

Gulf War illness is a serious condition that affects at least one fourth of the 697,000
U.S. veterans who served in the 1990–1991 Gulf War. . . .

Gulf War illness fundamentally differs from trauma and stress-related syndromes
described after other wars. Studies consistently indicate that Gulf War illness is not
the result of combat or other stressors and that Gulf War veterans have lower rates
of posttraumatic stress disorder than veterans of other wars. . . .

Evidence strongly and consistently indicates that two Gulf War neurotoxic exposures are causally associated with Gulf War illness: (1) use of pyridostigmine bromide (PB) pills, given to protect troops from effects of nerve agents, and (2) pesticide
use during deployment. (RAC 2008, 1)

How can we make sense of these dramatic shifts? Do the 2008 findings of the
Research Advisory Committee reflect a settling of the science? Has contestation
over Gulf War–related Illnesses ended? We draw on new interviews with scientists and veteran activists to try to determine how the contestation and science
of Gulf War–related illnesses has shifted, and whether the "gulf of difference"
between veteran illness sufferers and scientists and medical practitioners has, in
fact, narrowed.

DEFINING CONTESTED ENVIRONMENTAL ILLNESSES

Throughout our research on Gulf War–related illnesses, and on contested environmental illnesses more generally, we emphasize how laypeople contribute to
discovery and knowledge production, how diverse interests shape medical knowledge, and how, as a result of these conflicts, science and government often fail to
provide adequately for illness sufferers. Environmental factors in Gulf War–related
illness include not only the toxic substances to which veterans were exposed but
also inoculations and other medical treatments they received during Gulf War

service.[3] It is hard to disentangle the iatrogenic effects from other environmental effects, and indeed, some research focuses on the combinations of these and other toxic exposures.

Contestation can occur in any of the stages of defining an illness: when, where, and in what dosage an individual was exposed to a potentially causative chemical; whether a given chemical compound is present in an affected person's body; and whether a chemical compound identified as present in a body is linked scientifically to negative health outcomes. Even when an exposure is documented and chemical presence in a body is established, contestation can occur over whether some other factor might be causing the symptoms.

Gulf War veterans found themselves engaged in all these types of contestations. Veterans were eventually found to have been exposed to a wide range of chemicals, although most of the exposures were initially denied by the military: they resulted from the use of chemical weapons, radioactive ordnance, and preventive medical procedures. When the exposures were proved, the military shifted its official response to claim that exposures were too low to have caused any health effects. For example, one DoD report claimed that soldiers' doses of pyridostigmine bromide (PB) were one-tenth the dose used to treat myasthenia gravis, a neuromuscular disorder (Defense Science Board Task Force on Persian Gulf War Health Effects 1994). The same report admitted that although all soldiers were given PB, the DoD lacked any records of which soldiers actually ingested the tablets or of the actual dosage. By the late 1990s, as self-reported exposures were increasingly found to correlate with biological markers of exposure found in lab tests, official government responses focused on the lack of scientific data linking the known exposures to specific health outcomes.

Attributing physical symptoms to psychological stress offered government officials another way to contest veterans' claims, regardless of what was known about types and levels of exposures or links between known exposures and health outcomes. Scientific uncertainty has exacerbated the difficulties in conducting research on Gulf War–related illnesses, challenged veterans' abilities to make successful claims about their health, and given government agencies tools and arguments that can be used to deny veterans' claims. In short, the scientific uncertainty surrounding Gulf War–related illnesses made contestation more complicated.

IDENTIFYING SITES OF CONTESTATION

For our original study, we analyzed government documents (congressional hearings and reports from federal agencies); articles in medical and epidemiological journals; and coverage in major US newspapers, news magazines, and general-circulation science magazines. We also conducted ethnographic observation of the 1999 and 2001 conferences on Federally Sponsored Gulf War Veterans'

Illnesses Research and of the Boston Environmental Hazards Center (a center for Gulf War–related illnesses research operated by the VA Medical Center and the Boston University School of Public Health). We interviewed researchers, government officials, and veteran activists. The Boston Environmental Hazards Center provided access to their staff, activities, and meetings; facilitated our access to other VA programs; and helped us make contact with other Gulf War researchers and government officials.

To update our original study, we first revisited the literature. This update included a survey of all peer-reviewed research examining disputes over Gulf War–related illnesses, selected peer-reviewed scientific studies on the etiology and epidemiology of Gulf War–related illnesses, and major government reports issued between 2001 and 2008. We also completed new interviews with several scientists and veterans. The recent interviews were not intended to capture the breadth of opinions about the current state of Gulf War–related illnesses but rather to highlight our assertion that illness contestation varies over time and that dominant epidemiological paradigms are historically contingent.

GULF WAR ILLNESSES AS A CONTESTED ILLNESS

We first developed the concept of a dominant epidemiological paradigm in our original study by noting that social forces of disease discovery and knowledge production tended to solidify around particular explanations, much to the frustration of veterans. Veterans found themselves in opposition to an emerging belief system concerning the existence and causes of their disease. A dominant epidemiological paradigm is produced by a diverse set of social actors who draw on existing stocks of institutionalized knowledge to identify and define a disease and determine its etiology, proper treatment, and acceptable health outcomes (see figure 2.1). Although there are often competing paradigm for any scientific issue, one is usually dominant at a given point.

For new or poorly understood illnesses, contestation among various actors during the discovery process shapes the dominant epidemiological paradigm, but the paradigm rarely links an illness to an environmental contaminant, an iatrogenic treatment, or another problem of human action. Government, research, or other actors (e.g., journalists) may be responsible for identifying potential environmental causes, but it is typically laypeople who push such investigation further. The policies, public understanding, and scientific knowledge that exist before the discovery of an illness tend to result in a dominant epidemiological paradigm that fails to meet the needs of the sick population. If the gap between the dominant epidemiological paradigm's conceptualization of an illness and the sick population's conceptualization is great enough, those affected may mobilize, with the aim of transforming the dominant epidemiological paradigm. However, because the dominant epidemiological paradigm is inherently entrenched in and reinforced at a multitude of locations, even the most passionate efforts of challengers are often insufficient to alter it. The combination of embedded institutional tendencies and practices, cultural belief systems, routinely accepted ways of knowing, and vested interests perpetuate the existing understanding of the disease.

We trace the formation and evolution of the dominant epidemiological paradigm for Gulf War–related illnesses by examining the roles of the government, science, media, and activists in creating, perpetuating, and sometimes challenging, the dominant epidemiological paradigm. For Gulf War–related illnesses, the dominant epidemiological paradigm emerged when military officials denied that symptoms could be related to environmental exposures and DoD and VA physicians, unable to identify organic causes of disease, attributed complaints to war-related stress. The stress-based explanation discouraged attempts to investigate possible environmental causes. Veterans and some of their scientific allies strongly opposed this stress-based dominant epidemiological paradigm for a variety of reasons, including the fact that the stress explanation in effect blames the victim by placing the burden on patients to eliminate stress from their lives in order to get well.

A subtle but important shift occurred in the dominant epidemiological paradigm in the late 1990s, when some investigators began serious investigation into a "contextual-stress hypothesis," which recognized the possibility of environmental exposures working in conjunction with stress to cause illness. A 2000 Institute of Medicine report, for example, recommended new research on stress-environment interactions (Institute of Medicine 2000). Though many veterans would recommend against any federally funded research on stress at all (National Gulf War Resource Center 2001), official acknowledgment of the need for a better understanding of stress and exposure represented a minor victory.

Science and social problems are socially constructed (Spector and Kitsuse 1977; Best 1989), and different types of knowledge are "framed" for the public in different ways by different actors (Gamson, Fireman, and Rytina 1982; Snow et al. 1986). We follow Latour and Woolgar's (1987) notion of "science in action," which views scientific facts as social productions that depend on complex interactions between scientists, the public, notions of scientific legitimacy, and nonhuman actors, such as technologies. This view emphasizes that although the dominant epidemiological paradigm of Gulf War–related illnesses may be framed in purely scientific terms, the knowledge that supports it is actually constructed, contested, and conflicted in many different ways and may be used by different actors in pursuit of varying goals. For example, veterans attempt to frame their illnesses as both a result of service in the war and sufficiently serious to warrant treatment.

This emphasis on how knowledge is framed also highlights the media's interaction with the dominant epidemiological paradigm. We recognize the media's proclivity for monocausal explanations to social problems (Stallings 1990; Spencer and Triche 1994), for the simplification and noncritical acceptance of science (Nelkin 1995), and for framing issues in a manner that maximizes personal relevance to media consumers (Seydlitz, Spencer, and Lundskow 1994; Spencer and Triche 1994). We also draw on Downs's (1972) classic discussion of the issue attention cycle, in which media coverage of a topic passes through five stages: the pre-problem stage, alarmed discovery and euphoric enthusiasm, realization of the cost of significant progress, gradual decline of public interest, and the postproblem stage. Building upon Downs's notion of an attention cycle and Stallings's critique of the media's coverage of risk, we argue that the media's coverage of Gulf War–related illnesses eventually moved from a focus on disease etiology to a focus on the presence and extent of chemical exposures in the Gulf.

THE SOCIAL DISCOVERY
OF GULF WAR–RELATED ILLNESSES

As in most cases of occupational and environmental illness, symptomatic Gulf War Veterans were the first to identify their health problems as forming a pattern. Soldiers were aware of the potential for exposures in the Gulf because the history of the military's use of the defoliant Agent Orange, media coverage of Iraq's biological and chemical capabilities, chemical warfare in the 1980–88 Iran-Iraq war, and military vaccinations and training drills with protective equipment and gas masks.

Veterans returning from the Persian Gulf reported ailments not experienced prior to service. Media stories highlighted hardy people who found themselves unable to function at work or at home and who faced problems getting the government to recognize and treat their illnesses. Some veterans did not attribute their ailments to service in the Gulf until they learned of other veterans' illnesses from media reports. All the veterans we interviewed spoke of informal social networks and the importance of the media in sharing strategies for getting treatment after VA physicians refused to treat them. One veteran remembered: "Back in 1994 a lot of veterans were yelling in the newspapers. And every time something happened, the VA would get a workload. You know, they'd get this rush of complaints. If the U.S. government put out a list of possible complaints they could have had during duty in the Gulf War theater, I think that would have been a nicer way of doing it, not with all the veterans blurping up all over the United States."

Dissatisfied with their treatment by the VA and other authorities, veterans began organizing themselves, relying on existing organizations such as Veterans of Foreign Wars, Disabled American Veterans, the American Legion, and AMVETS. Groups specifically for Gulf War veterans formed, such as the National Gulf War Resource Center and Operation Desert Shield/Storm Association, though membership was small. The Internet was a major resource for collaboration, and veterans shared their stories with the media. Veteran activists regarded their actions as crucial to the research enterprise, as did researchers we observed at the Boston Environmental Hazards Center. As one researcher explained: "What got this thing up and running in the first place was the veterans' groups and individual veterans with incredible stories to tell that became public news stories. I would say that without that, you wouldn't be getting any of this, you know, the Gulf War–related illness work. Wouldn't have done any of this and wouldn't still be doing it."

Once disease sufferers identify an illness phenomenon, they often attempt to legitimize their views through government and scientific channels. Motivated by veteran dissatisfaction over DoD resistance and VA slowness to treat veterans, federal legislators began investigations of chemical exposures and pressed federal agencies to probe more deeply into existing research on potential toxic health effects. Interagency task forces were set up to coordinate research. The Institute of Medicine was mandated to provide an analysis of the existing body of research, and later the RAND Corporation received a contract to do the same.

Illness discovery requires scientists and physicians to recognize the new disease. Though some VA physicians and researchers dismissed veterans' complaints, others began to see patterns in the complaints and explored them further. Scientists researching Gulf War–related illnesses came from a variety of backgrounds and motivations. Some were federal employees assigned to do such research. Others were occupational- and environmental-illness researchers who saw this investigation as a logical extension of their work: some of these, in particular, were sympathetic to the veterans' complaints and believed they were not being taken seriously.

Investigative Challenges

More than many illnesses believed to have environmental causes, Gulf War–related illnesses are ambiguous and lack a clear definition. Some epidemiologists and physicians believed that the VA demand for a specific diagnosis was too strict, making it difficult for veterans to obtain recognition of their illnesses in the early period (Landrigan 1997). By the late 1990s, most scientists and physicians had abandoned the concept of a single Gulf War syndrome because of the multiplicity of exposures, the diffuse nature of veterans' complaints, and the lack of consensus on how to delimit the range of symptoms and illnesses. Epidemiological studies have identified different clusters of symptoms, and different studies have defined Gulf War–related illnesses in different ways. The 2008 RAC report, for example, outlines five different definitions. It observes that "seventeen years after the Gulf War, no case definition has been widely accepted as the preferred standard for defining the complex of multiple symptoms affecting Gulf War veterans" (RAC 2008). Some symptom clusters resemble chronic fatigue syndrome, fibromyalgia, or multiple chemical sensitivity, all of which are themselves poorly understood and subject to dispute (National Institutes of Health 1994; Davis 2000). The uncertainty further confounds the process of research, as there is no consensus on which of the many potential approaches, methods, and hypotheses to pursue. An epidemiologist pointed out: "I think it's very difficult for researchers. Even though we say we're totally objective, we state hypotheses, we develop a questionnaire where we, you know, do you permit five questions or fifty questions about something? An infectious disease scientist is going to look for infectious mechanisms. A neurotoxicologist is going to [look for other things]. So the scientists kind of design their studies in a way that they hope to find things that are in their field, what they'd like to find." The fact that researchers have examined Gulf War–related illnesses through so many disciplinary and methodological lenses has made scientific consensus difficult to achieve.

The Stress-Based Hypothesis

Despite the complexity of the issue and early resistance to disease recognition, the identification process eventually produced a body of literature addressing the prevalence and possible causes of veterans' illnesses. Though we emphasize lay discovery of these illnesses, the fact that most troops were given vaccinations against anthrax and pyridostigmine bromide to protect against nerve gases implies that the DoD anticipated exposure to biological and chemical weapons. The military received special permission to bypass the usual Food and Drug Administration approval process for these drugs (Rettig 1999).

Pentagon officials were also concerned about the health effects of oil-well fires, though an Army team concluded that negative health effects were unlikely (US Army Environmental Health Agency 1994). In addition, the military expected many cases of post-traumatic stress disorder (PTSD), as had occurred among Vietnam veterans. Centers were set up at several bases to detect psychological stress in troops returning from combat. The fact that many of the DoD's medical personnel were primed to treat psychological symptoms may explain their willingness to settle on stress as an explanation for soldiers' physical symptoms, even though very few returning soldiers exhibited classic PTSD symptoms (Wolfe et al. 1999).

Early research on the unexplained symptoms of Gulf War veterans seemed to support this stress-based hypothesis. When DoD medical professionals were sent to study previously deployed reserve units based in Indiana and Louisiana, the reports concluded that the cause of self-reported physical symptoms was psychological stress. Following presentations by experts who had been involved in these early diagnoses, a 1994 NIH technology assessment workshop supported the stress-based hypothesis, stating that veterans' symptoms were "the expression of post-traumatic distress," which "represents a psychophysiological response that needs to be evaluated" (National Institutes of Health 1994). The stress-based dom-inant epidemiological paradigm was strengthened by the Presidential Advisory Committee's 1996 report that attributed veterans' illnesses to stress.[4]

In the mid-1990s, however, a congressional investigation concluded that the United States had previously exported to Iraq materials used to manufacture bio-logical weapons. In response to this confirmation of Iraq's biological weapons capability and the testimony of veterans who believed they had been exposed to chemical warfare agents, Congress allocated money for VA investigations. Unlike the DoD's research program, the VA's research agenda was weighted heavily toward projects examining toxic exposures and their physiological and neuro-logical effects (PGVCB-RWG 1999). It also examined whether there was a higher prevalence of symptoms in veterans than in nondeployed troops and explored links to particular exposures. This work was hampered by unresolved debates over the definition of Gulf War–related illnesses, the question of whether these ill-nesses represented a unique syndrome or a series of unrelated symptoms, and the fact that the military had kept few consistent or complete records about what sol-diers were exposed to. By the late 1990s, most researchers did not believe that Gulf War–related illnesses represented a unique syndrome. However, some veterans groups continued to argue that there was a unique and distinct Gulf War–related illness and put their support behind researchers investigating that possibility, such as Robert Haley at the University of Texas Southwestern Medical Center. Others became involved in panels and committees at the VA and DoD, aiming to influence the direction of future research.

Early Findings

Relying on DoD and VA registries, early research found excess mortality among Gulf War veterans only for motor vehicle accidents, although these excesses declined over time (Kang and Bullman 2001). Other studies found no excess hos-pitalization (Gray et al. 2006). Veterans countered these findings by citing flaws in study design and noting that although many symptoms do not require hos-pitalization, they affect quality of life and may impede the ability to work. Most hospitalization research looked only at military hospitals, but these data may be misleading: veterans might have sought care at nonmilitary hospitals, either because they were dissatisfied with military care or because their spouse's health insurance allowed them to choose private care.

Veterans' claims were supported by studies showing an excess of self-reported symptoms among deployed versus nondeployed troops, including chronic diar-rhea, other gastrointestinal symptoms, memory loss, concentration difficulty, trouble finding words, fatigue, depression, PTSD, bronchitis, asthma, alcohol abuse, sexual discomfort, and anxiety (Iowa Persian Gulf Study Group 1997; Fukuda et al. 1998; Proctor et al. 1998). However, the validity of self-reported symptoms has been repeatedly questioned because physical examinations in major studies failed to find diagnosable medical conditions.[5]

Proctor et al. (1998) found increased symptoms in many organ systems in two Persian Gulf cohorts, as compared to soldiers stationed in Germany. When veterans diagnosed with PTSD were removed from the analysis, virtually no changes in results were noted. This finding supported the contention that stress alone was not the cause of veterans' complaints. Furthermore, the researchers found positive correlations between several exposures and symptom reporting for the specific organ systems in which the effects of exposure to toxic materials would be expected. Some epidemiologists view this work on self-reported symptoms and exposures as central to a new perspective on how to conduct research on environmental health.

Early research also investigated the possible effects of the nerve-gas antidote pyridostigmine bromide, depleted uranium, and oil-well fires, but by 2001, no causal links to Gulf War–related illnesses had been identified. The DoD-sponsored RAND Corporation summaries (Harley et al. 1999; Cecchine et al. 2000; Hilborne and Golomb 2001) and the Institute of Medicine's summary (IOM 2000) of the knowledge base concerning these and other exposures both concluded that there was no concrete evidence in support of the notion that any of these exposures caused Gulf War–related illnesses. Both reports note, however, that dose-response effects at chronic, low exposure levels are not understood well enough to completely rule them out, and they note poor record keeping as a major obstacle.

Researchers continued to identify biological markers that might provide evidence of exposure. In the late 1990s, researchers we interviewed at the Boston Environmental Hazards Center believed that studies of neurophysiological and neuropsychological symptoms were going in a promising direction. These researchers subsequently found subtle differences between symptomatic Gulf War veterans and control groups in neurobehavioral measures including attention, memory, and mood (Lindem, Heeren, and White 2003; Sullivan et al. 2003). Researchers also found significant differences in white-brain-matter volume (Heaton et al. 2007). Uncertainty existed, however, about whether some of these changes are markers for diseases or merely nonfunctional differences.

CONTESTATION: THE ONGOING CONTROVERSIES

When sufferers and their supporters challenge a dominant epidemiological paradigm that does not adequately meet their needs, they face many obstacles. We describe the most common below.

Missing Information, Misinformation, and Secrecy

Research on Gulf War–related illnesses has been plagued by insufficient or incorrect information, especially the lack of predeployment health assessments and exposure records. Without these data, exposure science is difficult or impossible. In lieu of predeployment health records, scientists relied on self-reported pre-deployment health information, an approach that is typically criticized for its lack of reliability and validity (National Institutes of Health 1994).[6] Veterans and researchers we spoke with all identified the denials and disputes over exposures as major barriers. One veteran remarked: "From a political standpoint, the biggest job for us is getting the government to recognize the findings that they don't want to hear about." A VA researcher commented:

> The government hasn't been real forthcoming with releasing information, and that's causing problems with the research. Right now we have a grant [from] the Department of Defense, looking at some people who were actually around where the detonation of chemical warfare agents occurred. And getting the information from them is extremely difficult. You feel like you're trying to do research with your arm tied around your back. . . . So I have to go scrap around and beg and go through all the channels to see if I can get this released, even though the Department of Defense has funded this study. Because I'm not in the Department of Defense, I constantly get the feeling that I just get the information they want me to have.

Until public disclosure about the presence of nerve gas at Khamisiyah, the DoD maintained that no exposures had occurred, thereby denying vital information to veterans and researchers. When the President's Advisory Committee asked the DoD to turn over the extensive logs of exposure data from the Gulf, the Defense Department was able to produce only thirty-six of an estimated two hundred pages (Shenon 1997a). Whether or not the DoD hid the missing logs, as some claim (Tuite 1997), the lost information is a serious impediment to research (National Institutes of Health 1994). Veterans often cannot be sure when or whether they were exposed to hazardous chemicals during the Gulf War. Although chemical alarms sounded daily and soldiers were trained to don gas masks upon hearing them, military commanders later told Congress that many were false alarms, though this information was not communicated down the chain of command. Thus soldiers may have believed they were being exposed to chemicals when they were not. In other instances, soldiers were exposed without their knowledge and with no chance to use protective gear. As the 1994 NIH Panel observed: "Although warfare has always been stressful and fear-inducing, the Persian Gulf War was the first combat experience in which the real threat of chemical and biological warfare was known to troops before entering the combat area" (National Institutes of Health 1994, 13).

According to many researchers we interviewed in the late 1990s, there was no serious dialogue between the researchers or research centers performing studies on Gulf War–related illnesses and the physicians treating the veterans. As one epidemiologist noted: "I know in the veterans' eyes it's a real issue. They have a lot of complaints about their medical treatment and their clinical care that they come and voice to us. But as a resource center we're not directly responsible for taking care of them clinically, and so we, I tried to help and direct them into proper channels within the clinical care side of it, people that I know here. But there is a division or separation, and so we could spend our whole life trying to clinically get them treated." Consequently, researchers told us, uninformed clinicians were not asking their patients questions that might have provided clues to etiology. Because of these omissions, veterans may not have received the best possible care, and valuable research data were not gathered.

Distrust, Disputes, and Fragmentation

Many veterans whom we interviewed distrusted government research on toxics. They knew that for decades, the government denied the existence of diseases among "atomic veterans" and civilian workers involved in nuclear weapons production (Caufield 1990) and among Vietnam veterans exposed to Agent Orange. The Agent Orange Act, providing compensation for Agent Orange–related illness, was not passed until January 30, 1991. The Institute of Medicine (1994) did not link Agent Orange exposure to Hodgkin's disease, non-Hodgkin's lymphoma, soft-tissue sarcoma, chloracne, and birth defects in veterans' children (such as spina bifida) until 1994, sixteen years after the first congressional hearings and twenty-four years after veterans were exposed. The government did not validate Agent Orange connections to diabetes or to birth defects in Vietnamese children until 2000 (Aldinger 2000). As the director of a veteran's group noted: "How long did it take those exposed to the atomic bomb? . . . They actually had people and they wanted to find out what effect this stuff had on them. They tested it out—radiation. . . . So there's a pattern, it looks like to me, that, hey, if we wait long enough, those of you who are sickest are going to die off and we don't have to spend all this money to give you the benefits."

After the Gulf War, sick veterans complained that officials offered only a psychiatric explanation for their symptoms and would not take seriously reports of toxic exposures. One remarked:

When . . . Gulf War veterans went to clinics and hospitals run by the Department of Defense and Veterans Affairs, they weren't met with open arms by many doctors. Many doctors thought that they understood readily what was occurring with these veterans. It was a short war; this must be mental illness or post-traumatic stress disorder. . . . And then, when veterans complained about being exposed to chemical weapons in the Gulf—seeing them, the alarms going off, reporting symptoms consistent with exposure to chemical weapons—these claims were not investigated seriously or with any sort of vigor at all by the Department of Defense. . . . When, after all that, these agencies now are tasked with investigating Gulf War Syndrome, do you think veterans are gonna believe the kinds of conclusions they come up with? Absolutely not.

Similarly, Dr. Michael Hodgson, then an American Legion medical adviser but later employed by the VA, remarked: "It is hard for me to believe that you can announce every other week that yet another ten or fifteen thousand may have been exposed to nerve gas and then convincingly tell veterans they don't have nerve gas disease" (Kolata 1996). Clearly, the historical context during the Gulf War influenced the dominant epidemiological paradigm, and its effect remains important in interpreting our recent interviews.

Disputes continue between government bodies: the DoD, the VA, the CIA, the Presidential Advisory Committee, congressional committees, the NIH panel, the Institute of Medicine committee, and HHS. At the center of these disputes is the DoD, accused by veterans' groups of concealing exposure information and strongly criticized by the Presidential Advisory Committee for mishandling information (often in surprisingly strong terms, such as: "DoD's slow and erratic efforts to release information to the public have further served to erode the public's trust" [quoted in Shenon 1996a]). This committee, in turn, was accused by veterans of censoring information that did not support stress as the cause of Gulf War–related illnesses. One of its researchers, Jonathan Tucker, claims he was fired for gathering information from veterans and whistle-blowers in his effort to show that the Presidential Advisory Committee overemphasized the stress paradigm while ignoring research into chemical exposure (Shenon 1996b). Presidential Advisory Committee members also disagreed significantly among themselves (Shenon 1997b).

Congress responded to the shortcomings of DoD and VA. Representative Christopher Shays (R-CT) requested in 1996 that the General Accounting Office investigate why federal studies failed to confirm the existence of Gulf War illnesses or their potential environmental causes, and the resulting report was quite critical (US General Accounting Office 1997). Shays chaired a House committee that chastised the Pentagon and VA for poor work and asked that they be removed from further oversight of Gulf War–related illnesses research (Shenon 1997c). Dissatisfied with VA research and treatment, in 1998 Congress directed the IOM to compare Gulf War veterans with other veterans, on the assumption that differences between groups of veterans would lead to a presumption of disease, treatment, and compensation, without concern over cause.

Because they view the government as the cause of the problem, veterans question the government's ability to perform objective science, and veterans' groups have argued that Gulf War research funding should not be managed by the DoD or VA (National Gulf War Resource Center 2001). A similar situation would be seen as a conflict of interest in other areas of health: if, for instance, corporations were responsible for researching occupational health. Even when veterans are invited to be part of panels and conferences, they often feel slighted. At the 1999 conference of federally funded Gulf War researchers, even though the conveners dedicated a panel to veterans' concerns, with veterans as speakers and DoD officials present to answer questions, poor attendance by researchers and officials suggested a lack of interest in veterans' perspectives. At a similar 2001 conference, organizers arranged the "public availability" session (a forum for laypeople to question scientists and officials) as a series of informal roundtables. Veterans in attendance told us they felt this was an attempt to fragment and silence them.

Struggles for Legitimacy and the Role of Stress

The struggle to legitimate both the study of Gulf War-related illnesses and the illnesses themselves creates tension and conflict for both veterans and scientists. Veterans want the government to recognize their illnesses as legitimate and to ensure eligibility for treatment and disability benefits. They also want a sign of official acknowledgment that they are not mentally ill. For many veterans, the reliance on a stress model, with the VA's accompanying cognitive behavioral treatment trial, represented a form of delegitimation. Many veterans feel that their illnesses are not legitimated as long as researchers claim that stress plays any role at all.

It is understandable that veterans would oppose the primary-stress perspective, which is framed around the idea that all wars are stressful and that soldiers have always returned with some stress-related illness (Hyams, Wignall, and Roswell 1996). That approach focuses on individual psychopathology and minimizes the effects of toxic substances and other environmental conditions. There is also public stigma associated with stress as a cause of physical health problems, as noted by Senator John D. Rockefeller IV (D-WV): "When you say 'stress' to the American people, when it's diffused through the media, they think it's something psychological, it's something of the mind, when in fact these people—maybe 50,000 or more of them—who went over there completely healthy and came back who are now very, very sick, and it's not just a stress syndrome" (quoted in Schmitt 1997).

Nevertheless, some might think that a primary-stress model would be of benefit to veterans. After the Vietnam War, veterans stricken by nightmares and intrusive memories, with the support of sympathetic mental health professionals, lobbied for the inclusion of a combat-related disorder in the third edition of the American Psychiatric Association's *Diagnostic and Statistical Manual*. The effort was successful, and the diagnosis of post-traumatic stress disorder was the result (Scott 1988). However, although the creation of PTSD validated the suffering of Vietnam veterans, many mental health professionals have concluded that Gulf War veterans do not meet the clinical criteria for the disorder (National Institutes of Health 1994).

Whether or not they meet the official criteria for combat-related psychiatric disorders, for veterans, the fundamental difference between the experience of Vietnam and that of the Gulf War is the attribution of responsibility. Vietnam veterans accepted a diagnosis of PTSD because it meant that they could get treatment and that the government was actually attributing their condition to their war experiences. In the case of Gulf War veterans, however, the government has linked veterans' illnesses to stress to *avoid* attributing their illness to wartime experiences and to prevent them from receiving government-provided treatment. Gulf War veterans view a PTSD diagnosis or other stress-related explanation as the government's attempt to place responsibility on the veterans for their own problems. One veteran formulated the problem this way:

> Many of the vets, in the early '90s after the war, were either diagnosed with major depression or post-traumatic stress disorder, or anxiety disorders and things like that, and they reacted ferociously, many, to these diagnoses, and suspected that physicians, especially physicians who worked for the government either in the military or VA, were trying to deny the legitimacy of their symptoms by suggesting that they were psychological in nature. So after a couple years, you couldn't say 'stress,' and you couldn't say 'mental illness' in a room of Gulf War veterans without really risking your health, and so the debate was hampered by that, because, you know, being exposed to oil-well fires I'm sure isn't good for you, being in a deep funk and being exposed to oil-well fires is probably worse for you.

For veterans, the fundamental issue was not whether stress exacerbated their exposures but whether the government would acknowledge that veterans were sick because of their exposures while serving in the Gulf.

A SHIFTING DOMINANT EPIDEMIOLOGICAL PARADIGM: THE CONTEXTUAL-STRESS HYPOTHESIS

Data from our original study suggested a shift in the dominant epidemiological paradigm from a "primary-stress hypothesis" (in which stress was seen as the primary causal factor) to what we termed the "contextual-stress hypothesis" (in which stress was seen as one in a combination of factors). The contextual-stress hypothesis establishes the link between poor health and psychologically stressful events (excluding PTSD, postcombat anxiety, or psychiatric disorders); it incorporates the effect of various environmental factors and seeks to understand how stress affects the body physically.

The dominant epidemiological paradigm is constructed and persists in multiple locations of science, government, academia, and the media, all of which contribute to maintaining the status quo. Hence, proposals of alternative paradigms incorporating environmental causes or other explanations must take on many different actors. The dominant epidemiological paradigm is not the result of a consensus meeting or of conspiratorial practice but of an affinity of perspectives among diverse actors. Perpetuating it may include some calculated efforts to withhold information and shape research directions, but mainly it occurs through an institutional logic of ordinary practices.

One barrier to alternative explanations is the determination of what counts as evidence. For veterans, self-reported symptoms and self-reported exposures are both important kinds of evidence. For the military and for most researchers, self-reported symptoms are seen as marginally acceptable evidence, and self-reported exposures are virtually never acceptable. Whereas Gulf War veterans give much credence to personal narratives of healthy people who returned from the war with illness, the military and researchers see these narratives as merely anecdotes that are contradicted by large epidemiological studies. When veterans uncover examples of military secrecy, such as the reluctance to admit that the United States blew up the Iraqi chemical weapons depot at Khamisiyah, they take these as proof of exposures that could have had toxic health effects. The military relies on its data that show no difference in the health status of Gulf War veterans regardless of proximity to the depot. Veterans also focus on the few scientific studies that report positive correlations between toxic exposures and health effects, despite widespread methodological criticism of those studies among scientists.

The case of Gulf War–related illnesses illustrates how external pressure from activists, as well as efforts within the government, can lead to a change in the dominant epidemiological paradigm. For example, a former VA employee reported that over a five-year period he saw the VA "moving from a defensive posture and a posture of denial to a posture of addressing veterans' problems and acknowledging that this isn't a matter of blame, that this is a matter of, 'we have a duty to help them get better.'" He explained this change:

> I think it was a combination of things. I think the average veteran was just saying, "Would you please acknowledge there is something wrong with me, and don't tell me it's in my head." The other is . . . despite the fact that we were being beaten up by certain corners of the community, particularly Congress, scientific panels were providing confirmation of what our findings had been up to that date, and I think that, even though there were criticisms by those groups too, it allowed us to be a little more bold, and also those committees taught us really good lessons. The Presidential Advisory Committee . . . was one because . . . they took to task VA and DoD for not doing the best job to reach out and take care of veterans and also the failure to communicate effectively.

In challenging the initial, stress-based dominant epidemiological paradigm, veterans began by seeking assistance from their congressional representatives. Some veterans felt that Congress was not as strong an ally as it was to veterans of other wars, because no Gulf War veterans were serving in Congress. Still, they maintained that their pressure on Congress led to many beneficial outcomes, such as the 1992 legislation requiring VA and DoD to create health registries, 1994 legislation permitting VA to provide benefits to veterans with unexplained symptoms, the allocation of $150 million for Gulf War–related illness research, and 1998 legislation guaranteeing presumption of exposure, similar to legislation passed that compensated people exposed to Agent Orange in Vietnam. Outside Congress, veteran activists reported much less success, as evidenced by the ongoing tension with the VA and DoD, and only minimal success within the scientific community. Though veterans' interests in studying exposure to depleted uranium and other toxic materials have resulted in concerted efforts by VA to fund research addressing their concerns, this research has failed to show health effects.

Veterans have also had mixed success with the media. At first, sick veterans were media heroes. As late as 1996, coverage of Gulf War–related illnesses was prominent, with a shift from the human interest story of sick veterans to a potential Pentagon cover-up. But by the late 1990s, according to our media-content analysis and the veterans we interviewed, the media was showing little interest in Gulf War–related illnesses.

Our original study found clear evidence of a shift in the dominant epidemiological paradigm from a primary-stress approach to a contextual-stress approach. At the time, it was still a paradigm in formation, without the firm consensus that would make it generally applicable. Unlike the primary-stress model, which viewed complaints as psychological symptoms, the new approach saw symptoms as real, even if inexplicable. We also concluded that in a contextual-stress approach, researchers understood the stress induced by potential exposures: for instance, the stress of experiencing chemical alarms, even false alarms, in the face of known and threatened chemical exposures. We also noted that more scientists were calling for studies of the interaction of actual exposures and stress reactions and taking more seriously the stress experienced by veterans over the inability to find explanations for their mysterious symptoms. In the clinical sphere, we argued that the new contextual-stress approach would discourage clinicians from immediately resorting to psychiatric consultations as the primary form of treatment and that the new paradigm called for a more multifaceted treatment program (Engel et al. 2000).

We also contended that the shift to a contextual-stress hypothesis in the dominant epidemiological paradigm had strong policy implications. Indeed, DoD eventually implemented systems for collecting better predeployment health data. We suggested that the shift to the contextual-stress hypothesis might raise awareness of the political and clinical costs of denying health problems in the first place. Finally, we argued that in response to both internal shifts and veteran pressure, the new dominant epidemiological paradigm was moving forward, especially in terms of clinical and policy developments, even without the scientific evidence to justify it.

SCIENCE THEN, SCIENCE NOW

Revisiting the case of Gulf War–related illnesses shows that the evolution of a dominant epidemiological paradigm is not simply a function of advancing scientific knowledge. In our most recent interviews, we were reminded how difficult research into the possible health effects of environmental exposures can be, especially when access to data is limited or the data are inadequate. The definition and understanding of Gulf War–related illnesses are still matters of debate. Obstacles to advancing the science originate from a variety of sources: not only the quality and availability of data but also the political and personal motivations of different actors and the complicated relationships among them. When the science on a contested illness is in disarray and unable to advance toward a shared understanding of a disease or condition, other forces may steer the evolution of the dominant epidemiological paradigm.

Early Scientific Disagreements

Even at the height of funding for Gulf War research, investigators disagreed over the research questions that should be asked. In 1995, the Research Subcommittee of the Deployment Health Working Group identified twenty-one priority research questions. The Research Advisory Committee's 2008 report, however, concludes that even though research was conducted addressing each of these questions, the overall strategy "falls considerably short of a well-coordinated federal program with a management structure capable of achieving identified research objectives. . . . Identifying funded projects according to which of 21 research categories they fall into is not the same as establishing and managing a research program to provide answers to priority scientific questions. The interagency group tasked with coordinating the Gulf War research effort appears to have served primarily in the role of cataloguing and reporting federally-sponsored studies identified as 'Gulf War research,' not as managers of an effective, well-coordinated federal research program" (RAC 2008).

This disorganization resulted in disputes among scientists that are best represented by an exchange in the *Journal of the American Medical Association* in 1998 and 1999. The dispute revolved around whether distinct symptom clusters could be identified in sick veterans (a question of importance for later work linking types of exposures to specific symptom clusters). Robert Haley, an internist and epidemiologist at the University of Texas Southwestern Medical Center, who challenged the dominant epidemiological paradigm by denying that stress is the cause of Gulf War–related illnesses, was attacked by colleagues who saw his methodology as flawed (Landrigan 1997; Gray et al. 1998). In the *JAMA* exchange, Haley praised a study by Fukuda et al. (1998) for finding two of the three symptom clusters identified by Haley, Kurt, and Hom (1997), but he criticized Fukuda's methodology as the reason that the third cluster could not be confirmed. Fukuda and his colleagues replied by noting that "our study was never intended to replicate or confirm the findings of Haley et al. We are skeptical of his study findings and conclusions because of substantial study design flaws already described by others" (Reeves et al. 1999, 329).

This exchange in *JAMA* also illustrates the nature of the debate over the role of stress. Fukuda and his colleagues remain open to the possibility that stress is involved and depict Haley as having a vested interest in denying any role for stress: "We agree with Haley that our findings do not necessarily implicate a psychological basis for symptoms reported by Gulf War veterans. However, unlike Haley, we do not have a particular etiology to champion. Given the nature of war, it remains probable that psychological factors have an important contributing role in the development of unexplained symptoms in some personnel after all wars" (Reeves et al. 1999, 329).

The exchange of letters also depicts how researchers may see other work only as it relates to their own, which is often aimed at reducing the complexity of possible explanations. One of Haley's goals was to tease out possible effects from multiple exposures. But other researchers were skeptical of any research that operated at such a level of complexity. One interviewee stated plainly that there would never be a comprehensive understanding of the causes of Gulf War–related illnesses: "I think there are commonalties, but we are never going to get the exposure models down because I think the exposures are too diverse. I mean, I've just never seen a public health study where you could have possibly multiple exposures. Are there? I don't know. I don't know that there were in the Gulf either, but I don't know how you'd prove that there weren't." Another researcher we interviewed also spoke of the complexity as an obstacle:

> What happens to people who engage in a military conflict when they're removed from their homes, when they witness great horrors, and when you throw into it, from our perspective, some environmental factors? And that's sort of what's interesting. . . . We study things in the way that we know them and the way we're most comfortable. So we're forced to in a way [to] reduce these things to ways we understand and know and know how to deal with. You know, war, like any other social experience, is very complex and it's hard to deal with complexity in a fashion that we're familiar with.

As these brief examples illustrate, at the time of our original study, the science on Gulf War–related illnesses was weak, disorganized, and sometimes contradictory.

Current State of the Science

The strongly stated conclusions of the 2008 Research Advisory Committee report imply that scientific uncertainty has drastically declined. Yet significant contradictions are still common in the literature. For example, Wesseley and Freedman argue that "no compelling evidence has been provided to support straightforward toxicological explanations for Gulf War illness" (2006). Gray and colleagues' retrospective report on ten years of research on this issue includes a warning against trusting self-reported data: "Because of self-selection bias, sensational media reports, and other potential confounders of self-reported information, registry data are limited in their epidemiological value" (Gray et al. 2004, 449). In a 2006 article, Gray, with Kang, went on to argue that research should be halted because there was no single, clearly defined Gulf War–related illness. Deahl's 2005 review of the scientific controversies dogging Gulf War–related illnesses research attempts to stifle scientific progress by arguing that "the very term Gulf War illness is contested, and the underlying cause of these symptoms and their relation to Gulf service remains the subject of a heated and often acrimonious debate," effectively bringing the debate back to its starting point in 1994 (Deahl 2005, 636).

At the same time, however, a number of independent studies were starting to detect causal evidence. In a breakthrough article in March 2008, Beatrice Golomb published the results of a meta-analysis of epidemiological research that found links between chronic health problems and at least one type of carbamate acetylcholinesterase inhibitor (AChEi). Golomb concluded that "increasing evidence suggests excess illness in Persian Gulf War veterans (GWV) can be explained in part by exposure of GWV to organophosphate and carbamate acetylcholinesterase inhibitors (AChEis), including pyridostigmine bromide (PB), pesticides, and nerve agents" (2008, 4295). Additionally, advances in neuroimaging identified concrete differences between symptomatic and nonsymptomatic veterans, including differences in white-matter volume in the brain (Powell et al. 2007).

The scientific argument for a contextual-stress-based hypothesis has also been strengthened by research demonstrating that psychological stress can alter the body's response to a toxin, making an exposed individual more likely to develop symptoms or a disease later on (Chrousos and Gold 1992; Kiecolt-Glaser et al. 2002). Animal studies (Friedman et al. 1996) and studies of soldiers (Keeler, Hurst, and Dunn 1991; Sharabi et al. 1991) have demonstrated that stress increases the biological effects of PB because stressful conditions allow PB to cross the blood-brain barrier. Other research has found that the combined effects of stress, PB, and pesticide exposure lead to a disruption of the blood-brain barrier and cause neurological effects that do not occur with any single exposure (Abdel-Rahman, Shetty, and Abou-Donia 2002). This research adds layers of complexity to the contextual-stress-based hypothesis, because stress at the time of exposure may be a cause of Gulf War illness even in sick veterans who, years later, display no psychiatric symptoms or PTSD.

Summarizing much of this research, the 454-page report of the Research Advisory Committee (RAC 2008) on Gulf War veterans' illnesses points to an emerging consensus on the cumulative effects of chemical exposures in the Gulf. The report argues forcefully that Gulf War illness is real, that it "fundamentally differs from trauma and stress-related syndromes described after other wars," and that "two Gulf War neurotoxic exposures are causally associated with Gulf War illness: 1) use of pyridostigmine bromide (PB) pills, given to protect troops from effects of nerve agents, and 2) pesticide use during deployment" (RAC 2008, 1). The report shifts attention away from debates about whether there is a unique syndrome associated with Gulf War service and focuses instead on the consistent findings of health effects in exposure-outcome studies.

It appears that the committee is attempting to make amends for the failure of science to validate veterans' reported symptoms. For example, the report acknowledges that for years the symptoms of veterans "were poorly understood and, for too long, denied or trivialized" (RAC 2008, 18). It also concludes that although veterans were aware that their exposures could have made them sick, Gulf War–related illnesses are not merely an artifact of this awareness.

The report attempts to downplay early scientific disagreements by noting that "in those early years, opinion camps formed on both sides of the issue. Both sides relied to a large extent on assumptions and conjecture to support their views, with little scientific data to settle the debate" (RAC 2008, 61). And, in what verges on an apologetic tone, the report acknowledges that veterans' cynicism toward the government is justifiable: "There is also a common perception that federal policy makers have not vigorously pursued key research in this area and that federal agencies have disincentives—whether political or fiscal—for providing definitive answers to Gulf War health questions . . . [that] parallels delayed federal responses to health problems stemming from hazardous exposures in earlier wars. . . . Although cynical, such views are reinforced by the slow progress made by federal agencies in addressing fundamental questions about the nature, causes, and treatments for Gulf War illness" (289).

How can we make sense of these most recent shifts? Do the RAC's findings reflect a settling of the science or an attempt to impose the appearance of certainty on an otherwise uncertain corpus of research? And if the RAC's report is accepted as representing the state of knowledge, does this mean that contestation over Gulf War–related illnesses is over?

THE SHAPING OF THE DOMINANT
EPIDEMIOLOGICAL PARADIGM

Our most recent interviews point to disagreements about whether the science is advancing. For example, one researcher and clinician observed: "The science doesn't seem to have settled in my view. There are those that would like to suggest it has, but on close look I think it is more perception than reality." The interviewee added: "But in my line of work, perception is everything." This interviewee also argued that the VA used the RAC report as a "political tool" to improve its image. Veterans influenced the make-up of the committee, according to this interviewee, and as a result the dissenting, skeptical voices in the committee's consensus-based decision-making process may have been left out. Moreover, "such a heavy emphasis on chemical exposures is to the detriment of other possible causes." The interviewee concluded that "RAC has not hindered advances in scientific understanding, but it certainly has not promoted them."

Another researcher we interviewed was more optimistic about the shift in thinking represented by the report: two years earlier, "You couldn't prove [Gulf War–related illnesses], no matter how many studies that were out there that showed exposure-outcome relationships, it wasn't true for some reason, and the DoD kept saying it, and VA kept saying it, and people kept saying it isn't proven." Then, according to this interviewee, "something happened to the zeitgeist. . . . [E]very other report has been denied. . . . This time there were editorials saying, 'We have to do something about the Gulf War Veterans.' . . . I have not been able to believe the change in public response to these guys in the last year. . . . For some reason now it's a fact. This moved from a crazy idea that some of us nutty environmentalists had, and people who were overly sympathetic to veterans had, to a fact! That's a fascinating shift."

Nevertheless, veterans continue to report that physicians within the VA are convinced that their symptoms are of psychological origin. One veteran we interviewed asked: "Do most doctors in the VA health care system even care? No. They only believe the reports they are given from the DoD, VA, and IOM." A researcher described the continued resistance of certain actors: "What fascinates me are the people who can't move, and you know I think that's kind of what happened to VA and DoD. I think there are some people there who've dug in their heels and said it's psychogenic, and now they can't take their heels out of wherever they've dug them into. They just got too much into that position."

This resistance is waning, however, according to one researcher: "There are some people who are still saying it's psychogenic, but I think they're being drowned out at this point. . . . People are not paying the attention to them that they did before. . . . They're viewing it that these guys blamed the victim. . . . So I think [the stress-based] paradigm is there, and I think there are people that still express that paradigm, but I think they're losing their legitimacy, and, you know, they were very powerful in the beginning."

Similarly, the chair of the Research Advisory Committee, James Binns, continues to challenge the notion that the absence of a definition somehow makes the condition imaginary: "This a real condition, that affects at least one-fourth of the 700,000 veterans who served in the 1991 war. And it of course is a complex of concurrent symptoms that typically includes persistent memory and concentration problems, chronic headaches, widespread pain, gastrointestinal problems, and other chronic abnormalities not explained by well-established diagnoses. It differs fundamentally from the trauma and stress related syndromes that had been described after other wars, and in particular of course the current war" (Collaborative on Health and the Environment 2009).

Binns adds that the RAC report makes an important contribution because "it looks at all types of evidence, which other previous studies, such as those done by the Institute of Medicine, have not done. The Institute of Medicine reports in fact have been quite restrictive in what they have looked at" (Collaborative on Health and the Environment 2009). By criticizing past IOM reports, Binns is already preemptively aiming to take the bite out of any future IOM reports that might criticize his committee's work. At least one researcher we interviewed eagerly awaits the IOM report because it promises "to offer much-needed criticism of the RAC report."

In the absence of a push from science to revise the stress-based dominant epidemiological paradigm, activists have continued to push change themselves. One interviewee explained the role of advocacy on the RAC: "The RAC's statutory mission was to impartially examine the scientific evidence on health symptoms and illness in Gulf War veterans. As this evidence became clear, the RAC was willing to make forthright statements about what the weight of evidence showed. The chairman of the RAC delivered the committee's conclusions to the secretary of the VA, members of Congress, and the press. His willingness to be an advocate for the RAC's conclusions has gotten them noticed in a way that would not have occurred otherwise."

More explicit advocacy was undertaken by Paul Sullivan, the previous director of the National Gulf War Resource Center and current executive director of Veterans for Common Sense, and Jim Bunker, current president of the National Gulf War Resource Center, who regularly attended meetings of the RAC, although they were not official committee members.

On the other hand, at least one researcher we interviewed felt that the role of veterans as activists has waned over the last eight years. He noted the major shift in funding away from Gulf War veterans' issues following the terrorist attacks of 2001 and the shrinking pool of veterans available to engage in activism. "Gulf War vets are the forgotten generation of veterans . . . [I]t was a successful war and a popular war compared to the Vietnam or Iraq war." Moreover, according to this interviewee, the 700,000 soldiers deployed in the Gulf War have been overshadowed by more than two million deployed in Iraq, and there is greater sympathy toward Iraq veterans because of popular disagreement with the war.

Other factors shaping the dominant epidemiological paradigm include historical and cultural changes. For example, although one researcher pointed to changes over time that lessened the influence of veterans of the Gulf War, another interviewee said that reports of poor care for soldiers wounded in the unpopular Iraq War helped the public understand that veterans of the Gulf War also suffered:

> People actually understand that these poor kids go there and have no idea what they're doing. I think there's much more understanding of that, and so I think there's a new sympathy for the warrior that maybe we didn't have back when we won the Gulf War and we certainly didn't have amongst the huge population in Vietnam. . . . I think it's brought people back to thinking about what could happen in an environment like that. It's brought people back to sympathy towards veterans . . . and people are willing to hear it now, and I really think it's because of the Iraq vets.

Reports of the treatment of veterans injured in Iraq has perhaps made the public more understanding of the hidden nature of casualties. One Gulf War veteran observed that people now respond to him differently when he wears his uniform in public, a change he believes to be the result of heightened public sympathy for veterans of the unpopular Iraq War.

Outcomes for Veterans

With regard to the treatment of Gulf War veterans, any significant progress resulting from a shift of the dominant epidemiological paradigm still appears to be far off. On the one hand, veterans are pleased with, and even feel vindicated by, the findings of the RAC report. According to Paul Sullivan, a Gulf War veteran and currently executive director of Veterans for Common Sense, "Gulf War Veterans I've spoken with, and me in particular as a Gulf War Veteran, are exceptionally pleased. We are very proud of the work that Chairman Jim Binns and the other members, and the Gulf War Veterans, who are on this Research Advisory Committee have done in the past several years" (Collaborative on Health and the Environment 2009). But one veteran activist commented, "I am sad to report that as far as the VA goes, the [RAC] report did little good. The secretary at the time sent it to the IOM, where it was laid to rest. The Congress is going to start hearing[s]. We are hoping this will get the new secretary of the VA to fixing the problems of the past." According to one researcher, it is the slowness of science itself that poses a challenge to veterans: "It didn't take us very long to figure out that this wasn't PTSD and they weren't crazy . . . but it took us a very long time to figure out what we thought it was. I think that our slowness as scientists to figure out what it was affected the whole course of what happened to the veterans. And I don't know how to speed that up, because science takes time."

CONCLUSION

Although science does indeed take time, it takes varying lengths of time depending on who the stakeholders are in the formation of a dominant epidemiological paradigm and what sorts of institutional, political, social, and other barriers impede challenges to it. But as veterans of the Gulf War attempted to transform their problems from isolated personal troubles into a shared social problem, their primary obstacle was not merely the slowness of science: it was their opposition to the dominant epidemiological paradigm. The dominant epidemiological paradigm is both a belief system and a process, and as such is subject to change. But the prevailing systems of scientific, government, and military power have made it difficult to challenge. Veterans have been only partially successful in their efforts, which have been made all the more difficult by uncertain and incomplete science and a sometimes distrustful and antagonistic relationship with government agencies.

For any illness, the dominant epidemiological paradigm is historically contingent, and thus our ethnographic work on Gulf War–related illnesses presents it at certain points in time and through the eyes of certain actors. By the late 1990s, it had shifted from a primary-stress hypothesis to a contextual-stress hypothesis, incorporating new advances in science and the opinions and demands of veterans and the public. The acceptance of this new paradigm may be cemented by emerging scientific findings pointing to specific chemical causes. But even as the Research Advisory Committee's 2008 report lends scientific authority and public support to the link between environmental exposures and Gulf War–related illnesses, contestation persists over what research counts as valid and how to interpret it, especially in debates about whether a unique Gulf War Syndrome exists. Finally, comments from the researchers, doctors, and policy makers we interviewed suggest that the statements made in a committee report have little power to change their minds, much less their practices. And many Gulf War veterans continue to suffer without effective treatment.

Some of these advances we note resulted from veteran activists' insistence that the government be held accountable and that it release information that could help advance the science. But cuts in funding for research and the long-drawn-out process of translating research into policy suggest that if veterans are not able to maintain pressure for justice and for effective treatment, the inertia of bureaucracy and the short attention spans of politicians and the media will impede change. Further research on the veterans' health movement might explore its continuing efforts to change the direction or scope of research and how advances in science or policy are affecting veterans and their access to medical care.

The severe consequences for ill veterans and their families of the slow progress of research and the protracted nature of contestation over Gulf War–related illnesses raise the question of whether science can be done differently. Could the VA and other government agencies have treated veterans differently from the beginning, giving greater credence to their claims of sickness to get them the best possible medical care? The causes and consequences of conservatism for the disciplines of science and for the lives of people affected by it deserve to be explored in greater detail.

Future research examining how nonscientific actors can use science to shift the dominant epidemiological paradigm, even in the absence of strong scientific support, would make a valuable contribution to the understanding of contested illnesses. Because the dominant epidemiological paradigm of any disease is always contested by various actors and institutions, it is always shifting, and there are numerous angles from which it can be approached. Because paradigms change slowly, and Gulf War–related illness is now a relatively old contested illness, future research might also explore how the dominant epidemiological paradigm changes over much longer periods. But for veterans who are still not well eighteen years after their service, the change will not come soon enough.

NOTES

This chapter represents an extensive revision and expansion of our earlier study: Phil Brown, Stephen Zavestoski, Sabrina McCormick, Joshua Mandelbaum, Theo Luebke, and Meadow Linder, "A Gulf of Difference: Disputes over Gulf War–Related Illnesses," *Journal of Health and Social Behavior* 42 (2001): 235–57.

1. We choose the term *Gulf War–related illness* in contrast to other descriptions like *Gulf War syndrome* because veterans suffer from a variety of symptom clusters. We do not believe that it is necessary to establish a unique diagnosis or unique symptom cluster to demonstrate the existence of a definable, examinable set of illnesses caused by exposures in the Gulf War.

2. Other government agencies that investigated Gulf War–related illnesses included the Centers for Disease Control, the Institute of Medicine, the National Institutes of Health, and President Clinton's Presidential Advisory Committee on Gulf War Veterans' Illnesses.

3. Here we adopt a more inclusive definition of environmental causes than we employ in our examination of asthma and breast cancer in part because of the need to recognize the possible interactive effects of toxins and medical treatments. Also, in breast cancer treatment, there is general acceptance that estrogen used in medical treatments (e.g., as used in hormone replacement therapy) is a potential carcinogen, even though environmental estrogens are not generally seen as risk factors. For asthma, there are no suspected iatrogenic causes.

4. By 2008, the scientific story was quite different. In its 2008 summary of research into Gulf War–related illnesses, the Research Advisory Committee concluded that

> research has not supported early speculation that Gulf War illness is a stress-related condition. Large population-based studies of Gulf War veterans consistently indicate that Gulf War illness is not the result of combat or other deployment stressors, and that rates of posttraumatic stress disorder (PTSD) and other psychiatric conditions are relatively low in Gulf War veterans.

Gulf War illness differs fundamentally from trauma and stress-related syndromes that have been described after other wars. No Gulf War illness–type problem, that is, no widespread symptomatic illness not explained by medical or psychiatric diagnoses, has been reported in veterans who served in Bosnia in the 1990s or in current conflicts in Iraq and Afghanistan. (RAC 2008, 4–5)

5. In addition, the 2008 Research Advisory Committee report concludes with reference to one study that "the reliability of self-reported exposures was unrelated to veterans' health status, that is, symptomatic veterans report exposures with the same degree of reliability as healthy veterans." The report also concluded in reference to a Boston Environmental Hazards Center study that "contrary to expectation, veterans who believed they may have been exposed to nerve gas showed no tendency to 'over report' health problems . . . [and that] media coverage . . . had very little impact on veterans' reports of chemical agents and other exposures in theater" (RAC 2008, 35).

6. Government realization of the lack of predeployment health data has led to numerous proposals for improved data management, including improvements in the monitoring and recording of possible exposures (Institute of Medicine 1999).

7

The Health Politics of Asthma

Environmental Justice and Collective Illness Experience

Phil Brown, Brian Mayer, Stephen Zavestoski, Theo Luebke,
Joshua Mandelbaum, Sabrina McCormick, and Mercedes Lyson

Asthma rates have risen so much in the United States in recent decades that medical and public health professionals speak of an epidemic, particularly in urban centers. The number of individuals with asthma in the United States grew by 73.9 percent between 1980 and 1996, with an estimated 14.6 million people reporting suffering from asthma in 1996. This is widely believed to be a real increase, not an artifact of diagnosis (Sears 1997; Woolcock and Peat 1997; Goodman, Stukel, and Change 1998; Mannino et al. 2002). Since then, asthma prevalence rates have reached a plateau, at roughly 7.7 percent of the United States population (22 million) (NCHS 2008b). From 1980 to 2004, hospitalizations for asthma rose 20 percent, and by 2004 there were 1.8 million asthma-related emergency room visits a year. The estimated cost to society from asthma is greater than $11 billion a year (Pew Environmental Health Commission 2000). As the number of cases has increased, medical and public health professionals and institutions have expanded their treatment and prevention efforts, environmental and community activists have made asthma a major part of their agenda, and media coverage has grown.

The belief in psychogenic causes of asthma, once widely accepted, has given way in the last two decades to a focus on environmental conditions, both indoors and outdoors. Some environmental groups and community activists concerned about asthma have entered into coalitions with academic research centers, health providers, public health professionals, and even local and state government public health agencies to investigate environmental causes. This remains, however, a contentious debate. These disputes, which are important because they influence public health prevention and government regulation, provide fertile ground for the development of the theories and methods discussed so far in this book.

Most public-health education and intervention efforts focus on removing asthma triggers found inside homes, such as mold, roach droppings, and tobacco smoke. These factors are amenable to short-term action that can reduce the frequency and severity of attacks and thus limit emergency room visits. Although public health professionals and organizations also recognize that outdoor air pollution contributes to asthma, they have less capacity to act effectively to reduce it, which involves regulation of emissions and changes in air-quality standards at the local, state, and national levels. Still, many public health agencies and programs increasingly understand that indoor environmental conditions are related to social inequalities, and they seek an intersectoral approach to improve living conditions, taking into account housing, transportation, and economic development when dealing with health interventions and illness prevention.

Activist groups, which do not provide direct medical and public health services, can place a different emphasis on air pollution. These groups define themselves as environmental justice organizations and view asthma within the larger context of community well-being. They emphasize the unequal distribution of environmental risks and hazards according to race and class and call for the mitigation of environmental factors that they believe are responsible for increased asthma in their communities. Such groups combine general education about asthma with political action to reduce local pollution.

We posit that asthma has become for many people a "politicized collective illness experience," particularly when community-based environmental justice organizations show people with asthma how to make direct links between their experience of asthma and the social determinants of their health. We are interested less in how the illness shapes the individual experience than in how community-based organizations work to create a collective identity based on the experience of asthma. Collective identity links social and physical realities and tends to be a function of shared grievances that might result from discrimination, structural dislocation, shared values, or other social constructions. Through the process of collective framing, these organizations transform the personal experience of illness into a collective identity focused on discovering and eliminating the social causes of asthma. This collective framing leads to the politicized collective illness experience (see chapter 2). Changing the perception of asthma by those who suffer from it reveals a new and more empowering path of response.

The approach outlined in this chapter integrates three important areas of medical and environmental sociology—illness experience, environmental justice, and lay discovery of environmental health effects—in order to explore two community environmental-justice organizations working to reframe the etiology of asthma. We begin by pointing out why asthma is significant for health and social policy. Then we examine the social discovery of asthma and its environmental correlates, the political and economic conflicts surrounding asthma research and regulation, and the transformation of the dominant view of the triggers of asthma. Building on those bases, we explore how activist groups have used the issues to build a collective "politicized collective illness experience," in which people with asthma make direct links between their experience of asthma and the social determinants of their health.

METHODS AND DATA

We focus on two community environmental justice organizations: Alternatives for Community and Environment (ACE) in Boston's Roxbury neighborhood and West Harlem Environmental Action (WE ACT) in New York City. Both have put significant emphasis on asthma education and organizing, and they maintain connections with academic researchers who study air pollution. We see them as influential models of an environmental justice approach to asthma activism. We also include data from our interviews with members of academic and community partnerships that are funded by one or more federal agencies.

We analyze these cases using content analysis of government documents and scientific literature in medical, public health, and epidemiological journals; sixteen participant-observations of ACE and two of WE ACT by a number of researchers; and twenty interviews with ACE and WE ACT staff, public health practitioners and researchers, and government officials. The ACE observations were mainly conducted at classes taught by ACE in public schools in minority neighborhoods in Boston. These classes provide basic information on the symptoms and environmental triggers of asthma and how to seek help. They also introduce students to concepts of environmental justice and offer them opportunities to get involved in community activism. A few observations were made of other public presentations by ACE staff at conferences and workshops. Observations of WE ACT included spending a day in the organization's office and another day with staff at a New York area environmental justice meeting. Unreferenced quotes come from interviews and observations.

ASTHMA IN HEALTH AND SOCIAL POLICY

The incidence of asthma is significant in the United States for a number of reasons. it has increased dramatically in recent decades; it varies by race and class; it challenges the notion of individual responsibility and focuses on social structural factors; and it leads to pressure on Congress for nationwide health tracking.

Although asthma affects people across all classes and is not restricted to dense urban areas, the poor and minority groups are disproportionately affected. People with asthma are more likely to be children age 5 to 14 years, black, and female (Mannino et al. 2002). In many low-income urban areas, especially minority communities, asthma rates are significantly higher than the national average. Whereas 8.2 percent of all U.S. residents have asthma, 11.1 percent of blacks have the disease (Akinbami and Moorman 2006).

Beyond these already telling statistics, we observed a large degree of community concern about asthma. In many poor and minority neighborhoods, it is one of the most visible and pressing problems residents face. Laypeople have become active in school-based programs, community clinic programs, novel public health initiatives, and activist groups that view asthma as related to social inequalities.

Activism has developed in response to the racial disparities in the incidence of asthma and the attention to air pollution as a trigger. In its focus on environmental and social determinants, asthma activism challenges the view that places the burden of asthma prevention on the shoulders of individuals. Because this approach requires sufferers or their parents to work to remove asthma triggers from their homes, they may feel that they bear primary responsibility for the problem. If their cleanup efforts fail to reduce symptoms, parents can feel responsible for their children's suffering. Moreover, this individual-level approach often obscures the role of corporate pollution and the failure of government regulation.

By contrast, asthma activism takes an intersectoral approach to health. Much can be done to reduce or prevent asthma through nonmedical action in the areas of housing, transportation, and environmental protection. The US Environmental Protection Agency (EPA), National Institute of Environmental Health Sciences (NIEHS), Department of Housing and Urban Development (HUD), and Centers for Disease Control and Prevention (CDC) have also adopted intersectoral approaches, including funding community intervention programs that have explicit antiracist foundations and that view social inequality as contributing to the asthma epidemic.

For example, the Seattle–King County Healthy Homes Project has focused on improving indoor air quality among low-income families using an explicitly justice-driven model of intervention (Krieger et al. 2002). This project includes elements of community advocacy, in cooperation with the Seattle Housing Authority, in efforts to empower families with the skills, knowledge, and access to care that will improve their living conditions. A similar project, the Southern California Environmental Justice Collaborative (see chapter 5), also works with communities of color, focusing on the need for a more comprehensive assessment of respiratory health risks that reflects the disproportionate hazard exposure experienced by minority groups (Morello-Frosch et al. 2005b). Likewise, Communities Organized against Asthma and Lead (Project COAL), based in Houston, Texas, brings local community and environmental health organizations together with environmental toxicologists to address asthma triggers in low-income housing (Motosue et al. 2009). Project COAL, like the other two projects, emphasizes the need for empowerment in public health interventions. Thus asthma has become an issue that has mobilized poor and minority people to identify social inequality and engage in widespread political action. Environmental justice approaches to asthma place ethics and rights issues in the center of health policy.

Asthma has been an important impetus behind improved health tracking. The United States has minimal national data-gathering compared to most industrialized nations. Such data are critical to assessing and dealing with asthma because they allow us to better understand inequalities of place (Fitzpatrick and LaGory 2000). Poor and minority people tend to live in areas of higher respiratory hazard exposure. The growth in geographic information systems (GIS) methodologies, the use of EPA's Toxic Release Inventory (a federally mandated reporting system that lists toxic emissions from individual firms, widely used in environmental hazards research), and other such geographically based approaches have increased awareness of place inequality.[1]

SCIENTIFIC INVESTIGATION OF ENVIRONMENTAL CORRELATES AND THE POLITICAL RESPONSE

Asthma activists, unlike many other disease sufferers, do not have to fight the government over the effects of environmental factors. Activist, public health, and government actors generally agree on the role of airborne particulates in inducing asthma. However, government efforts to enact stricter air-quality standards have met opposition from industry interests that have challenged both the scientific evidence undergirding new air-quality standards and the government's right to regulate air pollution in general.

Evidence dating back over fifty years suggests a link between asthma and air pollution (Dockery et al. 1993; Amdur 1996; Dockery 2000). Natural experiments have strengthened the evidence linking the two (Pope 1989; Friedman et al. 2001). Less is known, however, about the biological mechanisms that cause asthma and trigger asthma attacks. One study of schoolchildren in Southern California found that those who exercised outdoors in areas with high ozone concentrations were three times more likely to develop asthma (McConnell et al. 2002). Although recent research focuses on the link between air pollution and triggers of asthma (Barraza-Villarreal et al. 2008; Liu et al. 2009), many investigators continue to search for risk factors for asthma that are prominent in unhealthy residential environments associated with poor and minority neighborhoods (Williams Sternthal, and Wright 2009). As with smoking and its link to lung cancer, sufficient scientific data were not enough to adequately change social policy. Indeed, this failure points to a need for ongoing policy ethnography that allows the effects of science, policy, and activism to be taken fully into account.

The relationship between air pollution and asthma must be seen in light of a wide range of health effects from particulate matter. In total, airborne particulates have been estimated to account for more than 100,000 deaths annually in the United States from pulmonary and cardiac disease—more than from breast cancer, prostate cancer, and AIDS combined (Dockery 2000)—and these findings drive a range of research on the specific health effects of air pollution.

Regulatory standards based on epidemiologic studies have changed considerably over time and remain contentious. The EPA has been only marginally successful in reducing dangerous particulates. In accordance with the 1970 Clean Air Act (CAA), the EPA is required to constantly monitor air quality and to periodically evaluate its air-quality standards. Initially, the EPA regulated only large particles, referring to them as "total suspended particulates." In 1987, based on new research, the agency revised its standards regulate particulate matter down to 10 microns (μm) in size. In 1994, the American Lung Association filed suit against the EPA for failing to review the air particulate standards every five years as required by the CAA. In response to this pressure and the new evidence of adverse health effects, the EPA again revised its standards to include particulates as small as 2.5 microns in diameter (known as the $PM_{2.5}$ standard). Industry representatives who feared the high economic costs of reducing particulate matter in their airborne effluent feared the 1997 revisions. Immediately following the signing of the new law on July 16, 1997, a series of lawsuits against the EPA were filed. On May 14, 1999, in *American Trucking Association, Inc., et al. v. U.S. Environmental Protection Agency*, a federal appellate court concluded that the EPA had made unconstitutional delegations of legislative power. Though the appellate decision was a major blow for environmental regulation, in early 2001 the Supreme Court overturned the decision (Greenhouse 2000).

Following the 1997 EPA standard, the National Research Council published the study *Research Priorities for Airborne Particulate Matter*. In response to the claims made in the lawsuits, the study included a comparison of cost estimates with health effects, although the 1970 CAA did not require cost-benefit analyses. According to the EPA, the cost of 15,000 deaths that would be prevented by stricter regulation was higher than the challenger's estimates for the costs of compliance with the stricter standards. Industry critics of the new standards attacked EPA's ability to set the standards once again, this time charging that the EPA relied on "hidden data" and forcing the EPA to ask for a reanalysis of the data by the Health Effects Institute, an autonomous research group jointly funded by the EPA and the automotive industry. The second study reaffirmed the previous findings, but the EPA was forced to compromise yet again and postponed the adoption of the $PM_{2.5}$ standard until the next five-year review in 2002. In preparation for the review, the EPA installed thousands of air monitors across the country, strengthening the scientific evidence for the new standard (Greenbaum 2000).

APPLYING THE ENVIRONMENTAL JUSTICE FRAME:
ACE AND WE ACT

ACE began in 1993 as an environmental justice organization based in the Roxbury area of Boston and has since become nationally recognized for its work. One of its earliest actions was a successful mobilization to prevent an asphalt plant from being established in Dorchester. ACE had initially expected to focus on issues such as urban blight, not asthma, but a year of talking to residents showed that they regarded asthma as the most urgent community problem. ACE believes that to reduce asthma rates requires addressing housing, transportation, community investment patterns, access to health care, pollution sources, and sanitation, as well as health education. As one staff member notes, "Everything we do is about asthma."

WE ACT was founded in 1988 in response to environmental threats to the community created by the mismanagement of the North River Sewage Treatment Plant and the construction of the sixth bus depot in northern Manhattan. WE ACT quickly evolved into an environmental justice organization with the goal of improving environmental protection and public health in the predominantly African American and Latino communities of northern Manhattan. It identified a wide range of environmental threats, including air pollution, lead poisoning, pesticides, and unsustainable development. WE ACT has now extended its reach beyond West Harlem to other northern Manhattan communities.

Combining Social-Structural Approaches
with Environmental Justice

Many urban asthma coalitions have developed in recent years to treat, prevent, and educate people about asthma. Some of these programs talk openly about the racial and class inequalities in asthma incidence, pointing to poverty, racism, poor living conditions, inadequate sanitation, and unequal access to health services. They call for housing reform in order to provide living arrangements that will keep children safe from dust, roaches, and poor indoor air. Many people involved in these programs frame their concerns in terms of environmental justice. Several programs train community health workers, reminiscent of the paraprofessional organizations of the 1960s and early 1970s, in which laypeople in the community were taught public health skills (Cohen and Legion 2000).

Despite that broad political understanding, most asthma projects focus on controlling indoor environmental factors. Given the extent of the asthma epidemic, it is understandable that many clinicians, social workers, and community activists want to do front-line work; and rapid interventions to change personal behaviors are often effective in reducing asthma suffering. Yet even if these programs reach a significant fraction of inner-city residents, they cannot offer any protection against air pollution from external sources, both outdoors and when outdoor pollutants enter the home. The Northern California Household Exposure Study has demonstrated the importance of this outdoor-to-indoor pathway (see chapter 8).

Environmental justice groups, by contrast, focus on sources of outdoor pollution and engage in local, intersectoral political organizing. Their efforts include reducing or eliminating the use of diesel buses, pressing for stronger air quality regulations, and curtailing hazardous plant emissions. Although some broad national efforts, such as changing air quality regulations, will take a long time, changes in public transportation can be implemented relatively rapidly, resulting in benefits to the entire population. ACE has been able to obtain changes in transit policy, such as controlling truck idling and reducing future diesel bus use. A community-based participatory research (CBPR) partnership between WE ACT and the Columbia University Center for Children's Environmental Health brought about positive outcomes for the West Harlem community, including converting New York City's bus fleet to clean diesel and EPA installation of permanent air monitors in "hot spots" (Vasquez, Minkler, and Shepard 2006).

Transit Issues

ACE encourages communities to take ownership of the asthma issue and to push for solutions. Central to this philosophy is the role of direct action and education, such as a campaign in which residents identified idling trucks and buses as a major source of particulate irritants. They organized an anti-idling march in October 1997 and began giving informational "parking tickets" to idling buses and trucks that explained the health effects of diesel exhaust.

Because ACE identifies diesel buses as a problem, it has taken up transportation issues more broadly. ACE ran a campaign targeting the allocation of transit resources by local and state (Massachusetts) government. Charging "transit racism," ACE argued that the estimated 366,000 daily bus riders in Boston were being discriminated against by the fact that more than $12 billion of federal and state money was being spent on the "Big Dig" highway project (routing central Boston's arterial traffic through underground tunnels) while the Massachusetts Bay Transit Authority (MBTA) refused to spend $105 million to purchase newer, cleaner buses and bus shelters. By demonstrating the connection between dirty buses and higher asthma rates, ACE successfully reframed transit spending priorities as an issue of health, justice, and racism. In 2000 the Transit Riders' Union, largely created by ACE, successfully lobbied the MBTA to allow free transfers between buses, arguing that the many inner-city residents who relied on multiple buses for transportation had to pay more than those in other areas who had free transfers on the subway. In the Boston area, buses are more likely to serve inner-city, low-income communities and communities of color, whereas the subway lines serve more affluent communities.

Similarly, WE ACT identified diesel exhaust as a major factor behind the disparate burden of asthma experienced in West Harlem. In November 2000, WE ACT filed an administrative complaint with the federal Department of Transportation against New York's Metropolitan Transportation Authority (MTA), claiming that the MTA advances a racist and discriminatory policy by disproportionately siting diesel bus depots and parking lots in minority neighborhoods. This complaint brought significant public-agency attention to the disproportionate impact of diesel pollution on this community. In addition, using publicity campaigns such as informative advertisements placed in bus shelters, public-service announcements on cable television, and direct mail, WE ACT has reached a vast number of community residents and public officials to let them know that diesel buses can trigger asthma attacks. Though these efforts increased public awareness of WE ACT, and its efforts to improve local air quality reduced asthma rates, the media campaign did not lead to a shift in New York's Metropolitan Transit Authority's (MTA) policy on regulating and retrofitting diesel buses (Vasquez, Minkler, and Shepard 2006).

Community Empowerment through Education

A key component of ACE's efforts is reflected in its Roxbury Environmental Empowerment Project (REEP), which teaches classes in local schools, hosts environmental justice conferences, and, through its intern program, trains high school students to teach others about environmental health. Classes designed to educate students about environmental justice use asthma as a focal point. For example, REEP teachers discuss the process for siting a hazardous facility in a local neighborhood; they ask the students why such a decision might be made and what they would do about it. Through their "know your neighborhood" strategy, they teach students how to locate on maps the potentially dangerous pollution sources in their community. Experience with REEP has helped some of its high-school interns get into college. ACE also participates in job fairs for students. On some occasions, ACE has brought Harvard School of Public Health air quality researchers to present findings to school audiences. Among other benefits, having research scientists share their relevant work with them demonstrates to children in underfunded and understaffed schools that their health and opinions are valued.

WE ACT's Healthy Home, Healthy Child campaign reflects a similar community-empowerment approach. Although WE ACT has a clean-air campaign in which interested residents are encouraged to participate, the organization believes that focusing solely on air pollution is a disservice to the community. Developed in partnership with the Columbia Center for Children's Environmental Health, the Healthy Home, Healthy Child campaign educates the community about a variety of lifestyle and environmental risk factors, including smoking, lead poisoning, drug and alcohol use, air pollution, garbage, pesticides, and diet, and about actions that residents can take to alleviate or minimize those harms. The campaign began by focusing on specific asthma triggers but soon expanded to include other key concerns such as reducing drugs and alcohol use and improving sanitation services. In addition, empowering local communities entails bringing science to the people. Both ACE and WE ACT have helped communities conduct different kinds of science. ACE's teen interns have conducted local air-quality monitoring, and WE ACT has collaborated with Columbia University scientists to deal with larger-scale pollution emissions.

Organizing with Environmental Justice Principles

Although its work has national implications, ACE's promotion of a new approach to asthma remains expressly local. Like other environmental justice organizations, ACE believes that if it became too nationally focused or too involved in government and academic meetings, it would forsake the individuals in the neighborhood who granted ACE its efficacy in the first place. ACE is aware that even if national $PM_{2.5}$ air quality standards are implemented, local injustices will always require action and redress. Local action can have national significance through action and research by citizen alliances with scientists at research universities. In influencing the way asthma and air particulate research is done, the organizations can shape how the findings are presented and, in some cases, the findings themselves.

Strategies and information can be shared among local groups even without national organization. ACE borrowed the concept of a "transit racism" campaign from the Bus Riders Union in Los Angeles, and WE ACT's challenges to the Metropolitan Transit Authority's bus depot sitings mirror ACE's actions in Roxbury.

Reframing Asthma and Creating a Collective Illness Experience

Organizations like ACE and WE ACT treat asthma as an environmental justice issue and thereby transform the personal experience of illness into a collective identity aimed at discovering and eliminating the social causes of the disease. When people view asthma as related to both air pollution and to conditions in poor neighborhoods, their view of illness changes: their asthma narratives differ from those associated with other chronic illnesses, instead framing the disease in terms of environmental justice, housing, transportation, neighborhood development, the general economy, and government regulations. This broader view is reflected in the goals of one ACE organizer: "I think we have to look at how is it that our society has created such disparate environments for people to live in—from the kind of housing you have, to the kind of school you go to, to the kind of vehicle you ride in, to the kind of air that is outside your door. . . . I think that there's huge changes that are way beyond individual lifestyle changes that we need to look at about production of synthetic chemicals that may play a role, or about the way we're designing and building our cities, towns, and whatnot." This outlook enables people with asthma to place responsibility in part on social structural forces.

A common finding in qualitative studies of people with asthma is a feeling of powerlessness. Asthma has no definitive cure: sufferers can rely only on management to prevent attacks. For children, managing asthma requires reliance upon their doctors, parents, and teachers, which reduces their sense of individuality and exploration (Rudestam 2001). Children learn to associate various places with asthma exacerbation, leading many children and their families to associate local environmental hazards with their asthma and experiencing their home and school environments as threatening. When observing a child's difficulty in breathing during an asthma attack, parents themselves may feel powerless. Limited access to health care also leads parents to feel helpless to reduce their child's asthma suffering. Frequent trips to the emergency room are the norm for impoverished families seeking asthma treatment, resulting in both poor disease management and a feeling of loss of control (Center 2000). Not only do they lack access to health care, but they also have little control of either indoor or outdoor sources of asthma triggers.

Community groups like ACE and WE ACT take the position that the medical establishment has a limited ability to address many factors in the experience of asthma, and they see their role as a bridge. One WE ACT organizer described the experience of many people with asthma in a medical setting: "I think that doctors think that there is very little that they can do . . . . They go through this checklist of risk factors at the beginning of a physical, which now includes, 'Do you wear seatbelts?' Like different questions assessing individual behavior and risk-taking behavior. They focus on things that they feel they can change somehow." Groups like ACE and WE ACT realize that doctors are often unable to address larger issues than individual behavior, this organizer observed: "Even if a kid has really terrible asthma, they're in the hospital, you know, once every two weeks. Sometimes doctors aren't trained to say, 'Do you have mold in your home—where do you live?'" They also recognize that even if medical examinations incorporated questions about the home environment, many other important factors shaping the illness experience would still be neglected:

> It feels like [asthma] has been taken out slightly from the context of everything else that is happening to people . . . and I don't think that that is the way that community groups really approach asthma. They see it in the way environment justice sees it, defining the environment where people live, work, play, and breathe. And so it's the underlying conditions of poverty and social injustice that are contributing to all

these things. And no matter whose fault it is, you can't just get rid of cockroaches and expect asthma to go away. For that matter, you can't just put in better buses and expect asthma to go away. It's all got to be approached in a social justice framework.

The environmental justice approach to structural factors can change the self-perceptions of people with asthma and hence their illness experience. An essay by a REEP intern illustrates the kind of transformation that ACE can engender in people.

> There are things in my environment that truly outrage me. The fact that people have to wait hours for dirty diesel MBTA buses on extremely cold or hot days, the fact that someone I know is being evicted from their home because they can't pay their rent, and the fact that a small child I see everyday has died of asthma in a community where asthma rates are 6 times the state average. These things should not be happening where I live or where anyone lives. Everyone no matter what community they reside in should have the right to a safe and healthy neighborhood. So what is environmental justice is a hard question but I know what it is to me. It is allowing everyone the right to have the best life has to offer from affordable housing to safe neighborhoods and clean air.

Involvement in ACE helped this young community member to draw the connections between a disease like asthma and a wide range of other political and economic circumstances. In painting this broad picture of the causes and experience of asthma, ACE and WE ACT create the foundation for an environmental justice-based approach to reducing the burden of asthma.

Through the educational programs of these organizations, people with asthma learn to manage their disease while beginning to see themselves as part of a collective of people who understand the effects of external factors in contributing to their illness. When they learn that even the indoor air quality in substandard housing is a socially determined phenomenon, they see themselves less as individual sufferers and more as part of a group that has unfair disadvantages. The environmental justice approach tells these people that they can act to change their social circumstances, and in that sense asthma becomes a stepping point to a politicized view of the world. For example, ACE got state, regional, and federal agencies to place an air monitor atop their Roxbury building, with a readout inside the office. They have used this monitor for their educational programs, showing students the relationships between their results on a pulmonary function test and current levels of outdoor air pollution. The ACE interns and many of the children they teach connect the experience of wheezing with the presence of bus depots and trash incinerators in their neighborhoods.

For a growing number of people and organizations, asthma has been transformed from an individual disease into the basis of a social movement focused on health inequalities. Building and maintaining this social movement is a growing concern for organizers, as noted by an ACE community member: "The other part of ACE that's really emerged probably in the past couple of years is our role as movement builders; building an environmental justice movement both locally and nationally. And the leadership development fits under that as well. But it has changed the way we look at our programs. Now we're trying to figure out how we not only take out interns and train them as educators, but train them as organizers."

People with asthma in Boston and New York are incorporating rhetoric from the environmental justice movement to address the social and political forces responsible for the disparate rates of asthma among urban minority communities. ACE and WE ACT look beyond medical explanations and solutions to the social forces shaping the urban environment. As one organizer noted: "I think our approach has been that if people are suffering from asthma, that's something we need to deal with now, today. And yes, part of that answer is a medical solution, figuring out how to get people the right treatment. But in the meantime, if there are things we can do to reduce the level of triggers, if we can figure out how to take more a pollution-prevention approach to figure out how to keep these things from getting into the environment, then we ought to do that."

Through community education and direct-action campaigns, ACE and WE ACT help people with asthma to overcome the stigma that frames asthma both as a weakness and as a result of living in an unclean household. Asthma activists use the destigmatization process to politicize fellow sufferers and gain allies in their effort to produce a healthy environment for their community.

Many people with asthma have arguably developed what we term a "politicized collective illness experience," in which their personal experiences of illness, symptoms, coping, and adaptation have become linked with efforts to assess societal responsibility for the causes and triggers of the disease as well as responsibility for treatment and prevention.

CONCLUSION

Much attention to the new asthma epidemic comes from laypeople who are concerned about environmental triggers. Their approach to asthma includes action in diverse social sectors, such as housing, transportation, and economic development. Because their view of the disease emphasizes race and class inequities, activists focus on political and economic action. Although they understand the need for attention to triggers in the household, they reject the view that individuals bear primary responsibility for asthma control.

ACE and WE ACT define themselves as environmental justice organizations for which asthma activism is only one aspect of their mission. They represent a unique type of health social movement organization because they are not centered on either a particular disease (as with environmental breast cancer movement groups) or on the health status of a specific group of people (as with the women's health movement). Their efforts show how laypeople's efforts can reframe health as a social rather than purely medical issue.

Because of the social justice ideology of these movements, which places issues of ethics and rights at the center of health policy discussion, government officials are pressed to pay attention. Asthma activists began with some advantages. They did not have to struggle for recognition of the epidemic: there was ample attention from medical, public health, and educational institutions and professionals, and there was an excellent science base documenting both the prevalence and the triggers of asthma. In addition, although WE ACT and ACE approach science and scientists differently, both groups have found creative ways to work alongside scientists while not placing primary emphasis on a biomedical approach.

In these campaigns, poor and minority people are using asthma rates as indicators of health inequalities. In cases of isolated community contamination, the intersectoral approach taken by asthma activists is difficult to adopt. But as more diseases come to be understood as phenomena linked to modern industrial practices and consumer lifestyles, illness activists stand to learn from the approaches of asthma activist organizations such as ACE and WE ACT.

The growing attention to social and environmental determinants of asthma also fosters a different approach to the illness itself, namely the creation of a politicized collective illness experience. This approach, together with support from public health and science allies, can lead to concrete changes in health policy, especially in terms of health tracking, academic and community collaboration, and stronger air-quality regulation. The Trust for America's Health (formerly the Pew Environmental Health Commission) has pointed to asthma as one of the central reasons why the United States needs a national health-tracking system and has garnered much scientific and government support for this approach. Health tracking involves collecting data that allow scientists to connect rates of disease with a range of factors, including environment, occupation, and lifestyle or behaviors. It also provides information about the rates of disease by geography and ethnicity, revealing whether clusters of diseases are occurring in particular communities or population groups. This combined information can greatly help in the development of strategies to reduce and eliminate disease and lower the cost of medical treatment (Pew Environmental Health Commission 2000). The passage of a 2004 health-tracking bill in Congress led to the National Environmental Public Health Tracking Program, headed by CDC, which funds state departments of public health and universities to develop a national health-tracking network, including the use of existing health surveillance systems and the creation of new biomonitoring initiatives.

Innovative academic and community collaborations, sponsored by federal grants, have developed in recent years, with asthma as a main focus because there are strong community organizations available to do joint work with researchers. And the growing power of the environmental justice activists, combined with much support from public health professionals and a solid base of research demonstrating the harms of airborne particulates, may lead to stronger air-quality regulation.

NOTES

Originally published as Phil Brown, Stephen Zavestoski, Theo Luebke, Joshua Mandelbaum, Sabrina McCormick, and Brian Mayer, "The Health Politics of Asthma: Environmental Justice and Collective Illness Experience in the United States," *Social Science and Medicine* 57 (August 2003): 453–64. Reprinted in David Pellow and Robert Brulle, eds., *Where We Live, Work, and Play: A Critical Appraisal of the Environmental Justice Movement* (Cambridge, MA: MIT Press). Used with permission of Elsevier.

1. GIS allows the geographic mapping of many kinds of information, allowing researchers to show spatial patterns.

8

Pollution Comes Home
and Gets Personal

Women's Experience of Household
Chemical Exposure

Rebecca Gasior Altman, Rachel Morello-Frosch, Julia Green Brody,
Ruthann A. Rudel, Phil Brown, and Mara Averick

Until recently, most work on environmental pollution focused on problems in the air, water and soil. This chapter offers a new theoretical framework, which we call the exposure experience, to examine the presence and effects of chemical pollutants in homes and inside bodies. To medical sociologists' work on "illness experience," our work adds a focus on the environmental experience of communities, the role of science in shaping people's experiences of their health and bodies, and a focus on embodied experiences that may precede the manifestation of symptoms.

For this study, our primary field site was the homes of middle- and upper-income people on Cape Cod, a rural coastal region of southeastern Massachusetts with high rates of breast cancer. Scientists configured air monitors to collect samples of chemical pollutants in the ambient indoor air of homes. They analyzed these indoor air samples, as well as house dust and women's urine samples, for substances that, in previous studies, were shown to be endocrine disruptors (substances that interfere with human hormones). In collaboration with the scientists, we interviewed the participants to understand what they had learned about indoor and embodied pollution through their involvement in this novel scientific work.

Biomonitoring science and personal exposure assessment measure environmental chemicals in the human body and household air and dust.[1] Public perceptions about environmental problems have shifted in recent decades from concern about outdoor environmental pollution to indoor contamination (Murphy 2006), and from rivers to streams of blood and urine. For example, the US Centers for Disease Control and Prevention (CDC) now reports on 212 chemical pollutants in the blood or urine of the U.S. population, including pesticides, flame retardants, and plastic additives (CDC 2010), and they expand the scope of their search each year.[2] These developments reflect the growing awareness that humans must protect themselves from the environment as much as we must protect the environment from humans: our indoor and outside environments harbor and transmit the waste and by-products of modern industrial production (Szasz 2007; Scott 2009).

Biomonitoring and household exposure information has become more widely available. In addition to regular reports from the CDC, some community-based exposure studies present participants with personal data as well as aggregate study results (Brody et al. 2007a). Similarly, in response to government surveillance programs that report average exposures among populations, social movement organizations conduct exposure studies and publicize volunteers' results using interactive websites. Some projects have featured participants' results alongside pictures and biographies that put a human face to the rising tide of exposure data (Environmental Working Group 2003; Brown 2007; Washburn 2007a).

However, both types of studies come with substantial uncertainties, leading to debate about whether and how results should be reported. For many of the chemicals, scientists do not yet know what concentration levels pose health risks, and they often cannot "fingerprint" exposures to determine specific sources; nor can they recommend evidence-based strategies for reducing individual exposure when exposures are ubiquitous and products poorly labeled.

Though there has been a rapid increase in exposure assessment using these techniques, there has not been a parallel rise in social science that investigates their significance. Only a handful of scholars have begun characterizing how people respond to personal exposure data (Usher et al. 1995; Quandt et al. 2004; Nelson et al. 2008; Emmet et al. 2009; Morello-Frosch et al. 2009a), a field of study that the National Research Council identified as important.[3] Whether and how to report personal exposure information, then, are empirical as well as ethical questions.

In the context of a study that sampled for eighty-nine environmental chemicals in 120 homes and biological samples (Rudel et al. 2003), we examined how people assign meaning to their results. This study is among the first to investigate the experience of study participants who receive personal results from biomonitoring and exposure assessment studies, and the first to apply the tools and perspectives of medical sociology. Our framework for studying exposure experience adds to the medical sociology literature on illness. In addition, examining exposure science represents a unique opportunity to track changing public knowledge about the accumulation of synthetic chemicals and industrial by-products.

For the past two decades, research on social responses to pollution has typically examined specific contamination events, whether from acute disasters or chronic pollutant leaks or releases. Here, we study responses to pollution from previously unexamined, everyday household activities and products that have acquired what

Rachel Carson termed "the harmless aspects of the familiar" (Carson 1962): electronics, carpeting, cleaners, beauty products, and so on. Moreover, as we demonstrate, science—not just the direct experience of environmental problems—shapes participants' embodied health experiences. Indeed, science increasingly contributes to how people discover and understand environmental health threats (Murphy 1997; Fischer 2000), both aside from and in addition to their embodied or direct experience. This finding suggests future opportunities for social scientists to study diverse exposure experiences, how they vary, and how they are mediated by environmental science.

INDOOR POLLUTION
AS A NEW EXPOSURE EXPERIENCE

Early research on the embodied experience of pollution involved case studies of acute contamination crises, industrial disasters, and disease clusters surrounding one predominant exposure source. Social scientists found that such events disrupt community identity, social relations, and connections to place, and they prompt widespread fear and anxiety (Brown and Mikkelsen 1997; Couch and Kroll-Smith 1991; Erikson 1994; Edelstein 2004). They attributed such responses to the historical absence of knowledge that could address communities' concerns and help them develop strategies for remediation (Erikson 1994). However, over time, knowledge about environmental problems has evolved through increased media coverage and research that has deepened collective understanding about interactions between humans and the environment (Szasz 1994).

Couch and Kroll-Smith (1985, 1991) developed the concept of "chronic technological disaster" to characterize a different exposure scenario. They pointed to gradually developing environmental problems that are often not noticeable under routine conditions. Public responses to these equally insidious environmental problems were far more muted. Beamish (2002), like Clarke before him (1989), added to these insights by showing how assumptions built from an institutional, organizational, and popular preoccupation with large-scale disasters shaped the residents' exposure experience in ways that constrained them from recognizing and acting on more ambiguous, chronic environmental problems.

The relatively new "home front" of indoor environmental pollution generates a different exposure experience. For those living in contaminated communities, contact with the contamination source is powerful because it is immediate: for example, the chemical plume underneath their homes or chemicals entering through the kitchen tap. Biomonitoring, however, has made visible environmental contamination from seemingly benign consumer products and housing materials that has transgressed the boundaries of home and body, which is detected in urine samples and household dust collecting beneath the sofa.

This is not to imply that science and concerned citizens have overlooked the dangers of environmental contamination. Social scientists have documented that citizens and workers have long feared for their health and turned to science to assuage those fears (Levine 1982; Brown and Mikkelsen 1997; Gottlieb 2005). More recently, the expanded use of biomonitoring and exposure science has altered the relationships among exposed populations, science, and chemicals and led to a different exposure experience. During the 1980s, citizens' requests for personal exposure data often exceeded what science could offer them (Harris 1983). When exposure studies were conducted, they measured how community exposures differed from a control or reference population, but they rarely quantified exposure for individuals living in contaminated communities, and certainly not from products that they had brought into their homes.

In these cases, exposure science was used to verify or quantify exposure to an extant problem "discovered" by the community. However, other environmental problems, like ozone depletion, were less visible until scientists and activists went looking for them (Murphy 1997). Similarly, Fischer acknowledges that pollution risks are invisible and remain unknown until research makes them plain to the public and policymakers (Fischer 2000, 51).

Personal exposures to chemical pollutants in homes and bodies can be thought of as a "new species of [environmental] troubles" (Erikson 1994), in which science plays a paramount role in discovering and defining problems that often are not perceptible through direct experience. Rapid innovation in exposure assessment science has combined with advocacy-based strategies that treat access to scientific information as a public right (Brody et al. 2007a; Morello-Frosch et al. 2009a). Together, these trends alter how some people experience environmental pollution.

Although exposure science has expanded much in recent years, social science research has not kept pace. Prior research details an exposure experience characterized by disrupted lives, fear, and anxiety (Vyner 1989; Edelstein 2004). While these insights remain relevant, they were developed by observing responses to environmental disasters and catastrophes that differ from the exposure experiences we present here. Our research updates scientific understandings about the range of social responses to environmental health problems at a time when science increasingly shapes that experience.

Science, Exposure Experience, and Environmental Consciousness

Our exposure-experience approach builds on the study of human illness experience, a cardinal area of research in medical sociology (see, e.g., Bird, Conrad, and Fremont 2000; Lawton 2003). We present a framework for studying how scientific understanding and embodied experiences emerge through one another, a phenomenon that reflects what Jasanoff (2004) refers to as the coproduction of science and society. Until recently, the illness experience literature has tended to focus on direct experience with symptoms or with the health care system rather than how science intersects with and informs individuals' embodied and illness experiences. One emerging trend in medical sociology examines how technologies like medical imaging and genetic screening raise individuals' awareness of subclinical health effects or predispositions for disease in advance of physical symptoms (see, e.g., Cox and McKellin 1999; Robertson 2000). Though this research informs our work, these studies vary in the extent to which they bring science and technology into analytic view (Timmermans and Berg 2003) and thus offer few clues for examining the dynamic interaction between individual experience and science and technology.

We do not adopt a strict social-constructivist perspective on science; instead we acknowledge the objective reality of chemical body burden and the significance of the social processes that shape the meaning and significance of knowledge about chemical exposure. We draw from the literature on the public understanding of science, which informs us that the lay public relies on a wide array of knowledge and experience to interpret complex science (Irwin and Wynne 1996), often through an interactive and relational process rather than a purely didactic and cognitive one (Wynne 1996). From the work of Hilgartner and Bosk (1988) we expect that participants would consult three sources of social knowledge, with prior encounters with toxicants being paramount: interactions with professionals, researchers, family, and friends; knowledge gleaned from the media or social-movement discourse; and experiential knowledge, in particular experience with other environmental, health, or social problems. Most important, environmental sociology and psychology inform us that when dealing with environmental issues, individuals look to prior experiences for cues about how to respond (Couch and Kroll-Smith1991; Edelstein 2004). Therefore, we consider the role that past environmental experiences—what Edelstein (2004) terms "eco-social" history—play in participants' interpretations.

When we look at participants' narratives of their exposure experience, we attempt to understand how ecosocial history operates. Experiences from community relations, collectively experienced contamination episodes, and media or movement discourse coalesce into a set of assumptions, social cues, and social referents that individuals draw on to guide new encounters with chemical pollutants. These assumptions, in turn, inform how participants understand risks, anticipate government and societal responses, and respond to the situation (Edelstein 2004).

We further define the ecosocial and historical context as encompassing participants' past experience with pollution—or the lack thereof—and also the power relationship between the pollution source and the exposed population (Pulido 1996; Edelstein 2004). As the distribution of environmental pollution varies across populations and places (Morello-Frosch et al. 2002), we suspect that different communities have different ecosocial histories that filter and inform their responses to data about chemicals in their homes and bodies.

However, sociology also reminds us that certain implications follow from such a reliance on past experience to inform contemporary circumstances. Prior environmental encounters prime individuals and institutions to respond more readily to acute contamination crises—particularly those preceded by an attention-grabbing event, such as a fire, spill, or explosion—and to overlook or become habituated to evidence of more ambiguous environmental problems (Clarke 1989; Beamish 2002). In a study of public responses to a slow oil leak off the coast of San Luis Obispo County, California, that received widespread attention in 1995, Beamish (2002) found that residents, workers, and government officials, all witnesses to the leak, did not express dread or panic. Rather, they had a more measured response, and in some cases were unresponsive, until, over a period of forty years, the leak grew into one of the largest oil spills in US history. Hence prior experiences may channel attention away from chronic yet insidious environmental problems until they become disastrous.

We believe this latter scenario approximates the situation of receiving personal exposure results, where study participants learn about the build-up of chemicals in their most intimate environments. We explore here the implications of this interaction between science and past experience for study participants' embodied experiences of and responses to environmental health problems.

As environmental sociology has directed scholarly attention to the health and social implications of pollution, it has found common ground with medical sociology. This convergence is evidenced by a burgeoning literature that integrates the two areas, with science serving as a bridge (Kroll-Smith and Floyd 1997; Casper 2003; McCormick, Brown, and Zavestoski 2003; Zavestoski et al. 2004; Brown 2007). Our development of the concept of exposure experience builds on numerous articulations between medical and environmental sociology, such as the study of health-based social movements (Brown et al. 2004; McCormick., Brody, and Brown 2004), place-based health (MacIntyre, Ellaway, and Cummins 2002), environmental trauma (Couch and Kroll-Smith 1991; Erikson 1994; Edelstein 2004), and environmental suffering (Auyero and Swistun 2007). Similarly, our work is situated within the extensive literature on environmental health as an aspect of environmental sociology (e.g., Kroll-Smith, Brown, and Gunter 2000).

The Silent Spring Institute Household Exposure Study

Our qualitative study of women's responses to personal exposure information is one component of a collaborative, interdisciplinary research project to investigate possible links between environmental exposures and breast cancer (Brody et al. 2009). One portion of this effort—the Silent Spring Household Exposure Study (HES)—is designed to characterize common chemical exposures in everyday, indoor environments, which are poorly understood (US General Accounting Office 1999a). This research uses community-based participatory research methods that emphasize the right to know: thus study participants had the option of learning their own as well as aggregate results (Brody et al. 2007a). Participants in the original HES were drawn from an earlier case-control study of Cape Cod women diagnosed with breast cancer between 1988 and 1995 (McKelvey et al. 2003; Brody et al. 2007a).

The Household Exposure Study began with household air and dust sampling and urine sampling for 120 participants on Cape Cod, a region of Massachusetts with elevated rates of breast cancer (McKelvey et al. 2003). Samples were analyzed for eighty-nine chemicals that affect hormones, including alkylphenols, parabens, phthalates, polychlorinated biphenyls (PCBs), flame retardants, pesticides, and phenols.[4] Many of these chemicals are only partially regulated, and their health effects have not been scientifically determined. As a result, no up-to-date health-based guidelines for these chemicals exist to help participants evaluate whether their results are of concern. The researchers interviewed participants about building materials in their homes and their use of pesticides, cleaning, and personal care products. Researchers later resampled a subset of homes with elevated contaminant levels of PCBs, chlordane (a fumigant pesticide), and the flame retardant tris phosphate (tris). With the exception of tris, whose use is only restricted, all of these are banned in the United States, making their presence in the samples alarming. Blood samples were tested for PCBs in participants whose homes had high levels. The study was the first to report indoor measures for thirty of these chemicals (Rudel et al. 2003), and it was also among the first to report both community and individual-level exposure data to study participants for such a wide range of chemicals. It has since been repeated in two Northern California communities by a team consisting of researchers from Silent Spring Institute, Communities for a Better Environment, Brown University, and the University of California, Berkeley; and it has informed reporting by other researchers and the California Biomonitoring Program, the first state-based program in the United States.

Participants were asked during the informed-consent process whether they wanted to receive their results. Ninety-seven percent of participants said they did, and the results were reported in fall 2004. The report included a cover letter, a narrative results summary, and graphs (see the example in figure 8.1) that showed the concentration of chemicals found in each home compared to the distribution of results for all homes in the sample and to US EPA health-based guidelines, when available (as they were for about half of the chemicals).[5] The scientists enclosed a list of household products and industrial or household practices that were common exposure sources. Women whose homes were sampled a second time received follow-up results by mail in November 2005, and a member of the study team phoned each of them.

We interviewed a subset of women who had participated in the household sampling. Because Silent Spring Institute had drawn its HES sample from participants

A Guide to Reading Your Results

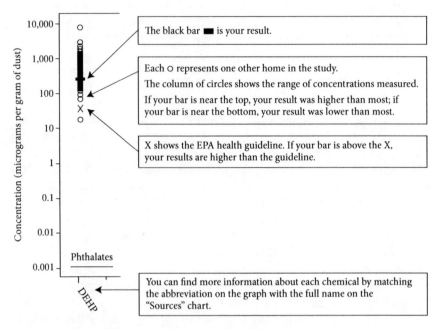

FIGURE 8.1. Instructions to participants for reading individual exposure results in Cape Cod household exposure study

in an earlier breast cancer study, the majority of participants were 80 years of age or older; so in order for our qualitative follow-up study to better represent women across the life course, we stratified all HES participants by age and oversampled younger women for inclusion in our interview sample. We selected thirty-seven women who had requested their results, who were still living in the area, and who had complete contact information. Of the women interviewed, eight were 59 or younger, fourteen were age 60–79, and three were 80 or older. Half the women interviewed had at least a college degree; 33 percent had some college or vocational education, and 17 percent had ended their schooling with high school graduation. All the women owned their homes. Although we did not ask how many were mothers, 80 percent had given birth. Seventy-four percent had been diagnosed with breast cancer, and others reported a range of family health issues, from Lou Gehrig's disease to other forms of cancer.

We conducted thirty interviews with twenty-five individuals between June 2005 and May 2006.[6] Interviews were conducted within six months of the women's receipt of their initial HES results. To refresh participants' memory, we mailed a second copy of their results just before the interview. Five women were interviewed again after their homes and urine were resampled. The interviewer was blinded to the participants' exposure data, unless they shared their results or requested assistance with reading the graphs.[7] The interview schedule included fifty-five semistructured questions about participants' interpretation of exposure results, impressions of the key findings, what the results told them about their home and health, and what responses, if any, the results prompted. Interviews lasted forty to ninety minutes.

WHEN POLLUTION COMES HOME

Study participants reported gaining a new or expanded understanding of their everyday exposure to environmental chemicals. Participation in the study led participants to make at least one but often several of the six following points:

1. Synthetic chemicals can be detected in household air and dust, and in human samples such as urine (e.g., "There's chemicals everywhere in this place!").
2. Most homes contain chemicals. Many extended this message to assume that most homes, including homes outside the study, harbored similar chemicals (e.g., "I just figured that was the way it was in every house").
3. Homes contain a variety of different chemical compounds. For example, one participant expressed surprise that researchers found sixty-seven of the eighty-nine target chemicals in sampled homes: "I didn't even know there were that many chemicals, but I guess there's a lot more than that even."
4. Even substances banned long ago, such as the pesticide DDT, were detected. The fact that chemicals could persist so many years after they were banned was a surprise to study participants.
5. Chemicals found in urine, blood, and household air and dust come from numerous sources. Many participants expressed surprise on learning that household cleaning products and beauty supplies were potential exposure sources for the chemicals detected. One woman's response is representative: "I never stopped to think about some of the things that I just automatically buy and use." Although several participants routinely avoided aerosol sprays, noting that they thought propellants could be "bad," women reported first learning from the study that chemicals found in indoor air and dust samples stem from nonaerosol forms of these products as well.
6. Many common household sources of chemical exposures are unregulated or understudied. Some participants questioned why epidemiological and toxicological data are lacking for many chemicals, why there were few EPA health-based guidelines for chemicals in the study, and why few consumer or household products are safety tested.

Perhaps more provocative than the revelations of what information participants gained was their tendency to identify information gaps resulting from absent or uncertain health data. Fifteen of the twenty-five study participants requested additional information about what the study results meant, asking whether the results signaled a problem, what defined an "acceptable" exposure, where the chemicals came from, and what they should do in response. Participants wanted more than a descriptive account of what was found and more than a comparative report of their results; they also wanted scientists' evaluation of the health implications of their data and recommendations for action. As one woman remarked, "Every home also has cornflakes in the kitchen, but that doesn't tell me anything." Another woman, who joined the study to understand her experience with breast cancer, noted that "I basically feel I got nothing" from the study. Yet in these cases participants were seeking information about potential health risks that does not yet exist.

The scientists' capacity to offer more health information was hampered by the limited availability of government health-based exposure guidelines, information about routes of exposure, or effective exposure-reduction strategies for many chemicals. A few participants expressed frustration, worrying that the scientists had withheld explanatory information. Their frustration festered even when participants requested more information and the scientists again explained the uncertainty of personal exposure information, and even when participants understood the social and political circumstances that created data gaps. As one woman noted:

> I think that if I said to her [the lead toxicologist on the study]: Specifically, where does this come from, and how did I get it? I'm not sure she would answer me; I don't know that she could answer me.
>
> Researcher: There's a lot that we don't know.
>
> Participant: Mmmm. And I don't like that. I don't like that at all.

In response to these circumstances, study participants sought information from others, not only the scientists but also friends and family (e.g., a friend with cancer, a daughter with a medical degree, or a son with scientific training). They shared study results with their physicians. Some participants consulted Internet resources or local libraries. One participant copied the results for her landscaper, who had applied pesticides to her lawn and garden. Yet these sources had few new insights to offer. Questions lingered. Participants' narratives reflected puzzlement over how to interpret levels and respond appropriately. The majority of interviewees also asked how other study participants responded to exposure data and whether their own queries were unique.

Most participants commented that the study offered them new information about exposures that were not a previous concern. This information in turn raised additional questions and comments that typically fell into three categories: the sources of the chemicals, whether the levels found in their homes were cause for concern, and what responses the scientists recommended.

Sources: "Where Is This Coming From?"

One theme in the interviews was a notable incongruity between women's perception of possible chemical sources and the range and quantity of chemicals found in their air, dust, and urine samples. Participants often said they were perplexed by the number of chemicals detected, despite the scientists' effort to inform participants about common household exposure sources. Eleven of the participants reported some variant of the following statement: "I don't use a lot of products," so "I have no idea where any of this was coming from." One woman remarked: "I'm surprised that they can find that many things by looking at your dust and looking at your air. I mean, that's amazing to me that they can actually find chemicals in your air in any amount whatsoever."

The discrepancy between data and perception can be explained partially by the unknown presence of many chemicals in everyday household, construction, and personal care products. Participants were unaware that chemicals can originate not only from sprays but also from carpeting, upholstery, electronics, plastics, pest control methods, landscaping products, and personal care supplies, many of which contain unlabeled additives.

Product use seemed unremarkable and unmemorable to most participants, which suggests that their use is a habitual constituent of consumer culture. Initially, when surveyed, many participants underestimated their product use. With additional questions and time for reflection, however, they would recall products used in routine housekeeping and personal care. One participant, on first scanning the list of common exposure sources provided to her, commented "I just, I don't use any of these things . . . when I look at it, I keep saying no to so many things. But, obviously, there is something. But, I keep saying, I don't have that, and I don't have this, and so on and so forth. I don't know." She noted that her home harbored chemicals at levels "higher than in most homes." Later, she raised several possible sources, but quickly rejected each one. Each possibility violated her understanding of what activities or products contributed to exposure. Similarly, another woman noted:

> Well, you know what you shouldn't use, like the sprays—too many sprays. That's the one thing that they [the scientists] spoke about a lot, were the sprays . . .
>
> Researcher: Like what kinds of sprays?
>
> Participant: Well, of course I don't use any. . . . Well, I don't use hairspray. I do use a bathroom spray. And, a countertop spray. Let's see what else. A window spray. . . . That's it. I don't have a lot.

Participants frequently attributed exposures to historical uses. Some realized that homes could harbor potentially dangerous substances no longer used in residential applications. For example, several participants noted the age of their homes and suggested that older homes harbor old contaminants (e.g., "It's a really old house, and God knows what it's been treated with . . . over the centuries"). Indeed, the age of a home does influence what chemicals are within it. With newer homes, the scientists did not expect to see high levels of lead, asbestos, or chlordane, because the United States banned household uses of these substances years ago. However, participants were less primed to think about exposures from contemporary sources. One participant attributed her exposures to the age of her house while a can of household insecticide sat, unmentioned, on an end table beside her.

Levels: "Is This High?"

When interpreting their results, participants paid more attention to the level of chemicals than to the number detected. Indeed, previous research has found that people read exposure levels as social indicators of risk that dictate their response (Clarke 1989). Historically, chemical regulation has also been attuned to levels: measuring the level of exposure, estimating the levels at which no health effect is anticipated, and setting limits for acceptable exposures.

When possible, participants compared their results to the government health-based guidelines depicted on the results graphs. Participants used guidelines to anchor their assessment of whether their levels were cause for concern. Results near or below the guideline were less noteworthy than those above it. Even though the scientists told them that many of the benchmarks did not reflect current scientific knowledge about potential health risks, most participants did not question the validity of these guidelines; some did, and a few asked whether and why the guidelines had changed over time.

In addition to calibrating their concern by the regulatory benchmarks, participants based their interpretations on comparisons between their samples and those of others. When asked if their results seemed "high," participants most often said no unless the amount reported in their home was considerably higher than reports for others. If their results fell in the middle of the range, or if a detected chemical was reported as being found in most homes, as was common, their concern dropped precipitously. Consider this exchange:

Researcher: Would you say that the results were high or concerning in any way to you?

Participant: [*flipping through results*] Well, I think that in some instances, they were high, you know . . . they're way up there. So I don't have anything to compare it to, you know, maybe they're wonderful. . . . So, I didn't get too alarmed because they look sort of middle range. And maybe if, you know, I'd come out up here [*points to higher end of the sample distribution*] or some place, and I was real nervous about that, then I probably would have read this [*pointing to the list of possible sources for each chemical*]. I mean, I'm interested, yes, but it didn't mean a thing to me unless it was something very, very bad.

When levels appeared "in the middle," participants perceived them as neither high nor as "raising red flags." When women scanned their graphs for levels that appeared abnormal, they often saw their data points clustered among others. In these instances, participants interpreted their levels as "average" or "normal." A typical response was, "I'm the common man; I'm right in the middle." For most participants, this perception of "average-ness" allayed concerns of health risk.

One participant turned the question back on the interviewer: "I'm just wondering if any of the levels are alarmingly high?" She observed that the levels of a particular chemical detected in her home were the highest of anyone in the study, much to her surprise. Like others, she looked for a threshold value, a social cue, to tell her at what level she should be "alarmed."

Though some women's homes may have had a large quantity of a particular chemical, or were one of the few homes in which a particular chemical was detected, unless the level appeared on the extreme upper end, women did not perceive the level as high and did not express concern. One woman's home, for example, was among only 2 of 120 homes in which a particular chemical was detected. Yet of those two hers was lowest. Her observation that someone else had a higher result allayed her concern.

Importantly, not all participants relied on levels to gauge whether their results warranted concern. One participant, when asked if the results seemed high, noted that her concern hinged not on the *level* of chemicals detected, but on the *number* of chemicals found and the ubiquity of exposure.

Responses: "Who Holds Jurisdiction over Chemicals in Homes and Bodies?"

Because measures of endocrine disruptors in air, dust, and urine are cumulative, the chemicals found are likely to have originated from many sources, some still unknown. As a consequence, exposure-reduction strategies for many of the compounds are also unclear or unknown. Along with their personal exposure data, participants were given specific suggestions based on the profile of compounds in their home. For example, if compounds from household pesticides were detected, Silent Spring Institute recommended that the participant consider eliminating the use of pesticides in her garden and home. Other recommendations included purchasing fragrance-free detergents and lotions and avoiding other scented products, like air fresheners. Another suggestion was to consider how to care for clothing: for example, to switch from using chemically intensive dry cleaning to wet cleaning for special garments and not to use mothballs.

While the scientists hope to investigate the effectiveness of these recommendations, they also understand they are partial and imperfect recommendations. Social scientists have documented the collective hope that we might "shop our way to safety" by, for example, selecting fragrance-free rather than scented cleaning products. Careful products choice creates the illusion of an "inverted quarantine," or self-imposed isolation from perceived toxic threats (Szasz 2007). However, because chemical additives or residues in consumer products are often unlabeled and unregulated, it can be hard to identify products to avoid. Moreover, many environmentally preferable products are more expensive and thus unavailable to some consumers. And, though there has been an explosion of new products claiming to be free of chemical compounds that have captured public or regulatory scrutiny (e.g., water bottles that do not contain BPA, or bisphenol-A), many substances are already so ubiquitous that we cannot possibly shop our way around all possible exposures to all possible chemicals of concern.

Participants sought to control or remediate exposures by changing consumption habits as recommended and by adopting alternative housekeeping strategies or technologies to manage exposures. On its website, Silent Spring Institute recommends cleaning with microfiber cloths to capture dust, removing shoes before entering the home to avoid tracking pollutants indoors, and choosing vacuum cleaners with a strong cleaning action and effective dust trapping (see www .silentspring.org/take-action/action-kits). Yet the scientists recognize that these solutions are partial, and they recognize the need to guard against the "technological fallacies" of environmental problems: the belief that chemical exposures are technical problems that can be "cleaned up" through ever more sophisticated scientific innovation, often at the expense of alternative, preventive courses of action (Edelstein 2004).

A subset of study participants learned that personal exposure-reduction strategies have limited effectiveness. For example, prior to enrollment in the HES, one woman eliminated all pesticide use in her garden and regularly consumed organically grown foods. She was surprised and disheartened to learn that pesticide residues were present in her urine despite these efforts: "It was overwhelming to know how many chemicals they found in my house, especially like I've already said, I've made really conscious efforts to eliminate so many things [pesticides]—my lawn, everything on the food that I eat. I have a water filtration system that cost me a thousand dollars to... to purify my water. I've made so many, many little things like that ... and to know that even so many years after my diagnosis, to know that I'm still being exposed. It's overwhelming."

Several participants who had their homes sampled twice recounted similar experiences. After receiving their first results, five participants reported making incremental changes. Several reduced their use of household pesticides or pur-chased fragrance-free detergents. Another removed old furniture and carpets that were suspected to be harboring chemicals of concern. These participants expected to see these changes reflected in their new results, but the results changed very little.

Other participants realized that several compounds found in their homes or urine came from compounds that were banned by the US government or had been phased out of household use, such as pesticides like DDT and chlordane and chemicals such as PCBs, which Silent Spring Institute found at trace levels in many of the homes they tested and at elevated levels in a few (Rudel et al. 2003). By interviewing participants whose homes had high PCB levels and searching an old poison-control reference that lists product ingredients, the researchers dis-covered that the likely PCB source was a wood-floor finish used in the 1950s and 1960s (see Rudel, Seryak, and Brody 2008).

Reactions to this information varied. One resident appeared concerned about her exposures and wanted to know how to reduce them. She also wanted to become involved as a volunteer with a local breast cancer organization. In the other household, in response to information that PCBs interfere with thyroid hormone functioning, one resident wondered whether the exposure might be related to her thyroid problems. She also explained that she "was old" and was not going to worry about this problem, but that she would explain it to her children so that they could decide what to do when they inherited the house. This finding highlights how banned substances persist in unrecognized exposure sources and points to the difficulty of removing such them.

Notably, participants recognized the limitations of individual responses and reported a desire to get involved in regional environmental health advocacy. Though we do not have enough data from this sample to explore this relation-ship fully, future research might investigate the ways in which self-discovery may mobilize individuals to participate in collective action. The relationship between personal exposure data and community organizing is now being explored as part of the Northern California Household Exposure Study.

Conversely, and far more commonly, we noted that participants attempt to control personal exposures by other means. Social scientists have observed that when physical mitigation strategies are not possible or fail to reduce a perceived threat, many people instead take symbolic measures to reduce threats (Vyner 1989). A variant on this theme, for some, is controlling the perception of chemi-cal risks. Some participants constructed symbolic boundaries around their social worlds, shoring up their homes and bodies against the chemicals thought to be lingering outside. These symbolic boundaries—whether physical or cognitive—separate person from pollutant, creating the perception of social distance that social scientists have found common among narratives about environmental quiescence, inaction, or normalization (see Princen, Maniates, and Conca 2002;

Norgaard 2006). For instance, one participant maintained that the pesticides sprayed outside her condominium were unrelated to the pesticides found in her home and urine samples:

> I did have some residual pesticides in my urine, and that surprised me because . . . whence might it have come? How long does it stay in your body? It's kind of a puzzle. . . . I know that there is a company that comes around maybe once or twice a year as needed to take care of insect invasion around the base of the whole building. We're on a level up. . . . So I have no pesticides here at all, never have.

Later, acknowledging that her condo association used a lawn service, she claimed, "I don't walk over the grass. . . . I walk on the walkways."

Three other participants also noted how such boundaries shielded them from potential exposures:

> Well, I don't know if I thought that you would find anything in my house. I didn't really think that. And the funny thing is, . . . maybe I wasn't a perfect student for the research. I spend half a year here and half a year in Connecticut. So, you could say I only have half a year of contaminants if you want to.

> You know, I can see why a lot of the sprays, of why they asked about how many sprays I use, which I don't use too many. Considering what you see on TV, in the ads you know, I don't begin to buy those things. . . . And, I don't use hairspray; the hairdresser does that. So, I don't use that. I'm trying to think of what other things. . . . But, there are so many you see on TV that I just don't use.

> I do have a cedar chest . . . and I keep a lot of sweaters that I don't use, and scarves, old scarves and hats and stuff, they just stay in there, and I've got some mothballs in there, but it's closed with a lamp on it, and it doesn't . . . it isn't in a room that's used. Upstairs. And mothballs are the only thing that I can think of that I do have in here, and they're probably disintegrated because I haven't put any in, in years.

Participants' Responses

Participants typically reported (and we observed) a measured, pragmatic initial response to reading their results. Most participants found their results curious or puzzling, but rarely alarming. Their responses differed from earlier case-study descriptions of encounters with uncertain chemical hazards (Edelstein 2004).

Participant: There was nothing here [in the data] that was a death sentence.

Researcher: Are you glad to have learned the results of the chemicals in your home?

Participant: Well, like I said, they weren't earth shattering.

Researcher: Right. So . . . [*probing*]

Participant: They didn't find anything, you know, bad.

There were a few notable exceptions; three participants described or displayed emotional reactions that more closely approximated responses to acute chemical disasters described by earlier social science research. For example, one participant reported her fear of "getting cancer" and living in a "polluted house."

Besides the fairly limited negative emotional responses, we observed an intriguing evolution from participants' recounting of their initial calm reaction to the flurry of questions during the interview. For many women, the research encounter unraveled their earlier conclusions and revealed a set of underlying assumptions about chemical exposures. Many realized that the study challenged their understanding of the "toxics problem." For example, one woman who initially reported that her results did not indicate cause for concern offered this comment at the close of her interview: "So, because now I'm doing this with you, this interview, maybe I think that would encourage me to look a little bit further now. Not be so complacent, with okay, gee, you did okay. So, you can write that off. . . . It's just that it seems to make sense to take it another step."

The Significance of Participants' Ecosocial History

Although we did not ask participants about their views on environmental pollution, they readily volunteered this information, typically by describing local or regional pollution sources. They reported being aware that they lived in a region with elevated rates of breast cancer, several sources of air and groundwater pollution, and a fragile ecosystem. The majority cited contamination problems on the Cape, especially at a local military base and Superfund site and two power plants (one nuclear powered), and an extensive history of pesticide application to cranberry bogs, wetlands, and golf courses. Similarly, participants recounted numerous contamination events outside the region, for example at Love Canal, NY, and in Woburn. MA, which made national headlines. Over half the participants referenced regulated or banned substances more readily than the other classes of chemicals in the study, which have only recently entered public debate (e.g., parabens, phthalates, and flame retardants). We wonder whether this finding has to do with an increased familiarity with the banned substances, which became part of popular discourse when regulatory scrutiny attracted public attention. Although many contemporary uses of household products and chemicals were *un*memorable, several participants recalled DDT stored in the garage, and another described applying chlordane around the foundation of her home.

These memorable "chemical encounters," and what participants learned about exposures from them, guided the assumptions and expectations they used to interpret study results. People invoked these experiences to interpret the levels of chemicals reported in their homes and bodies and to identify probable exposure sources and appropriate responses. When participants considered pollutant sources, they often looked outside their homes. The Cape Cod participants referred to the Massachusetts Military Reservation, where contamination of drinking water supplies resulted in regulatory action (US Environmental Protection Agency 2000). These events contributed to an assumption that toxic contamination occurs through concentrated military and industrial activities, accidents, and dumping, not the everyday use of household products. These experiences influenced the ways participants viewed the build-up of chemicals in their homes and bodies, channeling their concerns toward large-scale contamination and away from everyday, cumulative household exposures.

Finally, participants recounted instances where the government did act to ban substances and remove them from consumer products (e.g., tris flame retardants in children's sleepwear). It remains unclear whether and how these notable instances of regulatory action led participants to assume stronger regulatory oversight of household products despite the lack of historical precedents. However, prior toxic encounters led study participants to reexamine previously held assumptions about when and how humans are exposed to chemicals and what courses of action are most likely to reduce exposure.

SHIFTING PUBLIC AWARENESS

For study participants, pollution came home and got personal when they learned that toxic chemicals were found in unexpected places and from unanticipated sources, often from products that they brought into their homes and used on their bodies. By interviewing women as they processed new information about personal exposures, we observed how science challenges their existing environmental health knowledge and how prior knowledge shaped the participants' understanding of new personal exposure information.

First, participants perceived that harm or risk was proportional to the relative levels of chemicals detected in their home. They judged the levels by comparing their own results with those of others in the study and interpreted typical household levels as small in comparison with their perception of harmful contamination. Second, participants evaluated harm or risk based on sensibilities about the source of chemical pollutants. They assumed risks were linked to industrial, governmental, or military uses; to former household uses (e.g., pesticides sprayed around the foundation of a home, or asbestos tiling throughout a home); or to chemicals that are immediately perceptible (e.g., fumes). Finally, many participants felt they could control what chemicals entered their homes and bodies, although the study undermined this assumption for several women.

Though social scientists have documented that rapid innovations in environmental health and exposure science contribute to our expanding understanding of where and how humans interact with pollutants (Frickel 2004; Shostak 2005), fewer than a dozen scholars have documented how personal exposure research, including measurements of human body burden, affects people's understandings of synthetic chemicals and environmental problems (e.g., Casper 2003; Shostak 2004; Boswell-Penc 2006; MacKendrick 2007; Washburn 2007a, 2007b; Altman et al. 2008; Casper and Moore 2009; Emmet et al. 2009; Scott 2009; Wu et al. 2009). Participants' responses about their exposure experience underscore that a new category of science-mediated chemical encounters needs sociological attention.

Our research suggests that individuals' experiences have undergone a marked shift in recent years. Social scientists during the 1970s through 1990s noted the lack of shared or popular knowledge that could help inform and explain human encounters with toxic chemicals (Erikson 1994; Edelstein 2004). By contrast, participants' experiences in this study suggest that their shared understanding of chemical contamination resulted from a regional ecosocial experience and media coverage of "environmental crises" over the past two decades. The prevailing assumption among participants was that chemical pollutants are harmful when they exist in large quantities and when they are released into the environment by industrial or military accidents, large-scale use, or dumping. In contrast, personal exposure science illuminates far less dramatic and perhaps more insidious pathways for toxic contamination. One result was Cape residents' somewhat muted responses to their personal data, similar to results reported by Beamish (2002). We also found that older assumptions about the public-health significance of synthetic chemicals influenced participants' assumptions about exposures to everyday chemicals and their consequences (Beamish 2002; Frickel and Vincent 2007). Access to personal exposure information made those assumptions visible.

Integrating environmental health science into the study of individuals' embodied experience of health and the environment recognizes a broader trend in which science increasingly discovers and defines problems and thus mediates the experience of health and the body. This is an area ripe for more synthesis and theoretical development (Williams, Birke, and Bendelow 2003). Medical sociologists already recognize the importance of science and technology for embodied experience, with a particular focus on medical technologies that diagnose preclinical disease or disease risk (Timmermans and Berg 2003; Cox and McKellin 1999). These studies point to the ways that science and technology can medicalize and disembody illness experience, and, in the latter case, catalyze a new sense of embodiment or illness.

Reliance on prior experience by participants to interpret study findings is likely to persist in other settings. However, the specific social cues and references available to study participants will vary. Thus some of our findings about social cues that were significant to interpretation of exposure results may be more typical of women than men and may in fact be limited to this specific demographic group of predominantly older, white, middle-class women. Our research underscores the significance of participants' shared experience of living in a region viewed as a "contaminated place" and having a high incidence of breast cancer. Similarly, participants shared a generational or cohort effect. They were witnesses to the advent of environmental health disasters as media events (see Szasz 1994): for example, they recalled events at Love Canal and Woburn and the banning of DDT and other commonly used toxic substances. Omohundro (2004) calls for a research program on collective risk perception that accounts for the role of shared history and community identity, which she surmises play an important, though poorly understood, role in how environmental risks are understood and whether and how communities mount a response.

Certainly other contextual factors matter as well and must be considered along-side the findings presented here. For example, previous breast cancer experience is a contextual element in this study that would not be relevant in other populations, though we observed relatively little mention of breast cancer in connection with participants' interpretations of their exposure reports. Perhaps women in this study also demonstrate a cohort effect based on a shared set of housekeeping norms regarding cleanliness and the appropriate product for each household task. Studies like the Household Exposure Study reveal the potentially toxic consequences of these norms by implicating products used to produce or maintain hygienic homes, lush lawns, gleaming tile, plastic-wrapped leftovers, and vinyl-covered furniture.

Participant responses in this study may also have been influenced by the community-based participatory methods that were integral to the Household Exposure Study. The project works with a public advisory council, employs a Cape Cod outreach coordinator, and holds frequent meetings to keep study participants and community residents informed about the research design, progress, and results. These longstanding community relationships may contribute to the moderate emotional responses we observed: earlier research that shows that the method in which a risk message is delivered can be more important than its content (Furgal et al. 2003). If reporting occurs in partnership with affected populations, and communication lines remain open after the initial exchange, fears may be mitigated. Our observations square with a classic sociological finding that harm can follow as much from institutional responses to chemical pollution as from the physical insult (Freudenburg 1993; Erikson 1994). Thus it is important to bear in mind both the context of this study population and the reporting-back methods used when generalizing from our findings.

IMPLICATIONS FOR SCIENCE POLICY

The National Research Council (NRC) has called for more research on how participants in surveillance programs and personal exposure studies respond to results and the "mental models" that inform participants' interpretation of uncertain exposure data (Rudel et al. 2003; National Academy of Sciences 2006). This need has been reinforced by California's 2006 passage of the country's first statewide biomonitoring program, which requires participants to have full access to their individual results, followed by the introduction of similar legislation in other states such as Indiana, Washington, Minnesota, and New York. Our work responds to—and extends beyond—the NRC's call.

Our interviews indicate that study participants wanted their results. Their desire for this information parallels the increase of patient requests for medical information and participation in medical decision making (Charles and DeMaio 1993; Bury 2004). When participants received exposure information, they did not react with the alarm observed after acute environmental disasters. This response counters the position of some scientists and public health officials, who seek to avoid or limit communication of uncertain personal exposure information to protect participants from adverse emotional responses. We also found that participants wanted more rather than less information, including technical explanations about risks that were either unknown or remained uncertain.

Our observation that participants reconsidered their interpretation of study results during the interviews suggests that some would benefit from a report-back procedure that incorporates discussion. Furthermore, just as they compared their results with those of others, many women asked the interviewer about the responses of other study participants. With their questions, they sought to validate how their own responses and to learn about alternative courses of action. We hope that researchers, in collaboration with institutional review boards, will develop options for study participants to compare experiences while also respecting confidentiality.

Our results also suggest that scientists should attempt to contextualize study results and scientific uncertainty within the framework of participants' starting assumptions about toxic chemicals. Much of the debate about whether and how to report personal exposure information has focused on placing research findings in their proper "scientific" context by explaining the toxicological and epidemiological uncertainties. However, our research suggests that report-back protocols should also take account of the unique social and historical setting. One approach is to include the perspectives of peer-group or community members who understand how participants' historical experiences with environmental problems might filter their interpretation of new exposure data. In addition, involving community members could reveal how perspectives and experiences of the same environmental problems might differ within the community or study population, a possibility raised by Auyero and Swistun (2007) and Blum (2008).

By supporting community participation in reporting, our findings parallel those of the Canadian Northern Contaminants Program (Furgal et al. 2003), where risk communication occurs in the context of long-term relationships between scientists and communities, shared decision making, dense communication networks of scientists and community representatives, and reporting that is targeted to specific communities and subgroups based on their ecosocial histories (see also Usher et al. 1995). As we show below, our household monitoring in Northern California offers a very different demographic makeup, a different local context, and a more advocacy-oriented approach.

EXPLORING COLLECTIVE
ENVIRONMENTAL KNOWLEDGE

In this chapter, we report on the assumptions shared by participants in our exposure study. In the future, we hope to explore the mechanisms by which these shared assumptions are transmitted. Ethnographies by Auyero and Swistun (2007) and Blum (2008) on the contrasting experiences of residents within contaminated communities in Argentina and at Love Canal, New York, raise the questions of where and under what conditions shared ecosocial histories emerge. We also hope to elucidate the meso-level factors[8] that channel, transmit, or filter participants' regionally specific ecosocial histories. The results reported in this chapter reflect participants' experiences during a significant transition in public awareness of and legislative responses to toxic exposures. Over the last five years, local, state and federal policies have been enacted to address the hazards posed by toxic chemicals in consumer products (see Shapiro 2007; Altman et al. 2008). Awareness of their presence has also been reflected by an increase in "green consumption" (see Szasz 2007), as products and services marketed as less harmful (e.g., phthalate-free lotions, BPA-free bottles, and PERC-free dry-cleaning methods) flood the marketplace.

Silent Spring Institute's Household Exposure Study was carried out, however, before several "focusing events" (Speth 2004) trained the attention of the public, media and policymakers on the presence of hazardous chemicals in consumer products. The mass government recall of children's toys in 2007 and 2008 because of the possibility of lead exposure, as well as media, scientific, and regulatory scrutiny of the presence of endocrine-disrupting compounds, specifically phthalates and BPA in baby products, are two examples. They sparked Congressional action on the oversight of consumer products, particularly children's products. We speculate that these issues will influence how participants respond to biomonitoring and household exposure results in future studies.

The multitude of pollution sources and community factors (such as social class, level of education, and ethnic composition), also shape responses to exposure. To advance our understanding of these issues and refine our reporting methods, we repeated both the exposure study and the report-back approach with our partner organization, Communities for a Better Environment, in the Northern California

Household Exposure Study (Zota et al. 2008; Brody et al. 2009). The community of Richmond has a different experience of exposures to chemicals because it borders facilities associated with refining and port-related goods movement. As we anticipated, this community, with a history of contamination from numerous sources, compounded by government inaction, was less surprised by contamination in homes. CBE had been organizing for years to stem contamination from the huge Chevron refinery adjacent to the neighborhoods in our study, and the study was a strategic component of its activities. In addition to reporting exposure results to individuals, we hosted annual community meetings in which participants and other residents engaged with the data in order to compel the Richmond city government to regulate the refinery more effectively. In Bolinas, a rural community that we included in the study for comparison purposes, many participants had a history of environmental awareness and worked hard to keep toxic personal and household products out of their homes. They were surprised to learn that their homes, too, had significant chemical burdens and further surprised that homes in Richmond and Bolinas had similar levels of indoor pollutants from household products.

Just as responses in Richmond, Bolinas, and Cape Cod differed, we anticipate that public responses to personal exposure information will vary depending on the historical experience of the population and the social and temporal context for report-back. Our findings suggest that reporting strategies must be tailored to each community, because a community's ecosocial history shapes the range of social cues and scripts available for participants to reference, understand, and assign meaning to their personal exposure results. It is imperative for researchers, in partnership with communities and affected populations, to learn about the new, embodied awareness and experience of exposure in order to communicate personal exposure information effectively and to anticipate participants' responses. Through our efforts we hope to contribute to the advancement of environmental public health science while also participating in the development of the medical sociology literature on embodied health experiences where it articulates with science and the environment.

NOTES

Originally published as Rebecca Gasior Altman, Rachel Morello-Frosch, Julia Green Brody, Ruthann Rudel, Phil Brown, and Mara Averick, "Pollution Comes Home and Gets Personal: Women's Experience of Household Chemical Exposure," *Journal of Health and Social Behavior* 49 (2008): 417–35. Reprinted with permission of the American Sociological Association.

   1. We define environmental chemicals as materials extracted or synthesized in the industrial production of "goods and services that support consumer economies" (Geiser 2001, 15), including agricultural production and military applications.

   2. See the list of chemicals measured in the 2003–4 National Health and Nutrition Examination Survey (CDC 2005).

3. Another notable exception is the doctoral research conducted by the sociologist Rachel Washburn (2007a, 2007b).

4. These chemicals were selected because they are produced in large volume, found in common household materials and products, and suspected or known to disrupt hormones (Rudel et al. 2003).

5. EPA health-based guidelines were available for only thirty-nine of the sixty-seven detected target compounds. Many were outdated, and none took account of the potential for hormonal effects, which was the reason for inclusion in the study.

6. Two interviews involved pairs (one couple, one mother and daughter). In each of these cases, one person was the primary interviewee, and the other interspersed comments; the final count of individuals interviewed does not reflect the two additional individuals.

7. Interviews were more conversational and dynamic than traditional semistructured interviews. Silent Spring Institute researchers trained the interviewer in the interpretation of the data graphs. Several interviews required the interviewer to explain how to read the graphs and to discuss information about household exposures.

8. We thank Sara Shostak for suggesting this new direction.

9
———

The Personal Is Scientific,
the Scientific Is Political

The Public Paradigm of the Environmental
Breast Cancer Movement

Sabrina McCormick, Phil Brown, Stephen Zavestoski, and Alissa Cordner

Since the early 1990s, the environmental breast cancer movement has advanced a new public paradigm for causes of the disease. We describe here the framework, history, and strategies of the national environmental breast cancer movement (EBCM), or what one leading activist terms the "political breast cancer movement" (Brenner 2000).[1] Although now national in scope, the EBCM has its roots in three regions: Long Island, New York; the Boston and Cape Cod areas in Massachusetts; and the San Francisco Bay Area in California. Our case studies demonstrate the importance of understanding the fluidity of social movement actors and the concept of boundary movements introduced in chapter 2. They also provide a narrative of social movement formation in which a critique of traditional science emerges from the embodied perspectives of illness sufferers. Therefore, this social movement case study offers a new conceptual framework for social movement theory and illustrates empirical cases in which social movements have changed scientific processes and agendas as well as policy outcomes.

Breast cancer appeared on the public agenda in the 1970s and 1980s on the second wave of feminism. The disease slowly moved from being viewed as a private experience that could be overcome with a positive attitude and a supportive family to an illness that was politically charged, especially in terms of options and access to treatment. As women gained greater control over treatment options, a breast cancer advocacy movement emerged, focused on increasing research funding and finding a cure for the disease. Although these early activists criticized the medical control of their bodies, they did not challenge the biomedical model that focused on improving treatment and on individual strategies for breast cancer prevention (such as diet and physical activities) while overlooking root causes of the disease.

As the breast cancer movement was becoming more powerful, the mainstream environmental movement was starting to push regulators and decision makers to address the health effects of toxics. This effort opened the way for what is now known as the environmental breast cancer movement, which emphasized environmental links to breast cancer and challenged the mainstream biomedical approach to disease prevention. Its strategy epitomizes what we describe in chapter 2 as a new "public paradigm" that combines scientific and public engagement. Unlike typical scientific paradigm shifting, in which debate is limited to scientific conferences, journals, and consensus conferences, debates over the public paradigm of disease etiology and prevention occur in public. EBCM activists emphasize the precautionary principle, which places the burden of proof regarding the health effects of chemicals on industrial producers rather than consumers and declares that proof of safety should exist before chemicals are used (Raffensperger and Tickner 1999). The public paradigm for environmental factors in breast cancer also takes a strong political-economy perspective, blaming corporate chemical producers for their harmful products and environmental contamination.

Within this new paradigm, the environmental breast cancer movement works toward four goals: to broaden public awareness of environmental causes of breast cancer; to increase research into environmental causes of breast cancer; to create policy that could prevent environmental causes of breast cancer; and to increase activist participation in research. As noted in chapter 2, the EBCM crosses the boundaries between movement and nonmovement actors and between laypeople and professionals. The EBCM engages in this boundary work (Gieryn 1983) in four ways common to boundary movements. First, it pushes science in new directions and encourages public participation in scientific research and application. Citizen-science alliances play a central role here. Second, it mobilizes a range of actors who are not inherently social movement activists or organizations (e.g., foundations and government officials). A number of Long Island EBCM activists, for example, have worked closely with mainstream politicians to advance their agenda. Third, it crosses multiple social movements, as when Bay Area EBCM activists linked up with AIDS, women's health, and antitoxics activists. Similarly, Boston area activists found allies among those involved in precautionary-principle organizing. Fourth, it employs "boundary objects" as political symbols for constituency building and public education (Star and Greisemer 1989). These human and nonhuman objects are used by actors in multiple contexts and disciplines. Examples include mammography machines, genetic tests for breast cancer, patents on the BRCA-1 genetic sequence, pharmaceuticals, Breast Cancer Awareness Month, and Avon's Breast Cancer Walk.

We begin by offering an overview of the general breast cancer movement and identify several developments in science and public awareness that contributed to the rise of the environmental breast cancer movement in the early 1990s. The participation of movement organizations and actors in citizen-science alliances is a key example of boundary crossing.

EMERGENCE OF THE ENVIRONMENTAL BREAST CANCER MOVEMENT

In the past twenty years, the breast cancer movement has radically changed the popular perception of breast cancer from an individual disease, to be dealt with privately, to a politicized collective-illness experience. The mainstream breast cancer movement has addressed issues of breast cancer patient care, knowledge of and access to treatment options, social and political support for those affected by the disease, and research funding. National organizations like the National Breast Cancer Coalition (NBCC) and Komen for the Cure coordinate state and local activities, sponsor fund-raising and educational events, and work with the private sector to raise money. The private sector is involved in activities such as National Breast Cancer Awareness Month, an event that began in 1984 as a week to promote public awareness of breast cancer and mammography. Associated events now involve tens of thousands of people each year (see www.nbcam.org). The general movement's other successes include the production of a breast-cancer stamp, whose additional cost above normal postage is given to government research institutions, and the Shop for the Cure campaign, through which participating merchants and credit-card companies give a portion of their proceeds to breast cancer foundations.

Through the efforts of the general breast cancer movement, breast cancer research funding increased from $90 million in 1990 to more than $600 million in 1999 (Reiss and Martin 2000). Between 1992 and 2008, more than five thousand grants were awarded under the Department of Defense Breast Cancer Research Program, which funded $127.5 million in research in 2007 alone (CDMRP 2010).[2] The movement has also had great success in enacting federal legislation in support of prevention and treatment, such as the Breast and Cervical Cancer Mortality Prevention Act of 1990, the Breast and Cervical Cancer Treatment Act of 2000, and the Breast Cancer Patient Protection Act of 2003.

Despite these efforts, however, the causes and treatment of breast cancer are still subjects of debate. The dominant epidemiological paradigm for breast cancer is largely biomedical and focuses on individual factors like diet, exercise, age at first childbirth, age at menarche, and genetics (Thompson 1992; Kant et al. 2000). However, studies have also shown that such individual factors account for only a limited number of cases. The discovery of the BRCA-1 gene mutation led to a scientific focus on genetic causes, even though it has since been recognized that genetics accounts for only 5 to 10 percent of all breast cancers (Davis and Bradlow 1995). Activists also point out that the genome does not mutate rapidly enough to account for the recent rapid increase in breast cancer incidence.

These study results, coupled with mounting evidence suggesting environmental links to breast cancer, have led to divisions between mainstream breast cancer activists and the EBCM, which began in the early 1990s. The mainstream breast cancer movement generally accepts the dominant epidemiological paradigm. By contrast, even before the emergence of suggestive scientific evidence, environmental breast cancer movement activists linked the steady increase in breast cancer rates over the past fifty years (from 1 in 20 in 1964 to 1 in 8 in 2006 for women who live to age 80 [Evans 2006]) to the proliferation of chemicals in our environment. For example, EBCM questioning of the dominant epidemiological paradigm draws on emerging scientific evidence of the effect of endocrine disruptors on ecological and human health (Krimsky 1999). Endocrine-disrupting compounds can lead to adverse hormonal, reproductive, and neurological outcomes. Because this effect has been observed even at very low doses, these data challenge the traditional dose-response model widely used in the field of toxicology. Exposure to these endocrine-disrupting compounds affects hormonal and reproductive health and thus has a direct effect on breast cancer risk.

A growing body of scientific literature has elucidated potential environmental causes of breast cancer (Hunter and Kelsey 1993). Early studies supported an environmental-causation hypothesis; for example, Wolff and colleagues' 1993 study correlated the presence of DDE, a breakdown product of the widely used pesticide DDT, with increased risk of breast cancer. Later studies (Wolff et al. 1993; Hunter et al. 1997) showed equivocal results. More recent research indicates that when women are exposed to DDT before adolescence, their lifetime risk of breast cancer increases fivefold (Cohn et al. 2007). Research has assessed exposures over the life course using different types of evidence, such as studies of twins (Lichtenstein et al. 2000) and specific groupings or breakdowns of chemicals (Güttes et al. 1998; Dorgan et al. 1999; Høyer et al. 2000).

Although the EBCM has built on the successes of the broader breast cancer movement to focus on potential environmental causes and change how breast cancer is researched and publicly perceived (McCormick 2009), it has also criticized some of those successes. For example, for years discourse on breast cancer followed the position of the American Cancer Society, National Cancer Institute, and other parts of what the EBCM terms the "cancer establishment" that mammography is the most effective method of disease prevention. However, environmental breast cancer activists argue that once a tumor is detected through mammography, prevention has failed, since the tumor is likely to have existed in the body for several years. This stance is supported by growing scientific consensus that mammography is not very effective in reducing the risk of breast cancer mortality among women under 50 (Kopans 1991; Destounis et al. 2004; US Preventive Services Task Force 2009). EBCM activists also challenge the corporate control of public campaigns like Breast Cancer Awareness Month and have mounted a campaign to have revenues from breast cancer stamps shifted from the National Cancer Institute, which does not emphasize research on environmental factors, to the National Institute of Environmental Health Sciences, which does.

The activism that grew into the EBCM first began in Long Island, developed soon after in Massachusetts, and subsequently emerged in the San Francisco Bay Area. All these areas have higher rates of breast cancer than the rest of the United States, and public attention has led to numerous studies in these areas (Aschengrau et al. 1996; Robbins, Brescianini, and Kelsey 1997; West, Glaser, and Prehn 1998). In each of these locations, the development of the movement, research, and policy was influenced by media attention, the political climate and political connections, preexisting social movements, the response of local government institutions, and potential funding sources. A general movement framework unites the three locales into a national environmental breast cancer movement.

Exploring the EBCM provides insight into how multiple social movements and a wide variety of actors coalesce to form a new movement. Our research into this movement was central to the development of the field-analysis method presented in chapter 4. Analyzing the full field of movement actors and organizations allowed us to examine a movement and its effects in greater depth, making connections across diverse geographic, disciplinary, and organizational locations. Because of our engagement in citizen-science alliances, the EBCM example also provides a strong basis for understanding policy ethnography.

FIELD ANALYSIS IN ACTION

Chapter 4 describes our methodological approach of field analysis, using the EBCM as one of the classic examples. Here we delve more deeply into that example. We conducted twenty-nine semistructured interviews with EBCM activists and scientists. We selected people whose involvement and activism spanned the late 1980s to early 1990s, when the movement was forming. This sample provided both a local and a national picture of the movement.

We also conducted eleven ethnographic observations to supplement the interviews, primarily at Silent Spring Institute in Newton, MA. These included public meetings where the researchers presented their work and their participation in scientific review panel meetings, and conferences involving both scientists and activists. Although the interviews were the primary source of analysis, the observations provided a broader contextual picture. For instance, we observed how Silent Spring Institute brought its scientific work to lay activist audiences and how its representatives responded to critics at a scientific review panel. We also collected and analyzed printed materials from each organization to better understand their political stances and public activities.

We found that successful movement actors founded citizen-science alliances, which took different forms in each locale. State actors and the media have also influenced the outcomes of activism, and in some ways they can be considered movement actors in their own right. Through these channels, activists have inserted their perspectives into scientific systems. This detailed account allows us to see the fluidity of these actors in each "site of congruence" (Clarke 2001).

Long Island, New York

In the early 1990s, a few women in western Long Island noticed that they were surrounded by cases of breast cancer. They began to map breast cancer cases in their communities in a practice we term *lay mapping,* a form of popular epidemiology in which community members track disease cases by location to assess potential clusters or causes. One in Nine, a local breast cancer activist group, found that women with breast cancer were clustered in specific areas. At the same time, the Huntington Breast Cancer Coalition, another Long Island breast cancer organization, was mapping its own area and finding that case rates were higher than average. Once activists realized that rates in the area were elevated, they began to hypothesize about possible environmental causes. Groups interested in environmental causes of breast cancer, such as the Huntington, West Islip, and Southampton Breast Cancer Coalitions, among others, formed the Long Island Breast Cancer Network to span their multiple localities and promote public awareness about their concerns. Today Long Island is characterized by its widely dispersed network of organizations, a range of research projects, and multiple, small-scale use of geographic information systems (Burg and Gist 1998).

The hypothesis that more women on Long Island were getting breast cancer than women in other places was investigated by scientists at SUNY Stony Brook University's Medical Center, Department of Preventive Medicine. In 1993, they marshaled backing from other well-known breast cancer scientists and held a conference at which representatives from the Centers for Disease Control, Environmental Protection Agency, and National Cancer Institute were present. This alliance enabled the passage of the bill that planned and funded the Long Island Breast Cancer Study Project through the National Cancer Institute. The bill provided $32 million in federal funding for the study of potential environmental causes of breast cancer.

The Long Island organizations work on several fronts. Each group has mapped breast cancer cases and provides support services to women with breast cancer. The groups are funded by diverse local sources, and each organization has its own activist strategy. One umbrella organization, the Long Island Breast Cancer Network, unites and coordinates the groups' efforts, although it does not make statements or speak on behalf of participating organizations. Outside this forum, projects between organizations overlap only sporadically, because their areas of coverage and agendas differ.

Long Island activists were noteworthy in their ability to forge strong connections with Republican politicians on an environmental issue, typically Democratic territory. Bipartisan support for breast cancer activism probably facilitated this alliance. According to involved scientists and activists, these political connections and other activism efforts were largely responsible for a government public hearing on breast cancer held on Long Island.

EBCM organizations' relationships with local and state government on Long Island have been much more mutually supportive than in other locales. This difference may be due to the long duration of the involvement, which has allowed the development of personal relationships with influential representatives and of a broader base of voter support; it may also be due to local awareness of the federal funding supporting the Long Island study. The Southampton Breast Cancer Coalition has members who serve on research advisory boards and the New York State Department of Health's Research Science Advisory Board, which allocates funds generated by the breast cancer research check-off box on New York State tax forms. The group has gained financial and logistical support from local government, including funding for a GIS technician to conduct work on environmental hazards and breast cancer and an office in the town hall. Its fund-raising events have become so well known that they attract prominent officials, like the mayor of New York City. The media has also paid Long Island activists a good deal of positive attention. Many of them have appeared on TV shows such as *Oprah, Eye to Eye,* and *Primetime Live,* and group events are routinely covered in print and broadcast media.

Long Island breast cancer groups were not formally linked to environmental groups for some time, perhaps because of their Republican connections. Over time, however, they have engaged more in environmental advocacy and gained the support of environmental groups. For example, the West Islip group has fought against pesticide use on golf courses and recently gained approval for the first local ban on bisphenol-A. The Huntington Breast Cancer Action Coalition (recently renamed Prevention Is the Cure), which initiated one of the largest GIS studies on Long Island, focuses primarily on environmental causation of breast cancer. It promotes organic horticulture and urges residents to display pink flags in yards cultivated without chemicals.

Two research projects stand out for their great involvement of and effect on the Long Island community. The first is the Long Island Breast Cancer Study Project (LIBCSP), which comprises ten projects, including studies investigating potential effects of overhead power lines and looking for chemical contaminants in tissue samples. Activists from all over Long Island have sat on its project advisory boards. The second project uses GIS to map breast cancer cases and environmental factors in local areas, incorporating new technologies that improve on the original lay mapping. These research projects are noticeable examples of boundary crossing, spanning scientific disciplines and blurring boundaries between citizen and scientist roles and local versus expert knowledge.

The first results of the LIBCSP were released in the summer of 2002 and garnered wide press coverage (Winn 2005). The study found little support for a hypothesis that the chemicals under study were associated with increased breast cancer risk, but the researchers asserted that their null results were far from conclusive and called for further research. The press, however, pointed to this outcome as proof that collaborations between activists and scientists are unproductive for or even detrimental to advancing the scientific understanding of breast cancer causation (Kolata 2002; New York Times 2002). Activists and scientists both felt that this media perspective was unfair and might discourage funders from pursuing similar projects. Despite this controversy, further federal grants have been awarded to investigate environmental links to breast cancer through the Breast Cancer and Environment Research Centers funded by the National Cancer Institute and the National Institute of Environmental Health Sciences.

After the LIBCSP study was released and the controversy died down, local groups pursued independent agendas with varying degrees of scientific emphasis. The founder of One in Nine started a new group called Breast Cancer Help, focusing more on support and services. Prevention Is the Cure initiated a new agenda that included other illnesses linked to environmental exposures. The Great Neck Breast Cancer Coalition continued to collaborate with scientists by creating a new summer program for high school students to intern with breast cancer researchers.

The controversial public interpretation of the LIBCSP results and continued government and public interest in such projects demonstrate three important points. First, boundary-crossing activities are significant for both the public and science. Indeed, despite the early equivocal and controversial study results from the LIBCSP, community engagement in the project helped reshape scientific thinking about breast cancer etiology and catalyzed work in this emerging field. Similarly, activists and the broader public learned crucial lessons about the challenges and limitations of studying environmental links to breast cancer. Second, boundary crossing, in this case between scientists and community advocates, can make a social movement vulnerable to challenges and criticism from institutional actors such as the media. Third, boundary crossing in citizen-science alliances can break down the traditional roles of laypeople and scientists and hence has ramifications for public struggles over how to direct future knowledge-production efforts. Finally, scientific collaboration with activists can influence coalition building and the trajectory of movement strategies over time.

Massachusetts

Massachusetts EBCM activists gained state recognition in 1994, shortly after their fellow Long Island activists. Cape Cod has a rate of breast cancer 15 percent higher than the state average (Silent Spring Institute 2009). After several years of activism to raise awareness of this higher incidence, the Massachusetts Breast Cancer Coalition (MBCC) founded Silent Spring Institute in 1994 to study and educate the public about environmental causes of breast cancer, using a citizen-science alliance approach. Activists also achieved the passage of a bill in the Massachusetts legislature to provide $3.6 million for a three-year study to investigate why nine of fifteen towns on Cape Cod had elevated levels of breast cancer.

The first phase of the Silent Spring study was completed in 1997, with three important results: development of a GIS system that enables researchers to map cases of breast cancer against environmental data; a historical study of pesticide use and drinking-water quality on the Cape; and establishment of new field methods to study environmental estrogens (Silent Spring Institute 2007). Phase 2 of the project involved interviewing 2,100 Cape women to identify both individual- and community-level environmental risk factors, with the goal of collecting case-level data to supplement the findings of phase 1. Researchers examined home and wide-area application of pesticides to control mosquitoes, gypsy moths, and other agricultural pests. They also examined the prevalence of established breast cancer risk factors such as family history of breast cancer, reproductive history, and the use of pharmaceutical hormones. They measured dozens of endocrine-disrupting chemicals and mammary carcinogens in households, many of them for the first time (Rudel et al. 2001; Rudel et al. 2007) and estimated environmental exposure for each woman in the study, using GIS data (Brody et al. 2003; Silent Spring Institute 2007). Silent Spring's scientific work has shown how workplace and household chemical exposures from food contaminants, personal care products, cleaning products, and air pollutants may increase breast cancer risk (Brody et al. 2007b).

The Massachusetts Breast Cancer Coalition emerged out of the National Breast Cancer Coalition (NBCC), a nationwide organization that encompasses more than five hundred organizations and focuses on three main areas: research on breast cancer, access to medical resources for all women, and increasing the influence of women with breast cancer on policy decisions that affect them. It has strong political influence and exercises it in the legislative arena. The NBCC also holds national conferences attended by breast cancer activists of all kinds. The Massachusetts group has a stronger focus than the national group on environmental causation of breast cancer, the role of industrial pollutants, and the undue influence of industry in federal chemicals policy and regulation. Activists have at times mentioned this difference as a point of contention. While the MBCC wants to push a more radical and politicized agenda, the NBCC must attend to the interests and needs of a more politically diverse constituency. The Massachusetts affiliate has urged the national organization to take up environmental causation, with some success; for example, the third item on the NBCC's list of legislative priorities for 2009 was the enactment of the Breast Cancer and Environmental Research

Act. The NBCC noted in its 2008 annual report that "it is generally believed that the environment plays a role in the development of breast cancer, but the extent of that role is not understood" (NBCC 2008). This shift in focus is due at least in part to the MBCC's efforts to advance scientific study at Silent Spring and to educate the public about environmental causation at breast cancer activist events, such as the Race for the Cure in Boston.

The other main EBCM group in Massachusetts is the Women's Community Cancer Project, which takes a feminist view of all cancers. It has engaged in public protest and education, including the creation of a large-scale mural in Harvard Square. The more radical nature of its activism includes a critique of the so-called cancer industry, which reveals the corporate links between chemical manufacturers and the pharmaceutical industry, and action opposing direct-to-consumer marketing of cancer drugs.

As on Long Island, Massachusetts-area breast cancer groups take different stances toward the role of research in activism, according to their respective agendas. The Massachusetts Breast Cancer Coalition, for example, created Silent Spring Institute as a research arm of the movement. The Women's Community Cancer Project, on the other hand, is not involved in research. What both groups and Silent Spring Institute share is an orientation toward the precautionary principle and agreement that although other factors were important in supporting their work, engagement in research is a driving force behind many of the movements' successes.

These groups have engaged in boundary-crossing activities through their involvement in environmental activism, both collaboratively and independently. The MBCC has been and continues to be a key partner in the Alliance for a Healthy Tomorrow, a statewide environmental coalition. The MBCC has participated in forums for college, community, environmental, and health groups to educate laypeople, government representatives and their staff, and scientists about the precautionary principle and its applicability to diseases other than breast cancer. In this effort it has collaborated with Clean Water Action and the Center for Sustainable Production at the University of Massachusetts, Lowell, where the Precautionary Principle Project is housed. This project aims to advance understanding of the precautionary principle and to investigate ways in which the principle supports sound science as well as social and economic well-being. MBCC has participated in a number of campaigns aimed at incorporating the precautionary principle into state and local policy, including a 2001 bill in the state legislature on child-health legislation and local and statewide action to prevent pesticide spraying.

Although the creation of the Silent Spring Institute broke new ground in acquiring state government funding to support research, most interviewees attested to the lack of consistent support for their research agenda from state regulatory and public agencies. Although funding mechanisms were established by legislation, the Department of Public Health has controlled that money and challenged Silent Spring's research efforts since its inception. Silent Spring has been able to maintain funding by proving the validity of its research mission, but as a result, it has had strained relations with state government. In 2002, funding was cut when the state government incurred a massive budget deficit. Since then, Silent Spring has relied more on individual donations, grants from the National Institutes of Health, and private foundation support.

Building on its research findings from Cape Cod, Silent Spring Institute has made important contributions to various new areas of study. A major part of the Contested Illnesses Research Group's engagement with Silent Spring has been on new forms of methods of reporting biomonitoring and household exposure data to study participants. Chapter 8 describes women's experiences with the Cape Cod reporting, and chapter 13 discusses the broader framework for the right to know and reporting in other biomonitoring exposure and health studies. Silent Spring also published an important meta-analysis of mammary carcinogens in animals that was published in the journal *Cancer* (Brody et al. 2007b). Its innovations in gathering epidemiological data have led to a much broader understanding of chemical exposures that may be linked to increased breast cancer risk.

San Francisco Bay Area

Breast cancer activism in the San Francisco Bay Area began in the early 1990s. Its achievements include the inclusion of laypeople on state cancer research review committees in 1992. These initial efforts by activists to shape the breast cancer research agenda in California were enhanced when the Northern California Cancer Center, an independent research institution funded by various sources such as the National Cancer Institute, published statistics showing that the Bay Area had the highest rates of breast cancer in the world. Local breast cancer groups responded strongly to the publication and dissemination of these data, and activists began to focus on environmental links to the disease.

The major breast cancer activist groups located in San Francisco—Breast Cancer Action and the Breast Cancer Fund—have a national rather than local focus. The Breast Cancer Fund supports efforts to change detection, treatment, and prevention policies to recognize and focus on environmental causes. Breast Cancer Action focuses on education as well as regulatory and policy reform; its tactics include direct action, such as demonstrations, and coalition work with other political organizations, and campaigns to oppose pharmaceutical companies' direct-to consumer marketing of cancer drugs.

Groups with a more local focus have different emphases and objectives. EBCM activism in the Bay Area has been enriched by the perspectives of low-income, communities of color in the Bayview–Hunters Point neighborhood in San Francisco, which has a group of environmental justice activists affiliated with the Southeast Alliance for Environmental Justice. This organization mobilized as a result of an early study from the San Francisco Department of Public Health indicating abnormally high rates of breast cancer among African American women. These activists have loudly criticized the lack of racial-identity recognition in epidemiological research and institutional failings of risk assessment in the regulation of major pollution sources in their neighborhood (Fishman 2000). The involvement of environmental justice activists with groups like Breast Cancer Action has contributed to a multiracial perspective in San Francisco breast cancer activism overall.

Marin County Breast Cancer Watch (now Zero Breast Cancer), based just north of San Francisco, was one of the first Bay Area EBCM organizations and includes a strong citizen-science component. The organization originally received funding to conduct a study of adolescent risk factors for breast cancer and hired several researchers part-time in order to do so. Recently, it secured state funding to begin a study focused on potential environmental causes. Scientists and activists share an office, and scientists at nearby universities also work with the group.

These organizations were preceded by other cancer activist groups, such as the Women's Cancer Resource Center in the East Bay, founded in 1986. It was precedent-setting in providing services to women with cancer, such as educational workshops, a resource library, support groups, and a hotline. Its mission is to educate the public about cancer and to support women with cancer, as well as to engage in related activism. It now links its activism with the environmental movement as well.

Breast Cancer Action and the Breast Cancer Fund have been the most successful of the Bay Area groups at generating public attention and influencing policy change. These organizations began to push government to apply the precautionary principle as a part of San Francisco's city planning policy in the mid-1990s, after having joined in 1992 with the National Alliance of Breast Cancer Organizations to push for lay involvement in research proposals funded by the California Breast Cancer Research Program. Their approach became a model for the well-regarded citizen participation in the Department of Defense's Breast Cancer Research Program and has included some research on environmental causation. The Breast Cancer Fund has also advocated stricter standards for chemicals regulated under the federal Food Quality Protection Act. It works closely with the National Institutes of Environmental Health Sciences and the Food and Drug Administration to revise or develop new clinical trial protocols. Breast Cancer Action has collaborated with the San Francisco Department of Public Health Breast and Cervical Cancer Services and various community and health organizations to organize town-hall meetings on breast cancer in low-income communities of color. Representative Nancy Pelosi (D-CA) has helped these organizations by supporting funding for breast cancer research and publicly recognizing their efforts. Other local representatives have offered symbolic support by creating days of recognition for their events.

Marin County activists have faced more challenges from the local community, such as being prohibited from holding meetings in government buildings. Despite these challenges, Zero Breast Cancer gained massive support from NIEHS and other government agencies through its involvement in the Breast Cancer and the Environment Research Centers (BCERCs). Four such centers were founded across the United States in 2003; one is based at the University of California, San Francisco. Zero Breast Cancer, the Breast Cancer Fund, and the Bayview–Hunters Point Health and Environmental Assessment Task Force collaborate with researchers on studies related to chemical exposures and breast cancer risk. These seven-year projects represent possibly the largest investments ever made by the federal government in environmental breast cancer research, and California's BCERC was the only research center with activist involvement. This reflects a culmination of the citizen-science alliances built up over nearly fifteen years.

Although EBCM activists in Long Island and Massachusetts have occasionally focused on access to health care, activists in the Bay Area are the only ones who have made it central to their advocacy efforts. A recent change in federal policy attests to their effectiveness. Although federal funding supported access to mammography for low-income women, it provided no financial assistance for breast cancer treatment. With strong support from Bay Area activists, in 2000 the Breast and Cervical Cancer Treatment Act was passed, guaranteeing treatment to low-income, uninsured women diagnosed with breast and cervical cancer through the National Breast and Cervical Cancer Early Detection Program.

In addition to raising money to fund research, Bay Area activists have distinguished themselves from the East Coast advocacy groups through their radical approaches to direct action and raising public awareness about the breast cancer illness experience. They have used street theater, protests, sit-ins, and graphic displays, including a series of large posters and billboards of young women with mastectomies, shown nude from the waist up. These displays (like the model Matschuka's self-portrait of her nude torso with a mastectomy, shown on the cover of the *New York Times Magazine* in August 1993), have created controversy both within and outside the movement.

Historically, activists in the Bay Area have been closely connected to environmental activism. In 1995, Breast Cancer Action became a founding member of the Toxics Link Coalition and helped organize the first Cancer Industry Tour, an annual tour of polluting companies' headquarters and facilities with the message "Stop cancer where it starts," to draw attention to the corporations operating in the Bay Area whose products and profits are linked to breast cancer. One head of a breast cancer group in the Bay Area described her organization as having a stronger connection with environmental groups than with the general breast cancer advocacy community. There is also crossover in leadership between breast cancer and environmental organizations. Some Bay Area groups have always had a strong environmental component. For other groups, a transition occurred as they became more concerned about environmental causation, as noted by an activist in Breast Cancer Action: "We adopted a policy in 1998 about not taking money from known environmental polluters or pharmaceutical companies or anybody profiting on cancer. In the process of doing that, we realized that our alliances were not going to be with breast cancer organizations. . . . [I]n conjunction with that we adopted a policy about when we would join a coalition, and we can't join a coalition which violates that policy. It makes it a little tricky, but not in environmental work. So we began seeing our alliances more in the environmental field and in the broader women's health field."

Other research on the EBCM has highlighted its anticorporate stance, showing how activities and positions that originated in Bay Area organizations have spread around the country. Susan Ferguson notes: "The impression today is that breast cancer is a growth industry, with Race for the Cure runs and walks in most major U.S. cities, the constant entry of new drugs and clinical trials to combat the disease, whole bookshelves devoted to the topic at local bookstores, and a cornucopia of tee-shirts, hats, pins, and pink ribbons" (Ferguson and Kasper 2000, 5). Activists believe that many corporations are getting good public relations out of donations to breast cancer efforts, which *Adweek* even named a "dream cause . . . [because it is] the feminist issue without politics" (Zones 2000, 119). This attitude exemplifies the split between the environmental breast cancer movement and the general breast cancer movement in the Bay Area. Environmental breast cancer activists have sometimes stood at the end of the Race for the Cure and handed out their own literature about environmental causation (Klawiter 1999). Similarly, although they joined in a coalition to support the Breast Cancer Summit led by the mayor of San Francisco, they also picketed the gathering to criticize the lack of attention to environmental causation (Klawiter 2001). By doing so, Myhre (2001) argues, they were acting as "outsiders within," a position that highlights the boundary-crossing nature of these movement actors and organizations. Although the EBCM has benefited from general breast cancer activism, in some ways the relationship between the two is tenuous.

Radical activists in the Bay Area criticize pharmaceutical companies, medical supply manufacturers, genetic testing firms, and other medical companies for making money from breast cancer, often by scaring women. These more radical activists point with dismay to methods like those of the gene-testing company that put an advertisement in the *Hartford Jewish Ledger* (because Ashkenazi Jewish women are more likely to have the BRCA-1 mutation) saying, "If you carry damaged breast cancer genes and you live long enough, you are almost guaranteed to develop breast cancer" (quoted in Zones 2000, 125). They simultaneously claim that pharmaceutical producers and doctors often downplay the side effects from breast cancer treatments, including the increased risk of uterine cancer from the drug tamoxifen. They also criticize the overuse of mammography, a position supported by the National Cancer Institute (Brown, Kessler, and Reuter 1990). As a part of their critique of the larger breast cancer movement, these activists point out that Imperial Chemical Industries (ICI), the parent company of Zeneca (which later merged with Astra to become AstraZeneca), invented Breast Cancer Awareness Month, and AstraZeneca retains approval authority over all printed materials used by participating groups and corporations. Tying the political-economy critique together with their belief in environmental causation, activists point out that while AstraZeneca profits from drugs used to treat breast cancer, the company also produces pesticides and other chemical products that may be causing breast cancer (Zones 2000).

DIFFERENCES IN CITIZEN-SCIENCE ALLIANCES ACROSS SITES

Citizen-science alliances in different regions have facilitated activist engagement in science and advanced movement goals in different ways. Activist involvement in science was implemented in each area largely according to the structure mandated by the funding source. On Long Island, for example, activist representation on breast cancer review panels was implemented through the Congressionally Directed Medical Research Program funded by the Department of Defense.

Despite funding victories at the federal level, the extent and effectiveness of activist involvement in breast cancer research have varied significantly among the three locations we studied. For example, although Long Island activists helped to secure federal funding for a major environmental study, their major funder, the National Cancer Institute, had virtually no experience with community participation in scientific research. Advocates were unable to persuade the researchers to investigate all the chemicals they felt were important. In contrast, Silent Spring Institute, whose research mission statement explicitly promotes citizen-science collaboration, has a more diverse funding base that has given the organization more flexibility in the direction of its research and in its ability to engage the community. In the San Francisco Bay Area, the national EBCM organizations, such as the Breast Cancer Fund and Breast Cancer Action, are not directly involved in research projects that entail primary data collection, in large measure because they focus on policy change and regulatory reform. This emphasis allows them to be more radical in their advocacy approach because they are not constrained by state or federal regulations that prohibit lobbying in conjunction with expenditure of research funds. In a different EBCM approach, advocates in Marin County collaborate closely with partners at the University of California, San Francisco, in education and outreach efforts and long-term cohort studies.

Overall, activists have sought to build citizen-science alliances that can change the attitudes and practices of scientists and provide a new value structure to guide breast cancer research. Silent Spring Institute represents a very powerful victory in Massachusetts. In New York, successful partnerships were more limited. In the Bay Area, Marin activists sought opportunities to engage in research projects and eventually became part of the Breast Cancer and the Environment Research Center. For the EBCM in general, members' increasing expertise has led to invitations from scientists to sit on boards advising on research, thus providing the opportunity to influence research direction and study design and potentially improve the knowledge base for environmental causation.

THE FRAMEWORK FOR ACTIVISM: PERSONAL, SCIENTIFIC, POLITICAL

Our overview of movement activism in the three major locales demonstrates the importance of the personal experience of illness in activism as a political and scientific tool. We now turn from organizational issues to the issue of embodiment to show how EBCM work affects individuals.

"The Personal Is Political" as a Starting Point

Environmental breast cancer activists start from the classic feminist stance that "the personal is political": that individual women's experiences can be viewed as a political issue. This position is seen in one activist's description of the launching of her organization: "I refused to accept the fact that one out of every eleven women will die of breast cancer. I remember reading [that] Gloria Steinem said, 'The day the revolution starts is when one person looks back in someone's eyes and says, "No, I refuse to budge, I refuse to accept that."'" In interviews, activists told us that clinical and support services are crucial but not sufficient. A central activity of the traditional breast cancer movement response is to organize support groups. In contrast, the EBCM emphasizes a model of action that facilitates empowerment in the political realm, beginning with awareness of corporate production of chemicals, government failure to regulate chemicals, and scientists' and funders' reluctance to examine the external causes that make women sick. This awareness was demonstrated by one scientist who had breast cancer: "I was diagnosed with breast cancer, and soon after that I went to a rally . . . where they asked women to come down out of the stands and stand in a chalked area that was supposedly to be the shape of Massachusetts, and so many people came out of the stands, I couldn't believe it. Young women, old women, black women, white women. And I was flabbergasted, and it was at that point that I said to myself, . . . 'When I went to medical school breast cancer was rare, . . . I don't have a family history. I suddenly have breast cancer. I'm looking around at hundreds of women who have breast cancer, and this isn't rare.'"

The Role of Activism in Advancing a Public Paradigm

All interviewees, both scientists and activists, reported a strong belief that activism and social movements are critical in advancing research, educating the public, and changing policy about environmental causes of breast cancer. One scientist said that activists "have been the catalysts. They're the drivers. The environmental movement, the women's movement, specifically the breast cancer activist movement, they're the ones that are driving the establishment of research about environmental factors."

The EBCM benefited from the feminist movement's successes in many ways, including the increased public attention to women's issues, tactics for activism, and ideological foundations. Feminism has drawn attention to the lack of women's involvement in science and the construction of knowledge that fails to take account of women's experiences and worldviews. Although most breast cancer movement activists do not articulate a direct link between their activism and the feminist movement, an implicit connection is often clear from their philosophical stance and organizations' mission statements. For instance, one founder of an EBCM group, who was also involved in a network of environmental organizations, called breast cancer a "wedge issue" for larger gender equality and environmental issues: "We want to share leadership, and bringing ourselves [women] into balance in this issue will help to bring the whole planet into balance. I do think that environmental health, using breast cancer as a wedge issue toward that larger issue, is the issue of the millennium."

An activist in another locale extended this assertion: "We're just a breast cancer organization; you'd think we could stay focused. But breast cancer touches on every aspect of health, the economy, politics, so we get to do it all." These quotations, coming from opposite sides of the country, exemplify the overarching approach that unites what Klawiter (1999) terms "cultures of action, " that is, different modes of action across diverse wings of a larger movement. That approach identifies breast cancer as an issue that transcends the boundaries of social movement organizations and goals, with broad ramifications for gender equality and larger sociopolitical issues.

Some activists explicitly noted that EBCM tactics such as public protest and obtaining an activist presence in scientific research were adapted from the AIDS movement. AIDS activists have used public protests to alter the social perception of AIDS victims as well as to generate more funds for research and activist involvement in research (Epstein 1996). Some activists who belonged to the AIDS group ACT-UP were also members of Breast Cancer Action, and several wealthy AIDS activists were also major donors to Bay Area breast cancer groups. The use of public education and social protest strategies in the EBCM varies across locales;

popular epidemiology and activist involvement in some aspects of research are widespread.

EBCM activists we interviewed felt that social movements were instrumental in the development of research into environmental causation. One long-time activist emphasized the difference between the activist and the scientific perspective: "Changes that have to happen around breast cancer and all the things that influence it are going to come from the ground up. They're not going to come from the top down. . . . If you think about it, activists were the first to argue for this, and some of the scientific community has been sort of dragged along."

Activists also clearly articulated their wish to advance changes in attitudes and practices outside of science: "I think the role of social movements is to push the 'establishment,' . . . whether it's the scientific community, federal government, drug companies, or whoever. . . . We as activists are pushing people to broaden the scope of what they consider to be environmental problems."

Empowerment and politicization for EBCM activists often involve using knowledge of individual environmental exposures to inform science. In this process, both social movement actors and scientists are boundary actors crossing into new arenas of research and advocacy to advance social movement claims. Citizen-science alliances can alter expert and lay roles. For example, scientists may collaborate with community groups to search for potential environmental causes of diseases, especially when traditional funding sources and regulatory and public health bodies oppose such connections. Epidemiologists may teach lay activists about scientific theories and methods. This exchange of knowledge is central to the NBCC's Project Lead, in which epidemiologists provide breast cancer activists with the scientific training they need to serve on federal grant-review panels for science (Dickersin et al. 2001). One Project Lead participant spoke about the attempts of breast cancer activists to find "a place at the decision making table" that would bring out "not just our intuition, and our native intelligence, and our common sense, and our perspectives as the patient [and] the affected community, but also [help us to really learn] the science and the medicine of breast cancer."

These collaborations between citizens and scientists have changed minds on both sides. Activists described drastic changes in their understanding of what science can prove in terms of environmental causation, the length of time necessary to conduct research, and the processes involved. They often became so well educated about scientific methods that they had specific recommendations for ways research could be improved in the future. Activists without prior experience in science found that their feelings toward scientists had changed from fear and anxiety to respect and comfort. One woman who had worked on high-level government advisory panels said, "The thing that I came away with that was most surprising was how much the scientists and the MDs have come to value the activist perspective on these panels. . . . [They are] not only just putting a face on the statistics. . . .

They appreciate that . . . you ask the questions, 'Why is this relevant? Who cares?'" Thus, participation in a citizen-science alliance was a transformative experience for activists, teaching them to appreciate the very different perspective of science.

As this boundary-crossing process changed activist perspectives about science and researchers, activists raised concerns about becoming too strongly aligned with the government or scientists and potentially losing their activist perspective. However, such co-optation was not common. One older activist, who had played a critical role in securing activist participation in research and who was one of the first to be involved, expressed her feelings as follows: "I remember sitting at an NBCC board meeting years ago, and we were talking about, I don't remember the issue, and we were voting against it. It sounded like individuals really wanted it, but we decided it wasn't a good idea, and I said, 'Go back to our beginnings even a couple of years ago.' I said that had this question been raised then, we would have been amongst the loudest voices saying we want this, and now we know it's not a good idea. [I] said, 'Oh, we've become educated. But we never want to lose our fire.'"

We might expect scientists to worry that their legitimacy would be threatened by working with laypeople, but this was not the case. Scientists involved in EBCM alliances described some initial fears but generally acknowledged a sense of mutual respect between themselves and activists. They often greatly appreciated the input from activists, in addition to activist support of scientific research projects. (Of course, the participating scientists may be a biased sample, a self-selected group who were previously open to activist involvement in research, but they came from a wide diversity of backgrounds and experience.) The acceptance of citizen-science alliances by participating scientists is an important step in strengthening the legitimacy of this type of research.

Despite these expressions of mutual respect and goodwill, apprehension and prejudice on the part of both activists and scientists against the other group were the most serious obstacles to alliances. The process of dispelling these initial fears and prejudices was described by one activist: "I think there is a respect for bright people, and I think the assumption often is that activists are going to be hysterical women. And I think once most scientists realize that we're not hysterical women, they find themselves, you know, intrigued. And they might come to the table with a lot of prejudices and worries, but I have rarely seen it continue to be a problem."

The learning process for activists entailed gaining more knowledge about science and learning how their own knowledge was valuable to science, as one activist attests: "I know that professionals like to build up their own vocabulary and their own aura and arena so that it can't be pierced by anyone because, after all, they paid their dues. But it's nothing more than communication and relationships. Everything is understandable and pierceable. The more people are willing to share their expertise, realizing that the others are not trying to replace their expertise or their judgment, I think the more effective we can be."

Another activist expressed the same spirit of collaboration while still empha-sizing the distinct roles of each group: "I just think that it's important that we all work together. Activists have a seat at the table, not because we want to be scientists, but because we need to push along some of the work that should have been done long ago." In the words of one scientist involved in the Long Island Breast Cancer Study Project: "There get to be fads in research . . . dogmas . . . of what an acceptable area of research is, and so one thing I find very helpful about having a diverse group of advocates is that it can sometimes help to . . . loosen up whatever the current dogma is and get people . . . out of whatever dogma trench they're in."

These quotations show how activist involvement in science can provide a new value structure for science. In breast cancer research, the biomedical model of the disease has predominated. Consequently, research has focused on individual factors related to treatment and prevention. By taking a broader view of breast cancer risk that highlights the political economy of disease causation, the EBCM is able to create a new value system for science. Movement actors push scien-tists to examine why they ask certain questions and not others, why they use certain methodologies, and, more important, how their research affects women with breast cancer. An activist provided an emblematic example of such ques-tioning: a lay member of a review panel listened to a scientist give an extremely high score to a proposal simply on the basis of excellent methodology. When the laywoman pressed the scientist on the actual relevance of the project, the sci-entist revised the score downward. The boundary crossing that occurs between lay and expert knowledge on research review panels can thus reshape paths of scientific inquiry.

CONCLUSIONS

Our EBCM case study shows how the movement developed out of a politicized collective-illness experience that highlights the environmental causation of breast cancer. The EBCM crosses the boundaries between science and advocacy, and between scientists and citizens. Our understanding of this movement demon-strates that scholars need to examine social movements in a more complex and historical fashion, paying attention to the multiple movement actors and organi-zations involved. The EBCM has influenced the production of science and policy by focusing attention on women's health issues and on improving environmental policy making and causation research. This introduction of political values into the supposedly value-neutral world of science can overcome the biomedical ten-dency to discount the relationship between environment and health; it can also reshape methods through which health and disease are understood by integrating local and lay knowledge into the research enterprise.

The shift in scientific focus from individual risk factors to a political economy of disease that highlights environmental links faces resistance from corporate and government institutions, but it can catalyze a corresponding shift in accountability for disease prevention. Despite challenges to the more radical and socially transformative elements of the EBCM, this movement has fused aspects of its diverse origins in the public health, environmental, and women's movements. The EBCM's successes include significantly increasing public awareness, expanding the funding for research on environmental links, and establishing a dialogue created with the scientific community through citizen-science alliances.

Our initial work on the EBCM brought the Silent Spring Institute into a long-term, innovative, and productive collaboration with Communities for a Better Environment in the Northern California Household Exposure Study, a partnership that might otherwise never have been formed. From the understanding we gained of the movements, we were able to foster a large research project and long-lasting, interdisciplinary collaborations.

Although local concerns and cultural variations make each locale of the EBCM somewhat different, sufficient similarities exist to justify viewing this as a coherent national movement. Social movements have an enormous range of facets. They attempt credible challenges to government authority, to medicine and science, to health charities, and to the pharmaceutical and chemical industries and related organizations; they contend for power and authority among various organizations within a movement; and they undertake activities to increase public awareness. Our study shows how these facets are interlinked in the EBCM.

Our case study also offers important lessons about the components of social movements. Social movement actors are flexible, and social movements are not discrete objects but changeable social phenomena. This view allows us to discuss not just social movements, but social change more broadly, in a more complex way. Boundary movements such as the environmental breast cancer movement are centrally concerned with democratic participation in science and with using research to transform social policy. Ordinary citizens in this movement have had the strength and ability to learn enough about science to help make decisions about scientific research and to collaborate in research enterprises. Thus the environmental breast cancer movement has empowered people affected by breast cancer to improve scientific practice, protect public health, and reshape the priorities of science and medicine.

NOTES

This is a reprint of an article published in *Sociological Forum*, © 2010 Eastern Sociological Society: Sabrina McCormick, Phil Brown, and Stephen Zavestoski, "The Personal Is Scientific, the Scientific Is Political: The Public Paradigm of the Environmental Breast Cancer Movement," *Sociological Forum* 18 (2003): 545–76.

1. Our terminology for this movement was discussed with movement leaders. They generally agreed that the term *environmental breast cancer movement* is appropriate. However, other terms are also used.

2. DoD's involvement in breast cancer research stemmed from concern that the Republican capture of Congress in 1994 would result in massive cutbacks in National Cancer Institute funding. Responding to strategic lobbying by breast cancer advocates, Senator Tom Harkin (D-IA) led a successful effort to place considerable funding for nonmilitary research in the Department of Defense, where budget cuts were less likely.

10

School Custodians
and Green Cleaners

*Labor-Environmental Coalitions
and Toxics Reduction*

Laura Senier, Brian Mayer, Phil Brown, and Rachel Morello-Frosch

In the fall of 2003, the Boston Urban Asthma Coalition (BUAC) and the Massachusetts Committee on Occupational Safety and Health (MassCOSH) launched the Green Cleaners Project, a coalition of organizations, including labor unions and school administrators, to address well-documented problems of environmental quality in Boston schools. Coalition participants wanted to ensure that discussions about environmental health problems in Boston schools and their remediation would include the broadest possible array of stakeholders, including parents, teachers and other school employees, school administrators, and community health advocates. Despite the expensive and capital-intensive nature of solutions to many of the environmental health problems documented in the schools, the coalition quickly won a major victory on one component of their short-term agenda: the replacement of common cleaning products with less toxic, "green" alternatives.

The Green Cleaners Project has brought Boston in step with a growing national movement to improve environmental health in schools. Over the past decade, community groups and advocates have pointed to increasing rates of chronic illnesses among schoolchildren, such as asthma, diabetes, and learning disabilities, many of which may be caused by or exacerbated by environmental conditions. The movement has also protested inappropriate school siting, both for new construction and for existing facilities that have been sited on toxic landfills or brownfields, or adjacent to polluting facilities. Movement activists have also sought to influence the design of new schools by pressing for the adoption of energy-efficient materials and green building standards (Center for Health, Environment, and Justice 2002).

Boston's experience in school health advocacy projects has also, however, exemplified many of the challenges in uniting participants in two important social movements: organized labor and the environmental movement. Alliances between labor unions and environmental organizations, or "blue-green" alliances, have historically faced formidable obstacles, typically articulated as a class divide that forces union workers to choose between job security and environmental reforms (Obach 2004a; Mayer 2008). Pressured by management to side with the political interests of industry, union workers have often found themselves in opposition to the agenda of the environmental movement. Yet despite recent, high-profile examples of cases in which the pursuit of goals on the environmental agenda has threatened labor union jobs, there is a much older tradition of labor unionists and activists working together with environmental health activists, such as occupational health specialists and sanitarians, on issues of importance to both constituencies (Gottlieb 2005; Mayer 2008).

The member organizations in the Green Cleaners Project are also participants in a regional blue-green coalition known as the Alliance for a Healthy Tomorrow (the Alliance), a larger initiative to foster relationships and political partnerships between labor unions and environmental organizations in Massachusetts. In this respect, the Green Cleaners Project operates within a tradition of cross-movement cooperation and shows the importance of health concerns as a common issue that, in favorable circumstances, may draw additional partners into the blue-green coalition and motivate both groups to work toward a common goal.

In reviewing the activities and strategies of the Green Cleaners Project, we identify factors that led to the early success of this coalition and may assure its long-term stability. We show, first, how the Green Cleaners Project team assembled a diverse group of stakeholders and, second, how they maintained cohesion by merging concerns about a high-profile school health issue with a precautionary approach to managing school environmental quality. Invocation of the precautionary principle facilitated the construction of a frame that represented the individual and common interests of all stakeholders.

Although numerous other blue-green alliances have sprung up across the country in the past decade (Gould, Lewis, and Roberts 2004; Obach 2004a; Mayer and Brown 2005), the Green Cleaners Project is unique in securing the cooperation and involvement of environmental and community health advocates, labor unions, and school administrators, and thus it displays a level of organizational complexity that blue-green coalitions frequently lack. We highlight the role of "bridge builders" who negotiated a shared understanding among the stakeholders about the importance of eliminating toxic cleaning chemicals from the school environment. Of the various healthy-schools networks forming around the country, this is the first that we are aware of that secured the active and early cooperation of school custodians—the parties most directly responsible for managing school environmental quality. Although this coalition could have been launched without custodians' support, their involvement was critical in the successful transition to safer cleaning products, and their participation can help advance the coalition's long-term agenda. The bridge builders also benefit from state policies that support the institutional adoption of toxics-use reduction policies and makes incentives available to groups working to implement such changes. Finally, the Alliance provides the support of a strong statewide coalition of community groups, environmental health advocates, and labor unions that has worked to build legislative support for precautionary policies and the use of environmentally friendly products.

BACKGROUND

In 1996, parents, teachers, and community activists raised a sustained protest over air quality problems in a Boston public elementary school. In response, the Boston City Council ordered the school department and the Boston Public Health Commission to conduct semiannual environmental assessments at all Boston public schools. These inspections were not begun until 2002. The first inspection report, released in 2004, reported that 90 percent of Boston schools had at least one major environmental problem, such as leaks, poor ventilation, dust and mold, and pest incursions (Jan 2004).

These issues are of concern because mold, dust, and pest dander all contribute to asthma and allergies, and Boston schools have high rates of asthma among students and staff. Asthma is the leading cause of hospitalization among children. Nationwide, it accounts for an average of 14 million missed schooldays each year and results in some $9 billion in health care costs; these costs may be expected to rise, as asthma rates are increasing (American Lung Association 2004). Moreover, asthma is thought to affect attendance and overall academic performance (Mendell and Heath 2005). Asthma rates in the Northeast are higher than the national average. School health records in Massachusetts show that 9.2 percent of the children have asthma (Knorr et al. 2004). Because this health burden is borne disproportionately by low-income communities and communities of color (Bloom et al. 2003), the disease is a particular organizing focus among environmental justice organizations (see chapter 7).

Cleaning products commonly contain ammonium compounds, several of which are recognized asthma triggers (Bernstein et al. 1994; Purohit et al. 2000). In a survey of health care workers in four states, including Massachusetts, cleaning products were the source of the most commonly reported occupational chemical exposures linked to asthma (Pechter et al. 2005). Cleaning products are known to affect indoor air quality, also a recognized factor in exacerbation of asthma (Shendell, Barnett, and Boese 2004). An unhealthy indoor environment in schools reduces the ability of staff to perform and of students to learn, making the reduction of asthma in Boston's public schools a priority for many stakeholders with complex and often contradictory interests.

Many of the environmental problems documented in Boston's schools are related to the age of the buildings, the choice of building materials, and their maintenance. These problems are difficult and expensive to fix. The task force therefore attempted to prioritize the issues and identify some that could be remedied cheaply and quickly. One measure was the replacement of conventional cleaning products with so-called green cleaners. The citywide task force also pressed for a policy change to require all of Boston's public schools to adopt integrated pest management, a strategy that relies primarily on nontoxic means, such as physical and mechanical barriers, to reduce insect and rodent incursions, thereby reducing the need for toxic pesticides. The school health advocates thus began with a focus on "low-hanging fruit," that is, problems that would be easy to identify, easy to reach agreement on, and easy to solve.

State-Level Efforts to Foster Precautionary Policies

Massachusetts has long been a leader in encouraging toxics reduction through statewide regulatory initiatives. The state Toxics Use Reduction Institute (TURI), established in 1989, has worked with state industries to find cost-effective and less toxic replacements for hazardous substances (Mayer, Brown, and Linder 2002; Mayer, Brown, and Senier 2008). In 1996, TURI established the Toxics Use Reduction Networking grantmaking program (TURN) to help community organizations and municipalities develop toxics reduction programs (Toxics Use Reduction Institute 2003). The following year, Massachusetts passed a rule requiring all state executive departments to follow an environmentally preferable products (EPP) program designed to eliminate potential environmental and health hazards in state office buildings (801 CMR 21.00, passed April 18, 1997).

A precaution-oriented philosophy has also been embraced by the Alliance for a Healthy Tomorrow. Founded in 2001, the Alliance was the first coalition in the United States to promote the precautionary principle (Mayer, Brown, and Senier 2008), which has four central tenets: taking preventive action (even in the face of uncertainty about the scope and extent of adverse events associated with exposures); shifting the burden of proof to the proponents of an activity; widening the range of alternatives assessed; and increasing public participation in decision making (Kriebel et al. 2001). In its campaign in Boston schools, the Green Cleaners Project team has drawn on state-level efforts to foster precautionary policies (e.g., through TURI) and a small but significant base of support in regional blue-green organizing and advocacy.

Recognizing that workers are exposed to toxic substances in the workplace that often also affect neighboring communities and the environment, the

Alliance is part of a growing type of blue-green coalition focusing on protecting human health in both the workplace and the environment (Mayer and Brown 2005; Mayer, Brown, and Senier 2008). Previous attempts to bridge the divide between labor and environmental organizations on issues such as global warming or energy policy have typically failed to find common ground and ended in dissolution of the coalitions (Obach 2004a). By focusing on health as a link between blues and greens, however, coalitions like the Alliance are forming long-lasting relationships and including a more diverse representation of environmental organizations, among them environmental health and environmental justice organizations. In their collaboration with the custodians' union in the Green Cleaners Project, Alliance members MassCOSH and BUAC have sought to establish a similar type of solidarity with workers directly affected by cleaning-chemical policies.

The Alliance has taken up the work initiated by the Green Cleaners Project team to lobby for the passage of legislation requiring use of safer products when they are available and cost-effective. The Safer Cleaning Products Bill, introduced into the Massachusetts legislature in December 2004, was designed to reduce asthma and other health threats from toxic chemicals in cleaning products by requiring schools, hospitals and other health care facilities, day care centers, public buildings, and public housing to use greener alternatives. The Green Cleaners Project may be seen as a test case for broader adoption of safer cleaning products, because if it is feasible for a bureaucracy as large as the Boston school system to amend purchasing strategies to adopt safer cleaning products, then it should also be possible for other large organizations to "green" their operations.

School and Health Advocacy in Boston

The Green Cleaners Project team is a special subcommittee of a citywide task force dedicated to remediating the school environmental problems identified in the 2002 environmental assessment inspections. This task force, known as the Healthy Boston Schools Project, initially comprised members of BUAC, MassCOSH, the Boston Public Health Commission, and the Boston Public School Department of Facilities Management. In the fall of 2004, BUAC was awarded a grant from TURI to review cleaning-chemical policy in Boston schools. In consultation with a MassCOSH program director, the BUAC director decided to use the citywide task force as the base committee for this review, with the addition of representatives from the Boston school custodians' union and the school department's purchasing department. The Green Cleaners Project team thus represented various constituencies, each with a different perspective on and different responsibilities for school environmental quality. Its internal cohesion therefore depended largely on bridge builders, individuals who play multiple social roles that often cross movement boundaries (Robnett 1981; Rose 2000).

Previous scholarship on blue-green alliances in the United States has high-lighted the capacity of committees on occupational safety and health (COSH) leaders to function as bridge builders (Obach 2004a). COSHes were established in the early 1970s, at a time when many unions needed to shift their focus from health and safety concerns to protecting wages and job security (Berman 1981). They readily maneuver among organizations such as unions, management, and academia and thus encourage cooperation among entities that might not other-wise collaborate (Gottlieb 2005). MassCOSH, like other COSH groups nation-wide, advocates for health and safety protection and social justice for workers (Berman 1981). In this capacity, it often works closely with union leaders, but it also engages directly with workers, community groups, and health, safety, and environmental advocates. It also represents nonunionized workers and thus func-tions as a surrogate union, at least with respect to workplace health and safety (Gottlieb 2005).

Founded in 1997, BUAC has sought to "promote collaboration between orga-nizations and residents concerned about the various factors that affect asthma, such as the environment, quality of health care, access to health care, and edu-cation" (Boston Urban Asthma Coalition 2006). BUAC's school subcommittee, comprising parents, teachers, and school employees, developed a healthy-schools platform that identifies conditions that may exacerbate asthma, such as build-ing maintenance. Whereas most interventions in childhood asthma focus on individual treatment and management, BUAC addresses environmental causes and triggers. Like the various projects run by MassCOSH, BUAC's approach encourages cooperation among multiple stakeholders, involving school admin-istrators, teachers, principals, custodians, and staff. This coalition may appear to not include any conventional environmental organizations, but the emergence of groups like BUAC is itself a sign of the changing face of the environmental movement. BUAC has an explicitly environmental agenda and coordinates many activities with environmental health and environmental justice groups in the area. Indeed, this "new conventionality" of environmental organizations is partly what makes blue-green coalitions possible.

Custodians in Boston public schools are organized through Local 1952 of the International Union of Painters and Allied Trades (District Council 35), repre-senting approximately four hundred full- and part-time custodians. Although the union president describes his current working relationship with the school department as cooperative and communicative, relations between the school department and the union have been difficult.

Lacking the organizational resources necessary to support a full-time health and safety committee, the custodial union worked with MassCOSH to address occupational health and safety concerns. In the early 1990s, the school depart-ment laid off approximately fifty custodians and in 1996 forced a "best and final" contract on the union that granted the school department the right to contract out custodial labor. In 2001, the school department proposed cutting more positions, leaving some small schools without a custodian on the day shift. During this round of negotiations, BUAC and MassCOSH became concerned about the effect that custodial staffing reductions would have on school environmental quality (especially with respect to waste management and partial implementation of integrated pest management) and collaborated with the custodial union president in an effort to preserve these jobs.

This attempt to forge a new relationship between BUAC and the custodial union, with MassCOSH continuing to provide assistance, paved the way for the subsequent collaboration on cleaning product substitution. BUAC and Mass-COSH's joint organizational resources and experience in previous interactions with state environmental policies and city-level politics made them appealing potential coalition partners for the custodians. By identifying the protection of custodial jobs as part of a larger mission to improve school environmental quality, activists at BUAC and MassCOSH also placed the issue of school environmental health in a broader context.

Framing School Health with the Logic of Precaution

This case study of multiorganizational advocacy for product substitution provides a window into how organizations negotiate a precautionary approach toward hazardous substances. Massachusetts provides institutional support for organizations to embrace toxics reduction, and there is popular support for further legislative initiatives. Nevertheless, persuading individual organizations to shift to healthier cleaning products requires stakeholders to reach a common understanding of potentially risky exposures and agree on acceptable solutions. Although the coalition partners certainly benefited from favorable political opportunities and were able to mobilize diverse resources in organizing their campaign, they also used specific discursive and rhetorical tools to align their stakeholders' concerns. The Green Cleaners Project developed a two-stage process, first demonstrating the gravity of a specific health problem and then linking its mitigation to an overall strategy of precaution. In doing so, they employed various strategies to show how the precautionary principle supported the needs and interests of different stakeholders.

Framing is a process by which social movement actors construct and maintain a common identity or arrive at an agreed-upon set of meanings that give purpose and direction to the existence and actions of a social movement organization (Della Porta and Diani 1999; Benford and Snow 2000). Collective-action frames are produced by social actors at various levels, from individuals to organizations to coalitions (Croteau and Hicks 2003). When stakeholders from multiple social movement organizations collaborate on a social problem, interorganizational frame alignment is necessary to negotiate differences in the construction of meaning both within and between movements (Benford and Snow 2000). Whereas individual social movement organizations use frame alignment to merge the concerns of individuals into an organizational frame, coalitions use frame alignment to merge the concerns of organizations into a coalition frame.

The literature on social movements and collective action contains few case studies on the actual process of frame construction; it tends to treat frames as static elements used by social movement actors to accomplish their goals. In constructing coalition frames, aligning diverse identities and goals is particularly challenging. The differences in identity and purpose between labor unions and environmental organizations typically drive apart the interests of the groups and may explain why some blue-green coalitions have been difficult to sustain (Obach 2004a). The Alliance has used the strategy of frame bridging (in which ideologically congruent yet structurally divergent frames are linked) to link environmental and occupational health. The larger coalition is thus able to draw on organizational and political support from both movements in a fundamentally new fashion. Because many of the participants in the Green Cleaners Project team were also members of the Alliance, this was a familiar strategy to them.

Frame bridging requires movement actors to agree on a common goal (Benford and Snow 2000); this agreement in turn requires specific and explicit rhetorical work to articulate a movement's goals and strategies. The Green Cleaners Project team's use of framing has both strategic and discursive properties. Strategically, frame bridging connects the interests of environmental actors and the custodial union with a specific purpose: implementing a pilot project to substitute cleaning products. It also has important movement-building implications, fostering ties across movement boundaries. In this way, the Green Cleaners Project is an example of how a social movement organization can have specific strategic goals that are reflected in a larger discursive project.

In a coalition of diverse partners, framing must also attend to the potential disconnect between individual organizations' strategic goals and those of the coalition. Furthermore, the strategic and discursive elements of a collective-action frame are not always perfectly aligned. In the Green Cleaners Project, tension arose between partners over the best methods of reaching the strategic goal of reducing asthma. Some stakeholders expressed skepticism about broadening the dialogue to include the logic of precaution. In particular, they disagreed about the extent to which the project members should invoke health problems as a rationale for endorsing a change in cleaning products, with some school administrators expecting proof of health benefits to justify a change, and the union president being reluctant to endorse actions implying that his members might face health consequences from past exposures.

While frame bridging created an opportunity to bring together specific stakeholders to facilitate a particular initiative, BUAC and MassCOSH also hoped to foster a larger project to address thornier problems of school environmental quality (e.g., mold and pest infestations). They knew that longer-term success would require building relationships between diverse actors and helping the partners appreciate that school environmental quality could be incrementally improved through short-term projects like replacing toxic cleaning products in schools with safer alternatives.

METHODS AND PROGRAM EVALUATION

The Green Cleaners Project team began by assessing products used for general cleaning, floor care, and graffiti removal. Products were screened for potential health and environmental effects. Nine of the seventeen products had potential carcinogenic, teratogenic, or corrosive effects and were identified as candidates for replacement. Based on this information, the project team developed a plan for the replacement of these products with "greener" alternatives.

Many of the chemical companies that produce cleaning chemicals and janitorial supplies now provide greener formulations of their regular product lines. The school department purchasing agent contacted the two companies that Boston schools regularly purchase from and ordered the greener version of all cleaning products currently used in Boston schools. A team from the facilities management department then visited the four pilot schools, removed all of the conventional formulations of the cleaning chemicals, and replaced them with the new ones. In the summer of 2004, custodians working in these schools received training in the proper use of these chemicals. Although the corporate representatives of the top cleaning-product companies typically offer training sessions to assist in the adoption of the new products, several custodians felt these corporate-sponsored training sessions to be brief and of only limited relevance in addressing the cleaning issues they faced in school environments.

With no mechanism for feedback between the custodians and product manufacturers, custodians sometimes modified the application of the green products to obtain better results and meet the demand for cleanliness. This practice may, however, compromise the safety and environmental benefits of the products or compromise product performance, if, for example, it involves applying products in heavier concentrations than the manufacturer recommends. The Green Cleaners Project team monitored the pilot program to gauge product efficacy and to make further recommendations concerning the use of green cleaning products. This evaluation included a paper-and-pencil survey of custodians in the pilot schools.

The Green Cleaners Project team also asked the Contested Illnesses Research Group (CIRG) to conduct a qualitative evaluation. Our team was happy to undertake this project, because we had a grant from the National Science Foundation to study coalition formation between labor unions and environmental organizations.

Acting as consultants to the Green Cleaners Project team, we performed the qualitative evaluation and then produced a report for the team summarizing our findings. This practice is in keeping with our commitment to community-engaged advocacy and consultancy and our obligation to report findings to research participants. Twelve semistructured interviews, ranging from forty-five to sixty minutes in length, were conducted between November 2004 and February 2005 with members of the pilot team and with custodians and principals at the pilot schools. Questions covered the origins of the project, the rationale for the pilot project, expectations for evaluating the program's overall effectiveness, custodial satisfaction, and the cooperative dynamics and challenges that coalition members had experienced.

Interviews were coded and analyzed for the major themes of this project. Coding began with a preestablished set of codes, drawing on themes found in a review of the literature on school environmental health and blue-green coalitions. The code list expanded to include themes and issues that arose during the interviews, such as framing of the health message and brokering of negotiations. We analyzed transcripts and submitted a short report of our findings to the Green Cleaners Product team, which was used in the overall evaluation of the pilot program.

The Green Cleaners Pilot Project is the first application of the blue-green model in an institution like education, where diverse stakeholders might be brought together to address concerns about protecting human health and the environment. However, because this type of collaboration between custodians, environmentalists, and children's health activists is rare, we are limited in the extent to which we can generalize from this study until further examples can be identified and analyzed.

RESULTS

The Green Cleaners Project team succeeded in persuading school administrators to shift to green cleaners for two main reasons. First, the team successfully bridged the typically oppositional concerns of multiple and diverse stakeholders, effectively neutralizing the objections or securing the support of those that might have made such a project infeasible. By enlisting the custodial union as participants in the pilot project, the Green Cleaners Project team was able to convince the union that the initiative to switch cleaning products would not threaten jobs, that it would strengthen the union's calls for better worker training in general, and that it would allow custodians to participate in decisions about their work environment. The coalition thus strategically circumvented potential opposition to environmental initiatives on the grounds that they would threaten jobs. Second, the team developed and maintained a strategic frame for this project that unified the health concerns of school staff, environmental health activists, and the custodians' union under the umbrella of the precautionary principle. The project ultimately addressed both the community's and activists' concerns about health and school environmental quality and the workers' concerns about workplace safety and training. These two strategies helped to secure the participation of the major stakeholders in this coalition and have laid the groundwork for future collaborations among this team on other issues in school environmental health.

Enlisting Custodians in Protecting School Environmental Health

MassCOSH's organizational role was vital to the Green Cleaners Project, and its program director was an essential bridge builder. She is a founding member of BUAC and also heads the BUAC school health committee and chairs Mass-COSH's Healthy Schools Network. Through her involvement with the Mass-COSH and BUAC school health committees, she had extensive knowledge of the environmental issues in Boston schools and strong personal contacts with decision makers in the school administration as well as with the leaders of the teachers' and custodial unions. Her previous interaction with the custodial union helped establish the communication necessary for successful bridge building. Her involvement in the Alliance allowed her to apply the logic and discourse of precaution as a central element in the construction of the coalition frame, and her leadership in the Alliance and in the statewide Healthy Schools Network enabled her to link a local campaign for school environmental health to wider initiatives. Thus from the outset, the Green Cleaners Project had advantages in city and statewide politics, both in terms of access to political officials and in familiarity with the advocacy efforts of one of the state's most visible environmental coalitions.

The MassCOSH program director was well aware that the custodial union needed an advocate to support its initiatives to improve worker health and employee training. For the custodial union, job security and wages are paramount; it lacks the bargaining power to make health issues a priority. The custodial union president had first met the MassCOSH and BUAC organizers at citywide hearings when the school administration proposed eliminating custodial jobs. The president expressed his members' longstanding frustrations in their jobs. He noted, for example, that his members bristle at the use of the term *dirty* to describe the schools: "When people walk into a building and they see like, the plaster falling down and stuff, they perceive that as being dirty, so they blame the custodian, so we should be involved to really explain what the problem is, instead. Because people just see certain things and say, 'Oh, that's dirt.' But what's causing that?" The custodial union has struggled to gain recognition of the structural problems that contribute to school environmental quality, such as staffing, funding, and capital plans for building maintenance.

The MassCOSH project leader understood and acknowledged this position: "There has been a lot of shuffling around and staff reduction, too. . . . Some of the small schools didn't have custodians for some of the key hours of the school day, so if a kid threw up, the teacher either threw something, like that kitty litter stuff, on it, and they would call a floater custodian to come and clean it, or it would wait until they had their part-time person after school come and clean it. And we just felt like that was a public health problem." The union president appreciated MassCOSH's support at these hearings to help him hold the line against further job cuts. He was willing to cooperate on the Green Cleaners Project because he perceived MassCOSH as an important external advocate that could augment the union's efforts to protect jobs and to advocate for members' health and increased worker training.

The school department's decision to shift to green cleaners included a renewed commitment to worker training and an agreement to form a standing committee for the periodic review of cleaning-chemical use in schools, which would include a representative from the custodial union. These two provisions were significant victories for the Green Cleaners Project team. School administrators interviewed for this project reported that the chemical manufacturers all offer a range of products that changes frequently. They had changed product formulations frequently in the past, but before this project began, they had not sought input or feedback on these decisions from the custodians. Although janitorial work has historically been considered semiskilled labor, over the past several decades, as the global economy has tightened labor markets and more and more organizations have contracted out janitorial services, the work has been transformed into low-skilled, low-wage "dirty" work. The reliance on part-time and unskilled laborers has often driven contract cleaning companies to select cleaners based on their potency and efficacy, in an effort to curb costs by avoiding the need for worker training (Gottlieb 2001).

The evaluation of green cleaning products in the Green Cleaners pilot project included several types of qualitative assessment of product performance and the custodians' job satisfaction. Several custodians identified practical barriers to using green products, notably lack of equipment or insufficient training. Custodians expressed some dissatisfaction with several of the new products, but on investigation it was discovered that the custodians were using the products inappropriately (e.g., at full strength rather than diluted). This finding highlights the importance of active participation by the labor union in decisions about product substitution, and the need for training in product use.

Previous studies of janitorial work have demonstrated that management often pursues a combination of strategies (including job speed-up or work restructuring) to deskill custodial work and to thereby justify harsh labor practices and low pay. Pressure by workers and labor activists for training for custodial workforces is therefore not motivated purely by concerns about occupational health but may also be seen as an effort to defend custodial work as semiskilled labor and thus to restore the dignity of the workers and their right to a living wage (Salzinger

1991; Gottlieb 2001). MassCOSH and the union made worker training and worker input into chemical performance and selection an integral part of the campaign. The presence of MassCOSH as a well-established labor advocate on the project team brought a strong pro-labor voice to the table.

Throughout the pilot evaluation, participation in decision making was a significant issue. School administrators preferred to see the review of cleaning products as a case of top-down decision making, whereas other partners, like MassCOSH and the custodial union, pressed for greater involvement by those using the products. In the words of one school department official, the discussion of shifting to green cleaning products prompted further discussion about school cleaning chemical policies "among ourselves [administrators], which is probably where it belongs anyway." The custodian association president rather pessimistically stated that regardless of the decisions made about the Green Cleaners Project, custodians would have to use whatever products the school department provided. This view was echoed by the custodians in the pilot schools, who universally indicated that they had no input into product selection. Without advocacy by the BUAC and MassCOSH partners, it is unlikely that any call for a review of cleaning products would have arisen from the workforce or been heeded by management. In some respects, then, the greatest success of the Green Cleaners Project team may have been in obtaining employee input into decisions.

Bridge building operates largely through communication, and in particular by communication across the labor-environmental divide. MassCOSH was able to persuade the custodial union of the benefits of adopting a precautionary framework for school environmental health not so much on the strength of claims about alternatives assessment and product substitution as because of the way it democratizes decision making about toxic exposures. This element of the campaign aligned with the strategies of the custodial union in bargaining for training and participation in decision making.

Maintaining a Comprehensive Coalition Frame

Framing is essential if a social movement organization is to communicate its goals effectively, both among its membership and to political decision makers. For cross-movement coalitions such as labor-environmental partnerships, identifying common ground is especially important. Collaborations that link diverse organizations often take modest initial steps whose feasibility and success demonstrate the potential of a long-term collaboration. The Green Cleaners Project team leaders articulated this strategy consciously. By focusing initially on a high-profile school health problem such as asthma, and targeting the substitution of greener cleaning chemicals as a simple solution agreeable to all stakeholders, the team sought to create a solid base for a coalition that would integrate the concerns of school administrators and teachers, custodians, students, and parents; establish

the merit of a precautionary approach to school health issues; and lay a foundation for future campaigns to improve school environmental quality.

The project leaders began their framing efforts by emphasizing the significance
of asthma as a school health issue, suggesting that traditional cleaning products
presented hazards to both employees and students. However, the sparsity of data
that link product substitution and improved health created some difficulties in
getting all parties to agree on a common set of evaluation criteria. Thus project
participants faced a challenge in establishing clear evaluation standards and setting goals that would show how switching cleaning products would clearly advance
the overall goal of improving school environmental health. Several members of
the project team, for example, said that they thought the ultimate decision about
whether the school system should shift to green cleaners should be made on the
basis of whether asthma was actually reduced among students in the pilot schools:
if such data were not available, then cost effectiveness should carry the day.

The project leaders had hoped to sidestep controversies over the lack of
data by including in the framing of the project an orientation toward a broader
prevention-based, or precautionary, approach. Although they believed they had
established the shift to a precautionary stance as the ultimate goal of the project,
several members of the committee (especially the school administrators) insisted
that because the project had begun with a specific discussion of asthma as a school
health issue, they should expect quantifiable evidence that the program was
improving asthma outcomes. This problem persisted despite repeated cautions
from other members of the team that the project did not include monitoring for
a decline in asthma incidence. These misconceptions suggested that the lack of
agreement on evaluation metrics persisted and that at least some members of the
team were in disagreement about the adequacy of a precautionary approach as a
discursive frame to address this potential health issue.

Members of the project team also disagreed about whether the potential health
risks associated with cleaning products should be the chief articulation of the coalition's central issue. Although the representatives from BUAC and MassCOSH
wanted to maintain a focus on health, the custodial union president expressed
concern: "If it's an issue, I have no problem making it a major issue, but if it's not
an issue, I don't really want to scare people about it. But I think if we just explain
that in the long term, these chemicals will be healthier, easy to use, you don't have
to worry if you spill it on you. I mean, some of the chemicals, like the strippers, if
you put it on your hand and didn't wash it off, you got a burn. Stuff like that. If you
use different chemicals, you might not have to worry about that."

This ambivalence represents a legitimate concern on the part of workers: some
of the union members had worked with these potentially hazardous products for
a long time, and the union head did not want to raise concerns about past exposures. In the end, however, he supported the product-substitution effort because

of the broader discursive framing of the campaign, which included the democratizing principles of participation in decision making. Moreover, he reported a
shift in his attitude over the course of the project. After the school department
announced that they would shift to green cleaning products, he reported his
pleasure at this outcome and his appreciation for the assistance the union had
received from MassCOSH and BUAC. On seeing how powerful health messages
and a precautionary approach can be in articulating problems, he described him-
self as being more open to collaboration with other healthy-school advocates.

The union president's initial ambivalence about conveying a strong health
message may have been communicated to the custodians, however, when they
were trained in using the new products. When a sample of four of the eighteen
custodians in the pilot schools were asked by researchers why they thought the
school system had shifted to these newer cleaning products, two recalled having been told that the products were safer or healthier for themselves and the
students; the other two replied that they thought the shift had been made to save
storage space or because the new products were cheaper. The two janitors who
were aware of the health-based rationale for product substitution also had more
favorable impressions of the new products. One of these custodians has asthma
and appreciated the new products because, unlike the old products, they did not
appear to induce wheezing. In contrast, the two custodians who believed the shift
had been made for other reasons were more critical of the products' performance
and indicated that decisions on shifting to green cleaners should be made on the
basis of cost. Custodians' lack of awareness about the importance of health in
making the shift to green cleaners may have influenced their assessment of the
new products, as their application often differs significantly from that of traditional products and requires more physical labor.

The connection between the strategic aims of the cleaning-products substitution project and the discursive project drawing attention to school environmental
health problems was perceived best by individuals who were themselves suffering
from health problems. Custodians who suffered from asthma were more likely to
connect the project with the larger goal of improving health, whereas custodians
who perceived themselves to be in good health and unaffected by the traditional
cleaning products viewed the pilot project as a simple administrative shift in the
materials they were instructed to use. Thus, if personal experience mediates the
acceptance of a coalition frame, organizers should decide which parts of the frame
or message need to be made explicit.

The challenge of constructing a coalition collective-action frame for this project demonstrates that even when all parties have a stake in creating and maintaining a healthy school environment, they may approach the problem from
different angles, with different understandings of the scope of the problem and
different goals for remediation. More opportunities for engaged and participatory

discussions of environmental quality early in the process could have helped in clarifying the goals and positions of all stakeholders, in enumerating and prioritizing environmental problems, and in developing a plan that satisfied the interests of all stakeholders. Candid and frequent discussion of how short-term projects relate to overall long-term strategies are also important.

INTEGRATING HEALTH AND WORKER TRAINING INTO A SUCCESSFUL LABOR-ENVIRONMENT COALITION

The Green Cleaners Project's alliance of environmental health and labor activists, workers, and school administrators is a model other school districts can follow to foster a healthy environment for students and staff. By building a coalition among multiple stakeholders, all of whom have a material interest in managing school environmental quality, the project leaders were able to mitigate or neutralize ideological divisions that have traditionally scuttled cooperative efforts between labor and environmental movement organizations.

The participation of such a varied group of participants demanded the construction of a robust coalition frame. The precautionary principle made a good basis for this frame because team members could match its tenets to the environmental health activists' interest in product substitution as well as to the union's objectives of improving worker training and expanding workers' participation in decision making. The Green Cleaners Project provides a model for building new forms of labor-environmental coalitions, with bridge-building organizations such as MassCOSH occupying a critical role in mediation.

The project leaders were careful in framing the issues in this project: first, they selected a high-profile health issue, student asthma, to stimulate a wider debate about school environmental quality; and second, they invoked a philosophy of precaution as a means of mitigating the problem. This strategy allowed them to gain the attention of school officials by invoking a well-documented student health problem, and then to fold in a latent concern about the effect of cleaning products on workers' health. It is unlikely that the custodial union would have been effective in challenging decisions about the selection of cleaning products because of its relatively weak bargaining position.

The second strategy, framing the issue from a precautionary standpoint, allowed the team leaders to sidestep problems of demonstrating improved health outcomes in the absence of quantifiable data. However, a tension emerged between the more strategically oriented frame of reducing asthma and the broader discursive framing in favor of precaution-based environmental health policies. Nevertheless, setting the initial objective of product substitution allowed project leaders to link this campaign to larger campaigns at the state and national levels that invoke precaution as a rationale for improving and protecting school environmental quality.

Constructing a coalition frame that is broad enough to address and support the individual and common needs of a variety of organizations is a delicate process, and the experience of this team points to some clear deficiencies in theories of frame development and maintenance. The project leaders relied on the logic of the precautionary principle because they believed its tenets could unify the disparate needs of the coalition partners. In practice, this meant that they relied on some elements of precaution in conversations with some coalition members more than in discussions with others, especially in the early, crucial stages of coalition formation. The fact that not all coalition members readily embraced all elements of the principle (the union president was initially hesitant, and school administrators were resistant throughout the process) might suggest that the attempt to bridge the frames of the coalition partners was not wholly successful, even though the coalition did achieve its goal of product substitution. Theories of frame bridging and alignment need to be expanded to help us understand how and when coalition partners activate or rely on particular strategic or discursive elements of the frame to build the partnership. More theoretical work is also needed to help us understand how and when a coalition can persist and succeed when not all members have embraced all the elements of a complex frame, and how and when it might fail entirely. Though here we have stressed the importance of framing over more structural elements, building solidarity between labor and environmental organizations involves finding both a common ideological frame and the structural means to allow the groups to work together. By building ties through the promotion of the precautionary principle, the coalition leaders tied the concept of prevention to the more concrete goals of democratic decision making and increased worker control over working conditions.

As existing school infrastructure continues to deteriorate and funding remains inadequate, school environmental quality will become a greater problem for schools nationwide. The model of collaboration between diverse stakeholders adopted in Boston can serve as an example for other health and safety activists. Concerns are growing about toxic exposures for service-sector workers (Gottlieb 2001). From the perspective of labor unions and worker organizations seeking new issues to emphasize in organizing campaigns (Clawson 2003), health and safety and the environment are becoming central issues (Gould, Lewis, and Roberts 2004; Obach 2004a; Mayer, Brown, and Senier 2008). Furthermore, by arguing that workers should have a voice in decisions about the selection of products they use on a daily basis, campaigns such as the Green Cleaners Project are also advocating for worker empowerment and a larger role in decision making.

This program also highlights challenges and pitfalls that may beset blue-green or school environmental health coalitions. Although the team had some success in integrating the concerns of school administrators, custodians, and environmental health groups, some stakeholders were absent from the discussions: other school employees, such as kitchen and cafeteria workers; teachers; and parents. All these groups are affected by and can influence the implementation and effectiveness of new policies. BUAC has been particularly successful in enlisting parent advocates, for example by training them to testify in support of various pieces of legislation. Parents should be briefed on the Green Cleaners Project so that they can advocate for healthier school policies locally and statewide. Although including additional stakeholders in the process could complicate the decision-making process, it could also strengthen awareness of school environmental problems and enhance the community's commitment to school environmental health.

MassCOSH as a Bridge Builder

Since the success of the Green Cleaners Project, MassCOSH has continued its work in lobbying for toxics-use reduction and expanded its organizing role by advocating for legislative and administrative policies and practices that protect nonunionized workers. MassCOSH has also sought to influence toxics-use reduction more directly by supporting small business owners who wish to adopt safer chemical practices. For example, it helped a women's cooperative group of house cleaners to purchase green cleaning chemicals in bulk for its members. It has also helped train cosmetologists in exposure-reduction practices to protect them and their clients from fumes in beauty salons.

Most of the work of MassCOSH, however, focuses on policy advocacy, and in 2005, MassCOSH again played a bridge-building role in a project to mitigate hazards to contractors who sand and refinish hardwood floors. In 2005, two house fires in the Boston area occurred while hardwood floors were being sanded and refinished. The fires resulted in the deaths of three Vietnamese workers who were working with highly toxic and flammable lacquer-based floor-finishing products. Many Vietnamese immigrants and refugees have settled in the Boston area, where a number have found jobs in the floor-finishing industry. Although some operate as independent contractors, others are employed informally, for low wages, and without the protection of a union or government oversight to ensure health and safety (Azaroff et al. 2011). Over the past decade, more than two dozen similar fires have occurred in the Boston area, leading to more than a million dollars' worth of property damage.

In response to these episodes, MassCOSH convened a working group that brought together chemical suppliers, distributors, and representatives from the community of independent contractors who work with these chemicals. This working group received consulting support from TURI, which evaluated the lacquer-based chemicals used in floor sanding and refinishing processes and identified safer, readily available water-based alternatives. They issued a white paper summarizing their findings, conducted education and outreach among the contractors who apply these chemicals (many of whom are Vietnamese and Cape Verdean), and convened a task force that would advise on the development of legislation to regulate the chemicals in use in this industry.

The task force meetings were important in bringing together representatives from the major chemical suppliers and distributors in a forum where they could all agree on the dangers involved in the continued use of the lacquer-based chemicals. In the absence of legislation banning the products, a joint pledge to withdraw them from the market simultaneously (so that no supplier or distributor would retain an unfair sales advantage) was an important step in protecting the health of the contractors. Perhaps predictably, some contractors objected, because lacquer-based chemicals allow them to work more quickly. But through the task force, suppliers, distributors, and contractors could agree on the hazards posed by these products and the process of withdrawing them, both to protect worker health and safety and to create a level playing field for the other stakeholders.

As in the Green Cleaners Project, MassCOSH played an important role as a bridge builder. The task was more complex in this instance, partly because of the decentralized and nonunionized workforce but also because the involvement of the business community was different. Many more small decision makers needed to be persuaded to change their purchasing practices, as opposed to a central purchasing office in a school bureaucracy. This project also marked the first time that MassCOSH worked directly with business owners (the chemical suppliers and distributors), and the project leader was initially anxious that those parties might attempt to stonewall efforts at product substitution. In the end, however, this concern was unfounded, perhaps because of the highly public and tragic incidents that triggered the task force's formation. Overall, MassCOSH's success in bringing together diverse stakeholders—academic health and safety experts from TURI, the chemical suppliers, the distributors, and the independent contractors—enhanced the task force's credibility. It has achieved unofficial recognition as a source of authoritative information on the hazards in the floor-sanding industry. The Massachusetts State Fire Marshal's office has appealed to the task force for advice in revising parts of the fire code, and a bill was introduced into the Massachusetts legislature in 2006 to prohibit the sale and use of the most hazardous chemicals used in floor finishing and to ensure worker training in the proper application of the safer formulations of these chemicals. The Massachusetts legislature passed the bill, and the new regulations took effect on June 1, 2010 (MA CMR 527 10.15).

CONCLUSION

MassCOSH's involvement in the Green Cleaners Project was critical in enlisting the support and participation of all stakeholders throughout the process and led to the achievement of three practical objectives. First, the project team leaders pressed the school department for a commitment to train custodians in the proper use of new products. The custodial union had long demanded improved training for its workers but had needed to subordinate these demands to its efforts to protect jobs and wages. Second, the formalization of an alliance of organizations making up the Green Cleaners Project, through the citywide school health task force, provided a mechanism for detection of health problems in the schools in the future and a forum in which these problems could be discussed and solutions could be entertained. Finally, the cooperation of the custodial union with labor advocates and environmental health activists laid the groundwork for future collaborations in which custodians can document the persistence or emergence of problems that threaten school environmental quality. Although there are other healthy-schools programs around the country, the Massachusetts project is among the few that include custodial unions as core partners.

Along with these findings, this case study raises some provocative questions about bridge-building and framing strategies that may be useful for blue-green coalitions and coalitions working to address problems of school environmental quality. The precautionary principle can serve as a frame flexible enough to meet the needs of environmental health activists while also fulfilling labor's desire for participatory decision making in matters of occupational health and social justice. This work also highlights the importance of bridge-building organizations in the formation of coalitions, especially ones that include labor activists and labor unionists. Our analysis offers approaches for examining broader and more complex coalitions than typical blue-green alliances. More work is needed to determine how, whether, and when coalitions decide to adopt the logic of precaution; how it affects the composition of the coalition; and how it contributes to a coalition's success.

NOTE

Originally published as Laura Senier, Brian Mayer, Phil Brown, and Rachel Morello-Frosch, "School Custodians and Green Cleaners: New Approaches to Labor-Environmental Coalitions," *Organization and Environment* 20 (2007): 304–24.

11

Labor-Environmental Coalition Formation

Framing and the Right to Know

Brian Mayer, Phil Brown, and Rachel Morello-Frosch

Labor unions and environmental organizations occasionally become allies in the fight for the protection of workplace and environmental health. An increasing number of collaborations between "blues" and "greens" in the United States have been identified by social movement scholars (Minchin 2003; Obach 2004a; Estabrook 2006; Mayer 2008). Unions like the United Steelworkers are redefining the labor movement's political agenda and working to build ties with nontypical allies, including the environmental movement. This collaboration may redefine the relationships between these two social movements and offer new opportunities for advancing workplace safety and environmental health through the linkage of two distinct narratives of risk.

Social movement organizations that work together in coalitions may be more likely to succeed than individual organizations (Gamson 1990; Rose 2000; Jones et al. 2001; Van Dyke 2003). However, the potential coalition partners for particular organizations may be limited to those within the same movement (Van Dyke 2003). This limitation may reduce the likelihood of success when issues or solutions affect a diverse array of social movement organizations. Cross-movement coalitions are more likely to provide a broad base of mobilization. In order to form coalitions with partners that have potentially conflicting identities, however, movement organizers must invest additional resources and energy in building bridges.

Relationships between the labor and environmental movements exist within a complex web of clashing interests, electoral politics, and attempts to form both short-term and enduring coalitions. Working-class activists often find middle-class activists to be unresponsive or condescending (Mix and Cable 2006). Class differences between the two movements often perpetuate the stereotype of a "jobs versus the environment" divide. In this class-driven model, unions and other labor organizations are interested primarily in protecting existing employment opportunities and, to a lesser extent, economic growth, which is often idealized by the labor movement as creating new jobs (even though economic growth is not always associated with new jobs and is instead driven by downsizing and outsourcing). Environmental protection and regulation, which can limit economic growth and employment opportunities, are perceived as threats to jobs— driving the labor movement to ally with industry in opposition to environmental organizations (Schnaiberg, Watts, and Zimmermann 1986; Kazis and Grossman 1990; Gottlieb 2005; Mayer 2008). However, fighting the traditional "growth model" has sometimes aligned labor and environmental interests more closely, as the practice of eliminating jobs in order to promote growth may also have detrimental effects on environmental protection and occupational health.

In these circumstances, labor and environmental organizations have sometimes been able to see past their differences and develop collaborative campaigns and coalitions to address problems of shared concern. Labor-environmental coalitions represent an ideal social-movement dynamic for study because of their frequently opposed ideologies and the inherent challenge of bridging across movements and socioeconomic classes.

This chapter examines the formation of a cross-movement coalition involving labor, environmental, and community organizations in New Jersey during the 1980s. The New Jersey Right-to-Know Coalition developed in response to community and worker concerns about the risk of contaminant exposure from New Jersey's sizeable chemical industry. Building on the political momentum from a related campaign in Philadelphia, environmental and labor activists in New Jersey made a crucial decision to join forces in their push for regulatory reform of the state's hazardous-material management system. Through this collaboration, they achieved a more sweeping reform than either movement could have achieved on its own.

Based on Van Dyke's (2003) analysis of the conditions under which cross-movement coalitions are likely to form, we examine the formation and initial campaigns of the New Jersey Right-to-Know coalition. We emphasize the importance of framing, both in the development of cross-movement relationships and in the internal dynamic of the coalition. We examine how diverse coalition partners orient and frame their approaches and ideologies to recruit partner organizations and overcome tensions. Because the labor and environmental movements are among the nation's largest and most significant, this study offers insights for understanding the emergence of other seemingly unlikely coalitions.

FORMING A CROSS-MOVEMENT COALITION

Studies of interaction between social movement organizations tend to examine organizational relationships within a single social movement (Van Dyke 2003). Examples include the organizational analysis of the civil rights movement (Morris 1984), the women's movement (Staggenborg 1986), and the environmental movement (Lichterman 1995). Even when interaction between movements rather than organizations is examined, analyses tend to focus on the "movement conflux" (Mottl 1980) or "loose coupling" between movement and countermovement (Zald and Useem 1987). These studies suggest that the dynamic relationship between movement and countermovement influences all aspects of organizational activity, from recruitment to campaign mobilization. This perspective offers only a limited understanding of coalition behavior because organizations from similar or related movements are more likely to share common elements. Further investigation is needed to understand how dissimilar groups, despite their differences, interact and develop collaborative relationships in cross-movement coalitions, and whether and how these collaborative relationships are sustained.

When organizations within a single movement must compete for limited resources, they are unlikely to engage in coalition building strategies (Staggenborg 1986; Minkoff 1997; Van Dyke 2003). Cross-movement coalitions are less influenced by competition for economic or organizational resources, as their constituent movements typically draw from different resource pools. Resource scarcity may in fact drive the formation of cross-movement coalitions, because conditions adversely affecting one movement's resources may encourage partnering with a different type of movement in order to access a different pool of resources.

In labor-environmental coalitions, each movement utilizes fairly distinct resources. Environmental organizations rely on voluntary memberships, grant support, and individual donations, whereas unions are supported by membership dues and hierarchical organizational structures. Union members may occasionally join environmental organizations out of individual interest, but the perception of a conflict of interest tends to discourage collaboration (Obach 2004a). However, unions are coming under increased financial pressure. Fifty years ago, they represented roughly one-third of the workforce, but today the figure is approximately one-tenth (US Bureau of Labor Statistics 2007). The resultant decline in financial resources generated through dues and political influence has substantially weakened the labor movement. Hence unions may seek limited political influence from collaborations with external, nontraditional allies.

Van Dyke (2003) uses resource mobilization and political opportunity theory to explain why cross-movement coalitions emerge. She finds that intramovement coalitions tend to develop in order to better raise and manage funds and other necessary organizational resources. By contrast, cross-movement coalitions form out of a sense of a shared collective identity rather than a desire to share resources. These findings point to the importance of identity and ideological bridge-building between various social movement sectors. They lead us to ask what aspects of union and environmental collective identities might be linked and to study the political contexts in which bridge building occurs.

Coalitions may be perceived by social movement leaders as too risky to pursue when individual organizations face limited local political opportunities. Thus whereas intramovement coalitions are likely to develop in response to local political threats (Gerhards and Rucht 1992; McCammon and Campbell 2002), cross-movement coalitions typically develop in response to broader political threats that challenge commonly shared values (Van Dyke 2003, 229). For instance, blue-green alliances are much less common in Republican-controlled states (Obach 2004). Whereas one might predict that unions and environmental organizations would collaborate against a common conservative political opponent, Obach's survey found that these organizations attempted to conserve political resources by limiting electoral collaboration and focusing on single-issue campaigns. Although cross-movement coalitions may be more likely to develop in the context of broad political threats, their durability in the face of shifting political opportunities is less clear.

Shifting political opportunities and resource scarcity may drive coalitions together, but the ties that bind coalitions are more likely to be developed over time through the deliberate actions of movement leaders. Frame analysis views social movement actors as having the agency to guide the development of their organizations (Benford and Snow 2000). Frames refer to interpretative schemata (Goffman 1974) that allow individuals or social groups to locate and situate social phenomena in a way that makes these phenomena meaningful (Snow et al. 1986). Collective-action frames are employed by movement leaders to "mobilize potential adherents and constituents, to garner bystander support, and to demobilize antagonists" (Snow and Benford 1988). Effective frames are those that most resonate with broader cultural values and are therefore most salient to potential adherents' and constituents' life experiences (Kubal 1998; Benford and Snow 2000).

By shaping and constructing these collective-action frames, coalition leaders bring together individuals from diverse organizations that may never have interacted previously. Collective-action frames also function within a social movement organization by establishing a common interpretation of an ideology or perspective that unites movement members (Snow et al. 1986; Johnston 1995; McAdam, McCarthy, and Zald 1996). Maintaining a coalition-based collective-action frame that consolidates internal solidarity while weathering external forces requires leaders to engage constantly with coalition partners and can often limit the development of new frames.

Benford and Snow's elaboration of frame alignment, and in particular frame bridging, "the linking of two or more ideologically congruent but structurally unconnected frames regarding a particular issue or problem," elucidates how multiple social movement organizations identify and use such a common discourse (2000, 624). This process of linking entails the highlighting and elaboration of ideological similarities between organizational frames in order to construct a collective-action frame for a coalition that provides cohesion between the partners' various ideologies.

Coalition leaders construct collective-action frames by bridging ideological divides, but their ability to do so is limited by external political opportunities and organizational resources. Shifting political opportunity structures can both enable and constrain the formation of cross-movement coalitions (Meyer and Corrigal-Brown 2005). Although the construction of a collective-action frame is a necessary condition for coalition formation, shifts in political opportunities often create new opportunities for collaboration, such as backing a particular piece of legislation or political candidate. Conversely, shifts in political opportunities can create opportunities for conflict.

A thorough understanding of why cross-movement coalitions form and persist must be informed by a grasp of resource mobilization, framing, and political opportunity. For studying labor-environment coalitions, the best synthesis may be the interaction between framing and political opportunities. The framing perspective alone fails to address the political context in which coalition leaders must construct a collective-action frame. Likewise, because cross-movement coalitions require careful attention to communicating across movement boundaries and accommodating differences, the political-opportunities perspective fails to account for leaders' agency in bringing groups together. By examining the interplay between political opportunity and framing, we can better understand the dynamics of cross-movement coalition building.

METHODS AND DATA

This study is based on ethnographic and historical research on the formation and political trajectory of a cross-movement coalition involving labor, environmental, and community organizations in New Jersey. Data were collected over a four-year period (2004–8), and sources include retrospective interviews, participant-observations, organizations' documents, and news media. A total of twenty-seven interviews were conducted with the organization that was formerly called the New Jersey Right-to-Know, today known as the Work Environment Council (WEC), and related organizations. Subjects were identified through past and present membership rosters and through a snowball sampling frame that ensured equal representation of labor, environmental, and community leaders. This approach helped in recruiting participants from labor organizations, whose members had the highest levels of turnover in participation in the blue-green coalitions. Many environmental leaders and activists in the coalition remained members and were therefore easier to identify.

Semistructured interview questions asked respondents to identify their organization's core agenda and strategic goals and to explain how these goals and actions fit into the larger context of the cross-movement coalition. Questions asked respondents to reflect on their decision to participate in the coalition and the level of organizational support they received. Respondents were asked to specifically identify the perceived costs and benefits to them of collaborating with nontraditional coalition partners. To supplement these findings, we conducted seven ethnographic observations of meetings, legislative hearings, protests, news conferences, and forums. In addition, we collected and analyzed both published and unpublished documents from the Work Environment Council.

Interview transcripts and observation notes were analyzed using QSR NVivo, which allows qualitative researchers to assign codes to segments of interview transcripts and observation notes and assists with the exploration of relationships within the data. Transcripts and notes were coded and analyzed according to a preexisting set of thematic topics, and new themes were developed through an inductive analytic process while coding the data. Extracts representative of these key themes are presented throughout.

CROSS-MOVEMENT COALITION CASE STUDY: THE NEW JERSEY RIGHT-TO-KNOW COALITION

The New Jersey Right-to-Know Coalition formed in 1982 as a grassroots response to communities' and workers' concerns regarding the use, storage, and transportation of toxic substances. Although coalition leaders constructed a persuasive collective-action frame and won an early victory, state-level shifts in political opportunity structures subsequently limited the strategies and tactics of the coalition. We examine the relationship between framing and political opportunities in the context of a failed attempt to advance what the coalition actors believed to be a logical transition from winning the right to know to pursuing the right to act on that information.

A Joint Community and Worker Right to Know

The history of the New Jersey Right-to-Know Coalition begins across the Delaware River in Philadelphia, where occupational health and community activism during the late 1970s developed in response to widespread fears that the area's petrochemical refineries were poisoning residents. Community organizers partnered with union health and safety activists and environmentalists to lobby for a legislative reform of Philadelphia's chemical management policies (Ochsner 1992).

Leading this collaboration was the Philadelphia Project for Occupational Safety and Health (PhilaPOSH), one of the first and largest examples of a committee on occupational safety and health (COSH). COSH groups were formed in the 1960s and 1970s to act as semiprofessional organizations that aided workers, union and nonunion, with issues related to health and safety. In 1981, the community-labor coalition backed the passage of the first community right-to-know law in the United States. The *right to know* refers to reporting requirements imposed on businesses using or storing hazardous chemicals. Databases are generated for public use on the levels of pollution and the potential health risks for particular communities.

Health and safety activists in the labor movement in Philadelphia were motivated to campaign for a right-to-know law by a growing frustration in trying to improve hazardous working conditions in settings where employees were forced to work with unlabeled materials that carried unknown health risks. Chemical corporations argued that providing information to workers and health inspectors would force them to disclose trade secrets; this argument prevented unions from negotiating with management over the issue. The right to know was viewed by industrial managers as a contractual issue, like wages and health care, to be negotiated behind closed doors between industry and union representatives.

Unable to win at the bargaining table, union leaders and health and safety activists framed the problem as a violation of a basic civil right to access information about health and safety. This transformation marked a shift away from framing the issue as a traditional dispute between management and union leaders and toward a broader social critique of corporate malfeasance. A growing consumer-rights movement, combined with an increasing public distrust of many corporate practices, made for a broad public demand for more access to information. An organizer from PhilaPOSH who was instrumental in the formation of the right-to-know campaign highlights the growing frustration with industry's reluctance to provide information on hazardous materials: "We would raise these kinds of points and all these kinds of problems, pointing out that there is no right, even at that late date, which was approaching 1980—no right of workers to even know what it was that they were working with. That the company could just say: 'You're working with "Super-Wizzy-Clean Number 5." And I don't care that your rash is all over your body and you can't breathe when you work with it. We don't have to tell you what it really is.' And essentially that was the deal. And people were incensed at that. Say, you mean to tell me that we don't have that right, right now? So it was easy to rile folks up. It was a real volatile issue."

Realizing that political and public sympathy for unions was declining after President Ronald Reagan broke the Professional Air Traffic Controllers Organization strike in August 1981, the PhilaPOSH activists worked with community and environmental organizations to broaden their base beyond unions. They formed a cross-movement coalition involving a variety of social movement organizations, including environmental groups. By promoting a collective-action frame that linked the rather narrow issue of the labeling of hazardous materials in the workplace to illegal industrial pollution affecting all of Philadelphia, the health and labor activists were able to recruit many powerful social movement organizations that had never campaigned in conjunction with labor unions before. For example, in March 1979, PhilaPOSH and the Environmental Cancer Prevention Center, a community education program, jointly organized a conference on toxic exposures that brought together more than 350 labor, environmental, and community organizers, many of whom were meeting for the first time. Many of the health and safety activists associated with PhilaPOSH had previously employed direct-action tactics as part of union strikes and boycotts and welcomed the opportunity to challenge the political influence of industrial corporations by employing nontraditional tactics, such as local community protests. Rather than work to improve workplace health by filing grievances and bargaining for additional safety measures, organizers decided to publicize the plight of the industrial worker and link workplace hazards to a major threat to public health.

The combined political clout of this coalition surprised the Philadelphia city council members and generated enough legislative support to pass the nation's first citywide right-to-know law. Unable to quell worker dissent solely through contract negotiations, local politicians and business elites were forced to concede the need for better management of hazardous-substances information.

As labor and community activists were achieving success in Philadelphia, several local environmental organizations in New Jersey were beginning to formulate a plan for promoting the passage of a similar right-to-know law in their state. Fearing an accidental toxic release from any of New Jersey's many chemical refineries, community and environmental activists wanted access to information about chemicals they might be exposed to.

Our interviews revealed strong feelings of frustration among the New Jersey environmental community around the time the Philadelphia right-to-know law was passed. Unable to convince state politicians to enact the type of sweeping community right-to-know laws that many environmental groups desired, several environmental leaders felt that winning local city ordinances providing the right to know on a smaller scale was sufficient to advance their agenda. Many of the environmental organizations involved were small, local groups that lacked the coordination to manage a statewide effort. They emphasized the immediate need to protect their families and neighborhoods, which translated into distinct political demands ranging from the complete elimination of all potential hazards to the provision of technical information on hazardous substances.

Interest groups in New Jersey, particularly environmental organizations, have traditionally had little influence over state politics because of their fractious and often contentious competition for organizational resources and political influence. Facing a Republican governor backed by corporate interests, largely from industrial chemical firms, many environmental activists expressed frustration with the lack of immediate response from state legislators. In this case, in contrast to Obach's (2004a) findings regarding the unlikelihood of blue-green coalition formation in Republican-controlled states, the challenge of facing a conservative government backed by the very industries creating the grievances galvanized activists from environmental and labor movements to seek each other out and work together. However, this decision to collaborate required several environmental groups to give up their local campaigns and shift their attention to the statewide efforts. Because previous efforts to organize a solely environmental or labor campaign to challenge the political influence of the chemical industry had failed at the state level, the would-be leaders of the blue-green coalition adopted an alternative organizational form and a new collective-action frame to convince local organizations to join the new coalition promoting the right to know.

Antitoxics activism in the early 1980s was largely conducted by middle-class environmental activists who feared toxic waste buried in their neighborhoods or the drifting of poisonous fumes from refining facilities upwind from their neighborhoods. Groups like the Environmental Lobby, the New Jersey Environmental Federation, and the state branch of the Sierra Club were among the most prominent campaigners. These activists framed the right to know as a basic right that should be granted to all individuals to enable them to protect themselves from toxic exposures. This framing typically labeled workers as part of the problem, lumping unions together with the chemical industry as a single antagonist. By framing toxic waste as "toxic trespass" perpetrated by industry with the silent consent of workers, these groups' initial campaign perpetuated the stereotypical "jobs versus the environment" approach to environmental organizing that led to the historical blue/green divide. While these environmental groups narrowly advocated for community-based right-to-know legislation, leaders in the nascent coalition-building effort decided to push for a bill that would include worker and community rights to access information on hazardous substances.

In early 1982, just as the possibility of creating a right-to-know law was gaining public attention, several state legislators entered the political fray. Sensing that New Jersey could be the first state where such a major shift in environmental policy occurred, politicians on both sides of the aisle began promoting their own versions of right-to-know laws. A junior state senator, Dan Dalton, had made environmental policy a centerpiece of his agenda and was quickly persuaded to champion the right to know. Recognizing the looming battle between industry and environmental groups, Dalton's legislative staff, together with counsel from several activist organizations, decided to try to gain the support of organized labor before the industrial firms could coerce unions into lockstep (Ochsner 1992).

This crucial decision was guided by the experience of the labor organizers from Philadelphia, who joined the New Jersey push for right-to-know legislation because many of the workers whose health and safety they had fought for originally at the city level lived just across the Delaware River in New Jersey and in some instances belonged to unions that represented workers in both states. Key environmental organizers, such as Jim Lanard of the Environmental Lobby, had experience in working on legislative agendas and political campaigns with labor leaders—though not in direct collaboration or resource sharing. However, their familiarity with the operations of the labor movement and its leaders in New Jersey proved useful in organizing meetings and persuading labor leaders to consider joining a coalition. For labor organizers from Philadelphia who had worked with community and environmental groups to pass their city right-to-know law, New Jersey represented a more realistic opportunity to establish a statewide right to know than they were likely to have in Pennsylvania. PhilaPOSH organizers brought their excitement and experience from the Philadelphia campaign to New Jersey and found the work of bridging relatively easy, as a labor organizer from Philadelphia elaborated:

> The deal we did in Philadelphia was the right to know, not only for workers, but for community residents who may want information. That was a first and that really struck at the heart of a whole lot of this stuff that they were hiding from people in general. Workers were of course on the front lines of trying to get that information and protect their numbers from exposures and sickness and cancers and dying and all that. But the community suffered just as well from what was in the air and in the water and from fugitive emissions and spills, leaks, and fires and what have you. So they had a stake in it. When we began working in New Jersey, it was fairly easy to convince [environmental groups] that it was their fight as well as the fight of workers.

In a state with a high level of chemical manufacturing and refining, the number of political actors directly or indirectly dependent on the chemical industry was significant, and politicians advocating the right to know needed union support to overcome political resistance. Major unions, such as the United Steelworkers of America; the Oil, Chemical, and Atomic Workers; the United Auto Workers; and the Communication Workers of America all sent representatives to a May 1982 meeting with environmental organizers and state politicians to discuss the dynamics of a joint worker and community right-to-know campaign. More than fifty thousand workers were represented at the meeting by thirty-two unions that agreed to participate in the fledgling coalition.

Mirroring the Philadelphia campaign's emphasis on worker health and safety, coalition leaders approached union locals with workplace-hazard organizing experience about collaborating with community and environmental organizations to pass a joint right-to-know law that provided an equal level of information to all parties. Initially, their campaign strategies varied with the constituency. Drawing on the antitoxics framing of campaigns against hazardous waste, coalition leaders used terms such as *toxic trespass* and *violations of rights* to describe residents' fear of not knowing whether hazardous chemicals might be stored or used at a facility in their backyard. The testimony below, from an environmental activist who had worked for years to address the issue of asbestos contamination, highlights the uncertainty and skepticism of many antitoxics groups: "My neighbors and friends are dying by the week. It is a tragedy. But where do we go? . . . How many of you are victims or potential victims? How many of you have been exposed to the water you drank that was supplied by an asbestos pipe? Or your children were exposed to asbestos ceilings in the schoolrooms or tile floors? How are we supposed to know?" Union organizers like Matt Gillen of the Amalgamated Clothing and Textile Workers Union took a different approach: "Powerful disincentives exist against the dissemination of hazard information. Liability pressures from workers' compensation costs, engineering costs, and lost sales all contribute to a tendency to withhold delicate information. Basically, what we are saying is that we don't think we can trust employers" (quoted in Engler 1992).

Although the fear and uncertainty discussed by many other environmental activists generated public interest, it provided few specific legislative solutions. The unions' perspectives emphasized fundamentally altering the work environment to revalue worker health and safety—an important goal among union activists, but one that lacked widespread public support. Organizers from key organizations such as PhilaPOSH and the Environmental Lobby built on these two articulations of the problem and merged them to frame the issue of the right to know as a fundamental right that was being violated by corporate interests in the pursuit of profit.

By creating conceptual bridges between these two frames and constructing a common discourse, leaders formed a cross-movement coalition. Both environmental and labor activists could claim that chemicals and substances stored and used in industrial facilities were the sources of contamination, creating a series of "toxic circles" (Sheehan and Wedeen 1993) emanating outward from manufacturing facilities and affecting workers and communities alike. Rather than identifying as either environmentalists or trade unionists, all coalition members could define themselves as potential victims of unsympathetic industries interested only in profit. The coalition provided common ground for understanding the disparate groups' similar experiences and grievances with the chemical industry and for agreement on the need for legislative reform.

Calling themselves the New Jersey Right-to-Know Coalition, New Jersey environmental leaders and former PhilaPOSH organizers developed a unified agenda to pass worker and community right-to-know legislation, posing the issue primarily as one of safety. They pointed out that exposure to hazardous substances in the workplace killed thousands each year, and they emphasized the risks to residents living near these facilities. They emphasized workers' lack of access to information about chemicals used and stored at their workplace. This point reformulated the common antitoxics approach that had heretofore prevented labor-environment coalitions: an approach that emphasized finding the source of pollution and eliminating it completely, regardless of who might be employed by a particular industrial plant or the effect on their jobs.

Environmentalists' concerns with toxic chemicals were expressed largely as fears of hypothetical situations: for example, that New Jersey might face a major problem like the discovery of buried barrels of toxic waste at Love Canal, NY (see Levine 1982), or groundwater contamination of trichloroethylene and other industrial solvents in Woburn, MA (see Brown and Mikkelsen 1997). Unionists in New Jersey however, did not have to rely on hypothetical situations to make their case. Workers' moving testimonials about the harm they suffered from toxic exposures worked both within the coalition to motivate community and environmental members to partner with the unions, and externally to motivate politicians to act. The political strength of the blue-green coalition hinged on the combination of two narratives of hazard, with the public-health concerns of environmentalists and community activists overlying the specific and substantiated incidents of industrial accidents and deaths among workers in New Jersey.

The unions' support offered a powerful rebuttal to industry arguments against the enactment of right-to-know laws. These focused on the economic costs of reporting requirements, as an industry lobbyist noted: "It is true that it is difficult to point to any single issue when a business leaves the state. But there are many nails that go into that coffin—maybe three, four, five nails—and we're saying this right-to-know legislation will be another nail" (quoted in Engler 1992). Union participation in the campaign for the right to know reduced the power of assertions that reporting requirements would lead to industrial job losses.

Community residents, preoccupied with unknown hazards such as groundwater poisoning, buried toxic waste, and air pollution, were at first not especially concerned with the chemical workers' plight. One member of the Right-to-Know Coalition commented: "Prior to that, I didn't think that workers either knew very much or cared very much about the exposures that they might have on the job. Or that they would feel that they could be empowered to do anything about it to address the situation. It's basically, okay, you take that job. You know you're going to be working with hazardous substances . . . that's tough. Take it or leave it. It didn't occur to me that people could actually affect the policy in a workplace." After being approached by founders of the New Jersey Right-to-Know Coalition and listening to the accounts of hazardous working conditions, however, this activist revised her perception of the relationship between workers and environ-mentalists: "Hearing those stories of working with substances that they didn't know about, . . . having their skin burn, their eyes burning, coughing, and seeing their fellow workers die . . . made an impact on me. I realized that this wasn't a hypothetical. These were real cases of bad things happening." Several other par-ticipants in the Right-to-Know Coalition recalled similar moments where their preconceptions of the "other side" were challenged through the sharing of per-sonal narratives and experiences.

Within the coalition, union health and safety activists proposed several mea-sures that gained the support of environmental activists. Antitoxics activists in particular supported the call for access to understandable information about chemicals of concern, as one noted: "To us, the sexiest part of the law was these hazardous substance fact sheets that would be produced that would be written in everyday language. They would be developed for common hazardous chemicals that would be in the workplace. But these very same hazardous substances are also in household products, in pesticides. And we thought, once and for all we're going to have a fact sheet for all the pesticides that we're concerned about." Union members provided similar testimony, sometimes dramatic. During a legislative hearing on the right-to-know bill, United Auto Workers representative Bill Kane "placed a small red tank on the speaker's table and opened a valve, [allowing] a colorless and odorless gas to leak into the room. As the gas seeped into the room, one state senator shouted, 'Mr. Kane, I have a right to know what this is!' Kane responded with the token reassurance of an employer, 'Don't worry. We've been using this for years and no one has died yet'" (Ochsner 1992, 185).

Creating the link between workplace and community exposure to hazardous substances was crucial to building the coalition, according to one activist: "So I saw workers and community people or environmental people who had never sat in the same room before. Never had a sense of who 'the other side was.' And it was interesting in the end, they were like, 'You don't really want to shut us down?' And 'Oh, you really just want it to be safer.' . . . But you know, somebody who is a straight environmentalist and they don't have any interaction with workers, they don't think about this stuff."

Highly publicized environmental crises in New Jersey, including the discovery of dioxin contamination in a former manufacturing site in Newark and a chemi-cal fire in Edison in early 1983, boosted support for the right-to-know campaign by increasing public awareness of and sympathy for workers. The solidarity and political savvy of the Right-to-Know Coalition helped maintain public and media attention on the proposed legislation during a year of political maneuvering and negotiations, until a bill was passed in August 1983.

The passage of the 1983 New Jersey Worker and Community Right-to-Know Act was a major victory for the coalition of labor, environmental, and community organizations. Besides helping to bring about sweeping changes in industry's chemical reporting practices, the campaign brought together many of the state's activist groups. According to one environmental organizer, "Getting the right-to-know law passed was a very good organizing experience. It was a very good coalition building experience. We saw the common ground of workers in the communities. Workers that are exposed to the chemicals right there in the workplace, but the fact that these chemicals also disperse out into the community through emissions or being made into products that are being consumed by people. We also realized that the government wasn't going to be the ones to protect us. We had to fight for these rights." By framing the right to know as a concern shared by workers and community residents, the coalition united two groups of activists, each previously unfamiliar with the grievances and organizing capabilities of the other. And by portraying both government and industry actors as antagonists, this collective-action frame motivated the previously polarized labor and environmental movements in New Jersey to collaborate.

Political Constraints on the Blue-Green Frame

Although right-to-know legislation made it mandatory for companies to identify workplace and public health hazards, it did not require the elimination or reduction of those hazards. The law did not empower workers to protect themselves; it only granted workers the right to not work with a particular substance if information regarding its content and health risks was not made available. Workers were not granted the right to make use of any information about chemical health hazards by accompanying and providing input to government inspectors or by participating in the survey of chemical use and storage that companies carry out to comply with reporting requirements. Recognizing these inherent limitations of the law, the coalition reconvened to formulate a new bill, one that would empower workers and community members to inspect workplaces and to negotiate preventive measures to reduce exposures. This expansion of the right to know became known as the right to act.

This new agenda represented a major change in the coalition's collective-action frame. During the right-to-know campaign, the diagnostic framing strategies focused on the shared victimhood of workers and residents perpetrated by unsympathetic industrial corporations. In advocating for a right to act, the diagnostic framing transformed coalition members from helpless victims to citizens with the power over private business decisions.

This modification of identity and purpose did not sit well with all coalition members, and, the coalition's unity began to falter. While some coalition members who endorsed the right to know saw the right to act as empowering workers and communities by allowing them to take action to mitigate identified risks, others thought it went too far. To test the viability of the right-to-act concept, the coalition arranged several "good neighbor" programs in which concerned community members living near a manufacturing facility were escorted through the facility to improve neighborhood-industry relations. Not everyone felt this public oversight of private business decisions was justified, as one participant pointed out: "So the local volunteer fire chief lived in my community, as close as I do to this [manufacturing facility], and came along on the inspection. Actually at the end of the inspection, he told me that he didn't think that we had any right to go in there and do what we did. Even though he participated in it and was happy to come along. But when it came down right to it, he didn't feel that we had the right to tell that business, to go in and look over, and tell them what we thought. That had just crossed the line of privacy and the right for somebody to conduct their business the way we want to."

Although the local fire chief does not represent the entire firefighter community in New Jersey, the firefighters' union was an important stakeholder in the fight for the right to know. Therefore, the reluctance of this union member of the coalition to shift from demanding information to demanding action is emblematic of a broader socioeconomic and political challenge for the coalition. Although coalition members agreed that the right to know was a fundamental right, there was no such consensus regarding the framing of the right to act, as it conflicted with the principles of free-market capitalism, which resists excessive public oversight of industrial production.

Spearheaded by groups such as the New Jersey Business and Industry Association and the Chemical Industry Council, industry lobbyists launched an aggressive campaign to defeat the right-to-act law immediately following its introduction in the legislature. The Business and Industry Association's membership newsletter bluntly stated: "We have one issue that dwarfs all others in comparison, and that is the [Right-to-Act] Act. . . . In its current form, it would be a nightmare for New Jersey employers." Recognizing their defeat in 1983 with the passage of the Right-to-Know Act, industry quickly developed a united front to attack the credibility of the blue-green coalition. One reporter captured that rhetoric at one of the first public hearings: "Representatives of some of the state's largest industries opposed the act last night, conjuring up images during testimony of uninformed gadflies passing through factory gates and running amok" (quoted in Engler 1992). Industry representatives resurrected traditional arguments that right-to-act regulations would decrease the global competitiveness of New Jersey's core industries and force companies to cut jobs.

Industry representatives charged the Right-to-Know and Act Coalition with interfering in private production decisions. The labeling of environmental organizations as "nosy neighbors" undermined the motivation of many coalition partners, as evidenced in this environmentalist's experience: "The chemical industry homed right in on this. . . . The right to conduct themselves the way they wanted to couldn't be opened up to input from the community or from workers. That businesses run their businesses, and workers have to do what they're told. And that the community doesn't really have any right to go in the door and come in and say, I think it should be this way. And so that next step, the right to act, was a much more difficult position to back."

Industrial lobbyists rarely question the right of workers to participate in joint health-and-safety committees or inspections: their objection was to inspections by community members. Though the coalition emphasized worker safety, the main target of industry opposition was the environmental side of the coalition, who were portrayed as proponents of an intrusion on a private business's right to operate as it saw fit, within established guidelines. While the coalition highlighted the small number of OSHA inspectors, the paucity of safeguards to protect workers, and the general lack of pollution prevention in the workplace, the Business and Industry Association and other industrial lobbyists emphasized the intrusion of nosy environmentalists into private business and the ignorance of lay citizens about the chemical industry. These attacks on the solidarity of the blue-green coalition fostered, among policy makers and the general public, a perceived disconnect between the need for right-to-act laws to protect workers against occupational death and disease and the proposed legislation allowing community inspection of chemical facilities.

The political assault on the right to act was heightened by a sharp economic decline. Jobs in heavy and light manufacturing disappeared throughout the United States during the recession beginning in the early 1980s, and this downturn remained on the public's mind throughout the Right-to-Know and Act Coalition's campaign. Industry appealed to both politicians and the public with a claim that right-to-act regulation would force industry and much-needed jobs out of New Jersey. Toxic hazards in workplaces, never highly visible to the general public, became even less salient. Without a major industrial disaster to highlight the plight of workers, the media focused primarily on the community aspect of the labor-environment coalition.

Ultimately, the right-to-act campaign failed. After a clear defeat by industry when the bill came to a vote, the blue-green coalition retreated to a stance of defending the right to know from counterattack and found other means of using information to improve community and workplace environmental health. The right to know remains significant in debates over the safety of storing chemicals onsite and the consequences of an accidental release or a terrorist attack. By emphasizing public and workforce rights to information on potential chemical hazards, the coalition continues to press the state and industry to eliminate or reduce the storage and use of hazardous substances. It has also used environmental monitoring as a tool for determining whether neighborhoods inhabited by poor and minority groups are overburdened with the presence of hazardous substances.

DISCUSSION

The formation of the blue-green alliance in New Jersey began with a realization that neither side alone could accomplish its goals. Environmental activists, who were fairly close to enacting local versions of the right-to-know laws, decided to suspend their own campaigns and partner with labor groups, which they had previously viewed as sympathetic to industry, to fight for a different type of right-to-know law. The decision had obvious instrumental value, in that the divided environmental community became concerned that it might fail in its political campaign without the support of labor groups. Behind this strategic shift was not only the changing nature of political opportunities in New Jersey but also the power of strategic framing, which enabled coalition leaders to build solidarity among the ranks of both the labor and the environmental movements. Furthermore, labor support would ensure the long-term sustainability of any new right-to-know law, making it less likely to be weakened or dismantled later. Philadelphia activists, who developed a strategy based on political necessity, knew firsthand the power of a health-oriented frame to convince other labor and environmental activists that they shared a common interest. These bridge builders used this framework to build relationships and establish a partnership that changed the nature of environmental and labor organizing in New Jersey.

The connections between workers' personal experiences and environmentalists' interests in eliminating toxics in their communities can be seen as a form of frame alignment. Benford and Snow's (2000) elaboration of frame bridging as a strategy used by movement activists to link two ideologically congruent but structurally separate frames is a useful explanatory model for the connections forged between occupational health and antitoxics activism in the right-to-know campaign. Many of the partners had never met each other and thus had little reason to coordinate political agendas or share resources within a coalition. They were motivated to collaborate by their shared objective of securing a collective right to access health-related information on chemicals. Coalition leaders built these connections by illustrating the links between hazardous working conditions and the release of toxic substances into the communities along the fence lines of the chemical facilities. Thus Right-to-Know Coalition leaders bridged two unique movement cultures and fashioned a new form of solidarity between workers and environmentalists.

External efforts to divide the coalition by picking off individual members, such as the firefighters' unions, failed. The chemical industry's divide-and-conquer strategy of job blackmail, successful in other labor-environmental interactions, failed to undermine the coalition's collective-action frame. Despite a political climate slightly unfavorable to the coalition, largely due to a Republican administration, the framing of the right to know as a basic civil right and the citation of a number of major chemical accidents as illustrations of the problem provided the political momentum necessary to achieve the passage of the legislation and ensure its long-term sustainability.

By focusing on the ubiquitous nature of toxic exposures and the shared need for access to information, coalition leaders constructed a collective-action frame that crossed movement boundaries. The coalition thus presented a united front to state officials and elected representatives, one that industry and corporate interests had not previously faced. A unique coalition frame compensated for the traditional division and distrust between union and environmental activists by emphasizing a basic civil right to health information. Twenty years later, this coalition frame remains the foundation for collaboration between labor and environmental organizations.

Political opportunity played a limiting role when activists sought to expand their range of actions. In demanding a right to act, the coalition questioned the sanctity of private property by promoting community oversight of industrial production. This move prompted a better-organized countermovement of business interests that led to the defeat of the campaign and threatened to divide the labor and environmental coalition. By identifying themselves as stakeholders who should be involved in the production decisions of industry, rather than as employees and outsiders who deserved to know about production decisions, the coalition altered its collective-action frame in ways that threatened its solidarity.

Many union representatives involved with the coalition feared that their membership would disapprove of their involvement with a campaign that so directly challenged the industries that employed them. Whereas advocating for the right to know involved demands for slight reforms consistent with existing laws, like the information provisions in the federal Occupational Safety and Health Act, calls for community inspections of private facilities had little precedent. Although workers in hazardous jobs would have benefited from such reform, the conceptual shift from the right to know to the right to act was too radical for many actors. Their fears were increased when industry presented a united and fervent front against the right to act. As the political tide began to shift away from the coalition, the vital support and testimonies provided by union members during the right-to-know campaign became sparse. Where the right-to-know campaign benefited from the real-world illustrations of the hazards associated with a lack of information for workers, the right–to–act campaign lacked clear evidence that worker health and safety would be improved by community inspections of industrial facilities.

To prevent schism, the coalition ultimately returned to its original collective-action frame, opting to defend the right-to-know law and ensuring its successful implementation. This retreat was also necessary in the face of the strong opposition from industry, which mustered persuasive arguments about economic damage and potential job losses.

Although political failures often lead to the dissolution of a social movement organization, in this case the individual and organizational members of the coalition accepted the right-to-act loss and opted to focus on enforcing the hard-won right to know. Understanding the dynamic between the agency of coalition leaders in the framing of the coalition's identity and purpose and the shifting context of New Jersey politics allows us to explain the initial success and longevity of this labor-environmental coalition.

CONCLUSIONS

Cross-movement coalitions pose a challenge to traditional interpretations of the social movements literature. As Van Dyke (2003) argues, the importance of collaboration between different movements has been ignored for too long. With the new, complex challenges posed by global issues such as climate change and pollution created by the expansion of the goods-movement industry, such coalitions are likely to become increasingly common. Understanding their dynamics and potential is essential for contemporary theorizing about social movements. Because cross-movement coalition dynamics frequently operate in ways opposite to what mainstream literature would predict, research into these mechanisms is needed. Framing plays a significant role in the formation of cross-movement coalitions and should be explored in conjunction with political opportunities and economic context.

Health concerns are likely to be the common ground upon which long-term labor and environmental alliances are built. The growth in environmental health and environmental justice activism offers new opportunities for fusion between these types of environmental organizations and progressive labor unions. Coalitions similar to New Jersey's are emerging across the United States and internationally. Domestically, groups like the Alliance for a Healthy Tomorrow (based in Boston, MA) have adopted a framework of precaution to meld occupational and environmental health activism. In the European Union, labor groups are working with environmental organizations to reform chemical safety management and address climate change.

Our approach to the study of blue-green groups is also relevant to the growth of other seemingly unlikely coalitions. Some of these involve environmental justice groups that are forming links with groups representing apparently disparate interests, such as transportation activism and smart growth (Bullard and Johnson 1997) and industrial ecology advocacy (O'Rourke, Connelly, and Koshland 1996). Other unlikely coalitions have formed between religious and energy-policy activists. These alliances involve groups with dramatically different starting assumptions. Our approach to cross-movement coalitions makes it possible to understand how such alliances are formed and maintained and thus to grasp the new dimensions of a society replete with many new combinations of social movements that cannot be understood by existing models.

NOTE

This is a reprint of an article published in *Sociological Forum,* © 2010 Eastern Sociological Society: Brian Mayer, Phil Brown, and Rachel Morello-Frosch, "Labor-Environmental Coalition Formation: Framing and the Right-to-Know," *Sociological Forum* 25, no. 4 (December 2010): 746–68.

12

The Brown Superfund
Research Program

A Multistakeholder Partnership Addresses
Problems in Contaminated Communities

Laura Senier, Benjamin Hudson, Sarah Fort, Elizabeth Hoover,
Rebecca Tillson, and Phil Brown

The National Institute of Environmental Health Sciences (NIEHS) has a long tradition of coordinating basic research programs with community outreach. It has sought to promote science that engages communities in numerous aspects of environmental health research, from the identification of exposures of concern to the development of research priorities, the collection of data and interpretation of research findings, and the implementation of effective interventions to reduce exposures and protect public health. One example is the Superfund Research Program (SRP), which is dedicated to funding multidisciplinary research "to provide a solid foundation which environmental managers and risk assessors can draw upon to make sound decisions related to [the remediation of] Superfund and other hazardous waste sites" (SRP, n.d.). In addition to supporting a diverse roster of basic and applied biomedical and engineering research, the SRP is committed to the timely communication of research findings to organizations and agencies charged with cleanup of hazardous waste and outreach to affected communities to ensure that research projects are relevant to their needs. In addition to the SRP program, the NIEHS portfolio of publicly funded research includes other research initiatives dedicated to community-based participatory research, health disparities, and environmental justice (Suk and Anderson 1999; O'Fallon et al. 2003; Schwartz et al. 2006).

Effective research translation and community outreach can support and enhance basic and applied research programs in two ways: first, by making that research more responsive to local needs; and second, by helping to address some of the nonscientific issues surrounding contaminated sites. Such programs bring academic researchers into frequent contact with the communities surrounding their research sites. Regular communication between the two groups may bring to light additional research questions that are of pressing interest to the community at large. Moreover, the cleanup of contaminated sites is often hindered by issues beyond the technical aspects of site remediation. For example, a legacy of mistrust often permeates the relationship between academic scientists, regulatory officials, and the affected community. This history of mistrust can introduce tensions and miscommunications that may slow administrative or regulatory decision making. Even in best-case scenarios, cleanup of contaminated sites is a slow process, and although communities most fear health or ecological consequences, they are often burdened by additional problems, such as loss of community cohesion or financial setbacks. Research translation and community outreach programs that operate in conjunction with basic research programs can mitigate some of these collateral effects.

Among scientists who receive funding from such programs, however, some confusion remains about how best to differentiate research translation from community outreach activities while coordinating these supportive activities to achieve their maximum potential. The two activities engage different constituencies and have different goals. Although each targets a different audience or stakeholders, a well-integrated translation and outreach program should recognize that stakeholders often share common goals. Programs should therefore seek opportunities to bring stakeholders together. Cooperation may not be easy, given that relationships among stakeholders around contaminated sites are often contentious and many biomedical and engineering scientists are not trained to recognize and address social problems. By creating opportunities for cooperation, research translation and outreach can begin to repair trust among stakeholders, which may pave the way for the speedier application of research results to site cleanup and reuse and empower the stakeholders in pursuit of their individual and collective goals.

This chapter reports on a recent project by the Brown University SRP, in which academic researchers and state agency personnel collaborated with community activists on the development of a legislative initiative to mitigate the financial impact of living in a contaminated community, giving temporary relief to residents while they were awaiting cleanup. This collaboration allowed the well-coordinated yet distinct outreach and translation activities of the Brown SRP to foster close collaborative relationships among academic researchers, state agency personnel, and community members. We situate this case in a wider context of social-scientific research on contaminated communities and the tradition of community-engaged outreach and advocacy with those communities. We show how the inclusion of social scientists in a research translation and outreach program can increase interaction and trust between professionals and the community.

STRESSORS AND STRAINS
IN CONTAMINATED COMMUNITIES

Numerous studies have documented the adverse effects of contamination on individual and community well-being. Communities burdened by toxic waste suffer not only deleterious physical and environmental effects but also psychological stress and loss of community cohesion (Erikson 1976; Brown and Mikkelsen 1997; Edelstein 2004; Checker 2005). Living with toxic contamination is inherently stressful and demands some kind of coping response. Contaminated communities are often subject to stigmatization, which compounds a range of anxieties that community members already hold about the effects of the contamination on their health and well-being (Brown and Mikkelsen 1997; Edelstein 2004).

Adverse ecological and health outcomes associated with toxic exposures are often first identified by people living in the contaminated communities (Brown and Mikkelsen 1997). When residents request assistance from their local or state departments of public health, they are often frustrated with the responses. They frequently come to question beliefs that are often taken for granted, such as the ideas that technology and science are benign and positive forces, that experts know best, that the marketplace has self-regulating mechanisms to prevent harm, and that the government exists to help the people (Edelstein 2004).

One of the most robust findings from social-science research on people living in contaminated communities is that animosity and mistrust frequently develop between residents and the staff of regulatory agencies charged with responding to contamination crises (Ozonoff and Boden 1987; Brown and Mikkelsen 1997; Edelstein 2004). Residents are also frequently frustrated with and distrustful of academic researchers, reporting that they have too often been the subject of research that ultimately had no direct benefit for them. Academics seeking to enter the community must be prepared to prove and maintain their trustworthiness (Israel et al. 1998). One way to do so is to partner with community-based organizations that already serve the community and are viewed as trustworthy (Arcury, Quandt, and McCauley 2000). Such partnerships may be more difficult, however, if the academic partner also has relationships with state regulators or health professionals, who are often at odds with the community.

The literature on public participation and stakeholder engagement emphasizes both the benefits and challenges of community engagement. First, involving the community often improves the quality of the information that goes into the decision-making process. This lay knowledge, or popular epidemiology, includes the initial efforts made by the community to identify contaminated sites, as well as community-driven projects to map the extent of human health effects and to research historic uses of the property that may shed light on the sources and extent of the contamination (Brown and Mikkelsen 1997). Decisions made with public cooperation often have higher credibility and greater public acceptance than decisions made through narrowly technocratic processes or directed entirely by regulatory scientists and government experts (Chess and Purcell 1999).

There are, however, significant obstacles to public participation, especially with respect to form of participation, assessment of outcomes, and participant recruitment. Chess and Purcell found that no single form of participation (e.g., workshops, community advisory committees, or public meetings) was clearly associated with increased participant satisfaction or confidence in decision making. Actual impact on decision making was associated less with the particular form of public engagement than with other factors, such as the expertise of those planning the effort, the agency's commitment to public involvement, and the history and context of the site. Chess and Purcell note that public-involvement processes are improved by careful planning, clarification of goals, tailoring the forms of participation to the community's needs, deployment of multiple forms of participation, and collection of feedback that allows organizers to modify a public participation plan if necessary (Chess and Purcell 1999). These guidelines are similar to those that motivate community-based participatory research (CBPR): research should build on the strengths and resources of the community; partners should work collaboratively in all phases of the research; research should integrate the quest for knowledge with action so that all partners might benefit; and research findings should be disseminated to all partners, including the community as a whole (Israel et al. 1998).The experience of the Brown SRP team confirms that the benefits of community participation can outweigh the drawbacks.

SUCCESSFUL STAKEHOLDER ENGAGEMENT

Brown University's Superfund research project, "Reuse in Rhode Island: A State-Based Approach to Complex Exposures," began in May 2005. From the outset, the project team sought to integrate three themes: land reuse in Rhode Island, complex chemical exposures, and a statewide approach. Accordingly, the Brown SRP includes biomedical research projects designed to evaluate responses in sensitive and susceptible individuals to complex mixtures of toxic substances, and laboratory-based engineering research to model novel strategies and processes for the remediation of complex polluted sites.

Rhode Island is burdened by a long history of industrial chemical use. Because it is densely populated, the state has a clear imperative to develop remediation strategies that enable the beneficial reuse of contaminated sites and mitigate development pressures that contribute to sprawl and encroachment on open space. The state is also a "small world" socially, with only slightly more than one million residents. Academic researchers, government officials, and community members inhabiting this world have common incentives and opportunities to work together on these goals of land rehabilitation and reuse.

Methods: Integration and Coordination
of Translation and Outreach

The Brown SRP includes two core areas of activity: a community outreach core and a research translation core. The outreach core works in partnership with community-based organizations to better understand a community's concerns about the remediation of existing sites and to prevent future contamination or exposure. The research translation core partners with state and federal health and environmental agencies to conduct educational activities and provide organizational resources for physicians and other health providers, lawyers, environmental remediators, community development corporations, and local businesses. It is supervised by a tenured professor in the Division of Engineering and staffed by a full-time state agency liaison who holds a PhD in engineering and who is responsible for facilitating relationships with state agencies.

The outreach core is chaired by a tenured professor with a joint appointment in the Department of Sociology and the Center for Environmental Studies, who supervises the work of graduate and undergraduate research assistants in projects with the community partners. In addition, the outreach core offers opportunities for students to work on service-learning projects with community partner organizations. Undergraduates who enroll in seminars in the Department of Sociology and the Center for Environmental Studies can undertake one of these projects in lieu of producing a conventional term paper for the course. Service-learning projects have filled a wide variety of needs for communities, from technical assistance to leadership development training. One student analyzed fare structures and automated ticketing in the Boston area's mass transit system and the effect that proposed fare restructuring would have on minority communities. Another student summarized scientific reports on the contaminants present in river sediment for a watershed advocacy organization. Two students worked with middle-school students to design and deliver an environmental education program and to train them in public speaking so that they could attend school committee and city council meetings and articulate their concerns about a proposal to build a new high school on a heavily contaminated site.

The Brown SRP research translation core has been designed to facilitate communication between professionals, whereas the outreach core aims to facilitate communication between professionals and the community. Although the two activities are conceptually distinct, efforts are made to foster integration and cooperation between them. For example, the director of the outreach core is also the codirector of the research translation core. This joint function enables cooperation between government agencies, professional groups, and community groups who share the

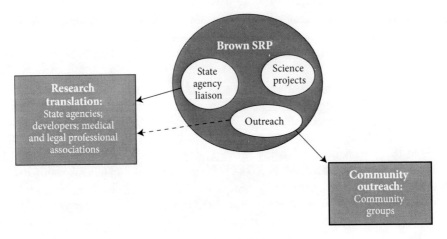

FIGURE 12.1. The Brown Superfund Research Program

goal of protecting human health and environmental quality (figure 12.1). Members of the research translation staff also work with community members, for example by inviting community residents to attend scientific workshops held by Brown SRP scientists; and outreach staff work with regulatory agency personnel to help them network more effectively with the communities affected by contamination.

The Brown SRP outreach core has established long-term partnerships with two community-based groups: the Environmental Neighborhood Awareness Committee of Tiverton (ENACT), a community-based organization campaigning for cleanup of waste from a manufactured gas plant in a residential neighborhood; and the Woonasquatucket River Watershed Council (WRWC), a nonprofit agency dedicated to the stewardship of a watershed basin that includes a Superfund site and several brownfields within it. In addition, the outreach core works informally with other groups throughout the state to build a statewide environmental justice network.

Both the outreach and the research translation teams have allowed the needs and interests of the stakeholders to guide the selection of their activities. The outreach core seeks to foster community engagement and public participation by engaging community groups in the identification of specific environmental hazards; providing leadership training by experienced advocacy organizations; and training community members in science, organizational skills, grant writing, media work, and government relations. The team has customized activities and interventions for each community group.

The research translation core adopted a similar strategy in working with regulatory agency personnel. The staff members sought guidance from agency partners on the technical issues they regularly confront. They have channeled this feedback to the Brown SRP principal investigators, who are planning future basic research projects to meet some of these needs. Both the research translation and outreach cores have thus assessed needs and designed activities that are relevant and useful to their constituencies. This partnership approach, coupled with regular and frequent personal communication, has helped to build trust between the cores and their constituencies.

A final and very necessary element of relationship building was an examination of communication. Several community environmental health groups in Rhode Island have had acrimonious relationships with state agencies, including litigation over the cleanup of contaminated sites. Because of this history, many participants at Brown, at the state agencies, and among the community groups harbored concerns about whether the team would be able to establish the sort of forthright communication necessary to build partnerships among the key stakeholders. The only remedy was a frank conversation among the Brown SRP leadership team, with outreach and research translation personnel present, at which all parties agreed on the importance of outreach and translation efforts to the overall success of the enterprise, and team members made explicit assurances not to violate confidences shared among the partners. These steps laid the groundwork for a positive working relationship. The success of a major outreach project in the first year of the grant was partly a result of the collaborative relationships the team had built.

Contamination in the Bay Street Neighborhood of Tiverton

In August 2002, a municipal crew working on a sewer interceptor project in the Bay Street neighborhood of Tiverton, Rhode Island, uncovered soil and sediment that were tinted a bright blue, characteristic of waste from a manufactured-gas plant. Testing revealed that much of the soil underneath the roads and extending onto private properties was heavily contaminated with cyanide, lead, arsenic, benzo[a]pyrene, and other toxic substances. The Rhode Island Department of Environmental Management (RIDEM) determined that the likely source of the contamination was the New England Gas Company, whose Fall River coal-gas plant was located just across the state line in Massachusetts. Waste from this plant is believed to have been dumped prior to 1955 on the Rhode Island side of the state line and later used as fill when the Bay Street neighborhood was developed.

The site occupies approximately fifty acres along the eastern edge of Mount Hope Bay (figure 12.2). In February 2004, the town of Tiverton imposed a moratorium on any digging or excavation that might expose the contaminated soil in the neighborhood. The moratorium area includes approximately 130 properties and affects more than two hundred residents.

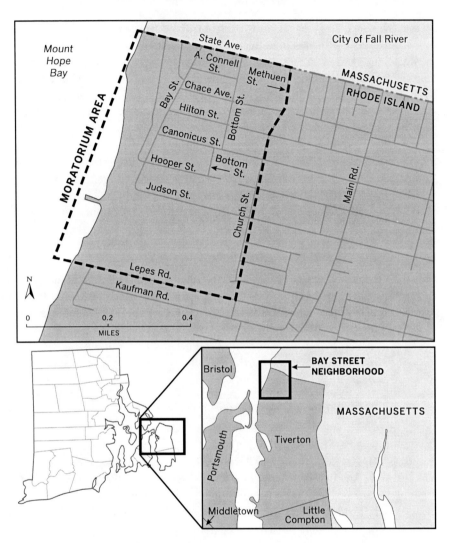

FIGURE 12.2. Tiverton, Rhode Island

Since the contamination was discovered, the values of the homes and properties in this working-class neighborhood have plummeted. As a result, home equity
loans and lines of credit are nearly impossible to secure. Unable to borrow against
the equity in their homes, residents cannot obtain loans for minor home repairs
(such as replacing a roof or a furnace) or more substantial renovations. Home-
owner equity is also an important financial resource for parents with college-age

children: the inability to use their home's equity as collateral for an education loan can limit the educational aspirations of future generations.

In response to these problems, a group of residents founded the Environmental Neighborhood Action Committee of Tiverton (ENACT) in the spring of 2003. Its purpose is to work with state and federal legislators and regulatory agencies to demand cleanup of the neighborhood. Negotiating a cleanup has been a lengthy process, however, and as an interim measure, they appealed to their legislators and to their partners at the Brown SRP outreach core for help in solving the problems residents face in securing loans for home repairs and improvements.

The neighborhood is not a Superfund site, but the Brown SRP team chose to work there because of its high profile in statewide discussions about toxic contamination and because it is heavily contaminated with complex mixtures of toxicants. It thus exemplifies the kind of scientific issues the Brown SRP was designed to address, as well as the kind of social and community-level issues that so often arise at contaminated sites. Even though none of the biomedical or engineering projects is directly engaged in remediation or assessment of the Tiverton site, the Brown SRP team saw this site as an opportunity to test the program's approach of working at the state level to address the multifaceted problems that exist at and around sites burdened by complex mixtures of contaminants.

Designing and Implementing a Loan Program for Residents

In the spring of 2006, two Brown undergraduate students in the Environmental Justice seminar (jointly offered through the Department of Sociology and the Center for Environmental Studies) undertook the design of a home-equity loan program for residents of contaminated communities as a service learning project. In cooperation with the state legislators who represent this district, they identified six possible legislative or administrative avenues to providing loans to families in the neighborhood. After reviewing the options with knowledgeable policy analysts, the legislators decided that the most promising and expeditious option would be to amend the legislation for the Rhode Island Housing and Mortgage and Finance Corporation (now called Rhode Island Housing), the self-sustaining affordable-housing agency charged with offering home equity loans in Rhode Island. The result was the Environmentally Compromised Home Ownership (ECHO) loan program, which makes loans of up to $25,000 available to homeowners living on or directly abutting a contaminated site. Loans are made at standard interest rates, all loans must be repaid, and Rhode Island Housing does not assume any liability for environmental cleanup.

Immediately before the legislation was due to be filed, the legislators became concerned that if the legislation were worded too broadly, the state would be deluged with applications for low-income loans from homeowners who were not in contaminated neighborhoods, or who had contaminated their own properties (e.g., through dumping or improper application of pesticides). The legislators

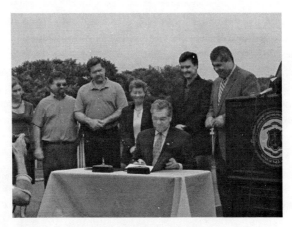

FIGURE 12.3. Rhode Island governor Carcieri
symbolically signs the Environmentally Compromised
Home Opportunity (ECHO) loan bill into law, July 21,
2006, one week after the formal signing. Behind him, from
left, are Sarah Fort (from the Brown University Superfund
Basic Research Program outreach core), Gary Rose
(ENACT treasurer), Bob Ferreira (ENACT secretary), Gail
Corvello (ENACT president), state senator Walter Felag,
and state representative Joseph Amaral.

raised this concern with the Brown SRP outreach team, who forwarded the
request to their research translation partners at RIDEM. The RIDEM Division of
Waste Management was asked to design a certification process for contaminated
properties. Because the site is not officially a Superfund site, RIDEM has oversight
of the site investigation and remediation; as a result, its staff were familiar with the
site assessments conducted to that point.

Within two business days of receiving this request, the research translation
partner at RIDEM was able to specify such a process and supply draft language for
inclusion in the loan bill. The final bill requires that a prospective borrower's property be certified as "known to be impacted by the release of hazardous materials or
petroleum," either by RIDEM through the state's waste management processes or
under the federal Comprehensive Environmental Response, Compensation, and
Liability Act (CERCLA, i.e., Superfund). Although the bill was originally drafted
to address the needs of Tiverton residents, other Rhode Island residents are eli-
gible for loans if their properties qualify for certification.

Through quick cooperation between the state legislators, the RIDEM, and the
Brown outreach team, the bill was introduced in the state legislature in June 2006
and signed into law on July 14, 2006. Members of the Rhode Island state and

federal legislative delegations were present for a signing ceremony, along with Brown outreach team members and many residents (figure 12.3).

THE DEVIL IS IN THE DETAILS: TRUST, FOLLOW-THROUGH, AND COMMUNITY WORK

The Brown case study provides an example of the importance of trust in academic and community partnerships. Academic researchers who want to work in contaminated communities must maintain the trust of their community partners (Israel et al. 1998). In social-scientific research, the concept of trust has several dimensions. *Role performance* refers to the type of trust that depends on academic or professional credentials. *Interest promotion* refers to the belief that each party has the other's best interests at heart (Mechanic and Meyer 2000; Hardin 2001). It is this form of trust that is most critical to functional partnerships and successful stakeholder engagement.

Social scientists have written extensively about trust as interest promotion, not only in its abstract theoretical dimensions but also in practical terms, as it is integral to the ethnographic method on which much social science research is based. Methods texts often describe the challenges of "getting into" a research setting, that is, gaining the acceptance of the subjects of the study (Lofland and Lofland 1995). Although academic credentials are certainly important in gaining entrée to a community group, regular face-to-face contact and personal interactions are indispensable in establishing trust as interest promotion. Making such contacts requires time and effort, but it is critical for establishing a working relationship with community partners in both community-outreach and research translation-initiatives.

Academic and community partnerships can be beneficial to both sides, but researchers must be prepared to encounter challenges and tensions. Academic researchers are not typically rewarded for building relationships: they are rewarded for publishing, teaching, grant writing, and professional service within the academic world. From the other perspective, as noted earlier, communities are often frustrated by experiences of entering into academic research projects that have brought them only meager benefits. Thus academic researchers who wish to partner with community groups, even in an egalitarian or participatory fashion, must be prepared to encounter skepticism or even downright hostility early in the relationship. (Learning to handle such responses without getting defensive is another example of an important skill that often goes unrewarded in the academic world.) Building partnerships is time-consuming and uncertain work: the project schedule or timeline should take these factors into account.

Aware of the skepticism with which communities generally view academic researchers, the Brown outreach team has taken particular care to follow the progress of the program, to monitor its implementation, and to try to resolve unforeseen difficulties. Although the ECHO program has been put in place and two loans have been awarded to neighborhood residents, awareness of the program is not yet widespread. Moreover, the program's focus on small loans may not be sufficient. Several people in the neighborhood had been forced into consolidating loans and paying astronomically high interest rates; the ECHO program was not originally designed to give these homeowners relief. In the fall of 2007, the Brown SRP team met with state legislators and staff from Rhode Island Housing and agreed to find a way to amend the ECHO program to allow for consolidation or refinancing of existing high-interest loans. Approximately half of the residents surveyed by the outreach team indicated they would be interested in refinancing.

The Brown outreach team is also working to spread word of this program to other states, in the hope that Rhode Island will become a model for national action to help other contaminated communities (a copy of the legislation's wording is available on request from Laura Senier). The team was invited to speak about this program at the National Environmental Health Conference in October 2006, sponsored by the Centers for Disease Control and Prevention and the Agency for Toxic Substances and Disease Registry. The NIEHS featured this program on its national SRP website and has sought updated information in order to increase awareness.

Meanwhile, in Rhode Island, residents and legislators agree that the ECHO program is but a first step. While the residents are grateful for the loan program and the opportunity to maintain their homes, they remain committed to their campaign for the cleanup of their properties and the restoration of their neighborhood.

Following our involvement in the ECHO bill, two other major legislative decisions brought some redress to the affected communities. In June 2009, pressure by the community outreach core and a number of environmental groups led the state legislature to bring to the floor a bill that had languished for two years. It raised penalties from $1,000 to $25,000 per day for companies that fail to heed RIDEM notices of violation. It passed unanimously, and although it was not retroactive and thus did not apply to Southern Union Gas (the successor to New England Gas), it was an important measure to protect other residents in the state. ENACT gained its most important victory in August 2009, when an out-of-court settlement resulted in a $3 million settlement for cleanup and $8.5 million in damages from Southern Union Gas. The cleanup was mired in technical and legal controversy, and as of May 2011 it still has not been completed. The Community Outreach Core is monitoring its progress by interviewing affected homeowners in collaboration with ENACT. In addition, the SRP team and ENACT will hold a planting festival to celebrate the end of the cleanup.

DISCUSSION

The Brown SRP outreach and research translation activities are designed to integrate the efforts of academic, community, and regulatory partners in the remediation of contaminated sites in Rhode Island. The Brown experience shows that the SRP can be a vehicle for bringing multiple forms of expertise to bear on such problems and that academic researchers can bridge the gaps that often exist between community groups and state regulators. This bridge-building function was best served at the outset by ensuring that relationships among the partners were well defined with respect to their core functions but flexible enough to allow both the research translation and the outreach functions to respond to new concerns and cooperate on common goals.

This close relationship between outreach and translation activities is fairly unusual among SRP grantees and has attracted some attention. Researchers and program staff from other institutions have asked questions about the role of the state agency liaison in helping to assess the needs of regulatory officials and agencies. The research translation team emphasizes the state-based approach as a key element in building credibility and trust among Rhode Island's professional and regulatory community. Other researchers have also inquired about the challenges and difficulties of working directly with community groups, often stating that they are hesitant to engage directly with the community because of the time-intensive nature of the work or concerns over political allegiances. While the Brown team has certainly experienced these difficulties, they have found that taking pains at the outset to define the relationships between the research-translation and outreach cores and their target constituencies paid off in the end by easing the anxieties that all parties had about working together. In particular, the social scientists on the outreach team. who have longstanding commitments to community-engaged research, have sensitized all members of the team to the importance of trust and cooperation.

Social scientists can contribute significantly to SRP and other environmental health research. First, as we show in our background section, social scientists have led the way in studying the social, economic, and psychological effects of toxic waste contamination. Second, social scientists are sensitive to the importance of establishing trusting personal connections with stakeholders, thus enabling interdisciplinary collaborations such as the ECHO program. Third, social scientists, especially medical sociologists and environmental sociologists, have a long tradition of successful collaboration with community activists that provides a model for their peers in the biomedical and engineering sciences to follow.

Since the passage of the ECHO loan program, the Brown SRP partners have cooperated on other projects as well. In the summer of 2006, RIDEM was ordered by a state court to convene a stakeholders' group to design a process that would ensure adequate community involvement in decisions about the remediation and reuse of contaminated sites. The Brown research translation partners at RIDEM invited the Brown outreach core director to participate on this panel. He pressed RIDEM to include members of the affected community groups. As a result, the stakeholders panel includes regulators, developers, business leaders, and members of various community groups who represent a diverse set of people and interests.

Centuries of industrial activity have left the United States with a substantial burden of toxic contamination. For more than two decades now, social-scientific scholarship has demonstrated that problems related to toxic sites extend well beyond the technical aspects of site remediation. Contamination has adverse social and psychological effects on individuals and communities. Remediation should seek to restore a community's sense of wholeness, safety, and integrity as well as clean air, soil, and water. Through its history of requiring research programs to engage with the public—through outreach and research translation activities—the NIEHS has acknowledged the ecosocial realities of contamination and has pushed academic researchers to connect their scientific inquiry to concerns about residents' health and social well-being.

The NIEHS's commitment to this tradition of community engagement is evident in its program known as Partnerships for Environmental Public Health. It has sought input on what academics, community stakeholders, and government officials need and expect from environmental health research. As of 2009, this program had begun to fund hypothesis-driven research in which community members are full partners. It may demand new approaches to engaging communities and the development of materials that will increase community awareness of environmental health. The NIEHS is already funding programs, in addition to the SRP, that address some of these goals: for example, research programs designed to investigate specific diseases or conditions (e.g., Centers of Excellence on Breast Cancer and the Environment, and a program on obesity and the built environment) or the needs of specific, vulnerable populations (e.g., the Centers for Children's Environmental Health or the Worker Education and Training Program).The partnerships program also established a special program providing an additional year of funding for existing NIEHS grants that involve community outreach. The expansion of these programs presents an opportunity to reflect on the lessons to be learned from integrating research translation and outreach with the demands of a successful basic science program.

The Brown SRP demonstrates how such an endeavor can succeed. A robust model of community engagement is critical on both the research translation and the outreach sides. Few basic science programs, even those with outreach components, have engaged communities or citizen action groups as directly as the Brown SRP has done. More often, their outreach activities are directed toward regulatory officials, health care professionals, or other professional groups. Communities are thus often defined as an audience for research findings rather than partners in the research process. Although arrangements such as these may be efficient at communicating findings to other researchers and agencies, it is questionable whether they fulfill NIEHS's expectations for its basic research initiatives: that they should combine research and outreach activities in a way that proactively engages multiple stakeholders. These goals are best served by vigorous outreach programs that seek to develop a reciprocal relationship between researchers and communities.

A second critical component of Brown's success is the integration and coordination of research translation and outreach activities, and the merging of these activities with the scientific goals of the grant: the remediation of contamination and land reuse. In keeping with the NIEHS mandate to make research an "accountable enterprise," the Brown SRP teams have collaborated with both regulatory agencies and community action groups. Clear lines of communication were established at the outset, with research translation staff assigned to work primarily with regulatory agency personnel and the outreach team working more closely with community activists. These lines of communication were flexible enough, however, to allow for cooperation and communication on goals shared by all parties. This collaboration led to success on an important outreach goal: to help a community coping with a profound and prolonged toxic contamination crisis. Although the scientific research at the Tiverton site has not been pursued to quite the same degree as the research translation and outreach activities, the site has highlighted the problems associated with complex mixtures of contaminants and suggested some new research questions that may be incorporated into future biomedical or engineering projects. Thus work on a specific outreach need can also focus attention on scientific issues that fit with the overall scientific themes of the program. Engaging with regulatory agencies and community groups ensures that the program remains grounded in the research questions that matter most to the constituencies served.

Outreach and translation mandates in basic research programs can offer investigators an opportunity to add value to all their activities. The Brown SRP demonstrates that although collaborating with a diverse roster of stakeholders may pose challenges, academic researchers can, in fact, build bridges among these groups to enable all stakeholders to participate creatively and cooperatively in solving the many problems surrounding contaminated sites.

NOTE

Originally published as Laura Senier, Benjamin Hudson, Sarah Fort, Elizabeth Hoover, Rebecca Tillson, and Phil Brown, "Brown Superfund Basic Research Program: A Multistakeholder Partnership Addresses Real-World Problems in Contaminated Communities," *Environmental Science and Technology* 42, no. 13 (2008): 4655–62. Reprinted with permission from *Environmental Science and Technology.* Copyright 2008 American Chemical Society.

PART THREE

Ethical Considerations

13

Toxic Ignorance and the Right to Know

Biomonitoring Results Communication: A Survey of Scientists and Study Participants

Rachel Morello-Frosch, Julia Green Brody, Phil Brown,
Rebecca Gasior Altman, Ruthann A. Rudel, Carla Pérez, and Alison Cohen

Tired of government inaction toward community concerns about refinery pollution in her neighborhood, Ethel Dotson, a fifty-three-year resident of Richmond, California, decided it was time to up the ante. Armed with ten vials of her own blood, she joined several other residents in front of California's Hazardous Materials Laboratory and demanded that officials test their blood for dioxin and other contaminants. "I have a right to know what's in my body," she argued (Sarker 2000). Dotson's demand that the state document "chemical trespass" (Doyle 2004) in her body reveals the scientific promise, as well as policy and ethical challenges, of the rapidly expanding field of chemical biomonitoring.

Biomonitoring, or body burden research, involves assessing the presence and concentration of chemicals in humans by measuring the original chemicals as well as their metabolites, or reaction products, in human tissues and bodily fluids (Pausentbach and Galbraith 2006). It has been used since the late 1800s as a means of assessing exposure to chemicals, particularly in occupational settings (DeCaprio 1997; Sexton, Needham, and Pirkle 2004; Morello-Frosch 1997). Between 1976 and 1980, biomonitoring studies by the Centers for Disease Control (CDC) documented significant declines in blood lead levels in the U.S. population, correlating with the introduction of unleaded gasoline (Jackson et al. 2002). Monitoring of blood lead levels in children was adopted to track the effectiveness of poisoning-prevention strategies and to detect exposures in homes contaminated with lead paint (Greene, Morello-Frosch, and Shenassa 2006).

As public health increasingly targets the environmental determinants of chronic diseases, biomonitoring is becoming a key source of evidence for claims that new prevention measures must be taken. These efforts rest on newly developed, highly sensitive analytical methods that can detect increasing numbers of chemicals, even in low concentrations. However, while animal and cell studies show the troubling biological effects of some of these chemicals, in many cases human exposure levels, exposure sources, health effects, and exposure-reduction strategies are not yet well understood. As a 2006 National Academy of Sciences report points out, although biomonitoring has advanced significantly, researchers, regulators, and decision makers face challenges in deciding how to interpret, report, and act on results that only partially elucidate links between environmental chemicals and health (National Academy of Sciences 2006). This chapter heeds NAS's call for research addressing these scientific and ethical challenges. Parallel issues are raised by other methods of personal exposure assessment, such as dust and air samples taken from an individual's home.

Biomonitoring now allows scientists to assess and characterize a wide range of chemical body burdens and potential health risks, including those that may have more than one route of entry into the body (e.g. inhalation, ingestion, and transdermal absorption) (Lioy, Freeman, and Millette 2002; Rudel et al. 2003). The tests measure three basic categories of compounds: biomarkers of exposure, effect, and susceptibility (Metcalf and Orlof 2004; Goldstein 2005). Biomonitoring technologies have also become more widely available, more practical, and less expensive. As a result, biomonitoring studies have proliferated in academia, state and federal agencies, environmental advocacy organizations, and nonprofit research institutes.

The visibility and policy effects of this new wave of biomonitoring have been profound. Scientific journals and the media have reported on studies such as those documenting the presence of flame retardants in breast milk (Hooper et al. 2003; Fischer 2005), pesticides in umbilical-cord blood (Whyatt et al. 2004), and endocrine-disrupting compounds (EDCs) in household air and dust and householders' blood and urine (Rudel et al. 2003). In 1999, the federal government began systematically tracking personal exposures in a representative sample of the US population (CDC 1999). When the results were released in April 2001, Richard Jackson, director of CDC's National Center for Environmental Health, predicted that biomonitoring "could be revolutionary for environmental health research in the United States" (quoted in Vastag 2001). These new exposure-assessment methods provide much-needed data to advance environmental epidemiology and track the effectiveness of environmental health policy and regulation. Recent CDC biomonitoring results have highlighted the effectiveness of antismoking efforts, including banning smoking in public places, and the surprising levels of exposure of women of reproductive age to hormonally active chemicals from consumer products (CDC 2005). CDC now issues body-burden reports every two years, expanding the number of chemicals tested, and is encouraging states to develop their own biomonitoring programs (Jackson et al. 2002; CDC 2003, 2005). In September 2006, California became the first state to do so.

Exposure assessment has always been one of the most methodologically challenging aspects of environmental health science and environmental epidemiology. Although biomonitoring is a direct indicator of human exposure to certain compounds and their metabolites, it generally cannot be used to identify their sources. As one biomonitoring study participant states: "None of these chemicals come with a return address." Moreover, these techniques can rarely predict health outcomes or identify potential effects undetectable in clinical research. Although lower costs have allowed researchers to expand the array of chemicals being studied, toxicological or epidemiological evidence of their potential health effects (Davis and Webster2002) and regulatory benchmarks for comparison (Wagner 1997) are lacking. Biomonitoring therefore raises a number of ethical questions.

We first review the evolution of exposure assessment science and the ethical issues associated with it. We then describe our methods for recruiting and interviewing individuals involved in biomonitoring research about their opinions and practices. Our results identify three approaches used by academic scientists and environmental organizations to communicate information about the effects of chemical exposures on health and to influence regulatory and policy change: clinical ethics; community-based participatory research; and citizen science "data judo." The first is biomedically driven, while the latter two emphasize prevention research and advocacy. Our results also reveal the ethical and administrative issues faced by scientists when considering whether and how to report individual exposure information to study participants. We report on guidance offered by government publications, professional association best-practice guidelines, and journal articles concerning individual results communication. We make recommendations based on our interviews with researchers currently collecting and reporting individual exposure data. We conclude with a discussion of ethical considerations for future work in this area.

EVOLUTION OF EXPOSURE ASSESSMENT SCIENCE AND ETHICAL ISSUES

There is little guidance for those conducting exposure studies on whether and how to report individual and community-level exposure data to participants. Occupational health specialists were among the first to grapple with the issue of biomonitoring and individual report-back. In the 1960s, the testing of blood, urine, and other tissues was a well-established practice for occupational health surveillance and research, although only a small portion of the many chemicals common in work environments were consistently examined, in part because of limitations in chemical analytic capacity (American Conference of Governmental Industrial Hygienists 2005; CDC 2005). Occupational health researchers typically conduct retrospective occupational cohort studies, in which morbidity and mortality records for a population of individuals working in a particular environment are analyzed to determine associations between exposures and adverse health outcomes. Historically, cohort members were not notified about individual findings, even though this information could have served as a basis for efforts to reduce exposures or conduct health screenings to reduce risks. However, in a speech delivered to the National Institute of Occupational Safety and Health in 1982, the bioethicist John Fletcher called on epidemiologists to "join other biomedical scientists who have the obligation to notify study subjects" (Schulte 1985, 359). The notification of individuals in a cohort study is now standard and is explained in OSHA's Hazard Communication Standards of 1983 and 1987 (Schulte 1985; Jonsen 1991; Schulte and Singal 1996).

Technical developments have enabled environmental health researchers to expand their previous focus on pollutants in occupational settings and contaminated environmental media, such as air or water, to contaminants in human tissues. Smaller-scale biomonitoring studies conducted by environmental advocacy organizations have been effective vehicles for promoting precautionary approaches to chemical regulation (CDC 1999; Jackson et al. 2002; Environmental Working Group 2003a). For example, policy makers in Europe and California used data from breast-milk monitoring to encourage a phase-out of certain PBDEs (polybrominated diphenyl ethers), flame retardants ubiquitous in electronic equipment, furniture, and other products (Environmental Working Group 2003). Biomonitoring has also been used to assess levels of other potentially hazardous substances, such as parabens in cosmetics and perfluorooctanoate (PFOA), which is used to manufacture Teflon for nonstick cookware and other domestic uses (Brody et al. 2007a).

Of the nearly 85,000 chemicals currently registered for commercial use, barely 10 percent have undergone basic toxicity testing, and these tests do not include assessments of carcinogenic, developmental, reproductive, neurological, immunological, or endocrine effects (Davis and Webster 2002). Exposure measurements are needed before researchers can evaluate links between exposure and health (Sexton, Needham, and Pirkle 2004; Stokstad 2004). The lack of causation data creates an ethical dilemma: if scientists cannot offer participants clear insights on health effects or the sources and pathways of exposure, should they notify participants of their exposure results or withhold the information? Moreover, the implications of test results are complicated by interactions of environmental exposures with individual and population differences in genetics, nutrition, health status, health-related behaviors, and exposures to other contaminants (Needham et al. 2005).

This issue was first discussed in the Department of Health, Education and Welfare's 1979 Belmont Report (National Institutes of Health 1979). The report's guidelines for protecting human subjects in research rest on three principles: autonomy, which includes the right to know (or the right not to know) as a basis for self-determination in acting on research results; beneficence and nonmalfeasance, which together encompass the researcher's responsibility to maximize good and minimize harm; and justice, which refers to the distribution of benefits and harm. Autonomy and justice argue for reporting individual results to study participants. Beneficence encourages researchers to consider benefits, such as empowering individuals and communities to take actions to direct their clinical care, reduce hazardous exposures, protect their health, and participate more fully in public health research and policy. Nonmalfeasance considers the possibility that reporting of results could create fear, stigma, and legal and economic complications (related to health insurance or property values, for example) and lead to unnecessary or counterproductive interventions (Brody et al. 2007a).

Although public health professionals have developed methods for reporting to individuals on regulated contaminants such as lead, study participants often are not informed of personal results considered by researchers to lack regulatory or clinical significance. Moreover, reporting individual data to participants has traditionally been a greater concern in clinical medicine: public health studies generally have dealt with community-level data, such as cancer registry information or environmental contamination data for food and water (Schulte and Singal 1996).

Biomonitoring also has implications for environmental justice. Communities that are socially, economically, and politically marginalized—from Native American communities in Akwesasne, NY, and St. Lawrence Island, AK, to African-American communities in Anniston, AL, and New Orleans—are beginning to conduct biomonitoring research to track exposures (cross-sectionally and longitudinally), record the extent of contamination, and pursue government funding, industry action, or legal remedies. However, some environmental justice advocates have approached biomonitoring with caution because of concerns that after-the-fact tissue measurements of chemicals cast these communities as environmental hazard detectors (Bhatia et al. 2005) and deemphasize the need to avoid such toxic trespass in the first place. Furthermore, some argue that this strategy can overemphasize the scientific aspects of environmental health problems, thus downplaying the roles of social inequality, economic exploitation, and racial discrimination in exposing these populations to environmental hazards (Sze and Prakash 2004; Morello-Frosch and Shenassa 2006). Because biomonitoring is both a powerful and a scientifically contested tool, elucidating its ethical and policy implications is critical for providing guidance to those who design biomonitoring programs and for those faced with the daunting task of interpreting uncertain data and making decisions about how to protect health.

METHODS

Our interest in this area stemmed from our own research, which involves environmental sampling of household air and dust as well as biomonitoring to assess the presence of endocrine-disrupting chemicals that may be linked to breast cancer (Brody et al. 2007b). Aggregate exposure assessment results were reported through peer-reviewed publications, media outreach, and public meetings, and individual reports were provided to study participants. To determine what information on report-back protocols was currently available to researchers and communities, we examined exposure reports published by government agencies, best-practice guidelines issued by professional associations, and journal articles reporting on specific studies. We assessed how documents presented exposure data and what information, if any, was provided to participants about interpreting and acting on the exposure data. We also examined how scientific uncertainty and data gaps were explained.

In addition, we conducted twenty-six interviews with scientists and community members involved in biomonitoring research. Interview protocols were reviewed and approved by Brown University's Institutional Review Board. Initially we contacted colleagues involved in academic and advocacy biomonitoring research and added to our sample researchers whom those colleagues recommended, through snowball sampling. We also drew on data from participant-observation at conferences and workshops where these issues have been debated and discussed. Uncited quotations and information come from those interviews and observations.

RESULTS

Frameworks for Communicating Biomonitoring Results

When considering whether and how to report individual data to study participants, scientists must weigh participants' right to know and the potential benefits of receiving the information against the possible psychological and practical harm of trying to make sense of data that may not provide a clear picture of potential health implications or guidance on how to reduce exposure (Schulte 1985; Jonsen 1991).We observed three distinct frameworks used by scientists for reporting biomonitoring results. The differences between these frameworks are summarized in table 13.1.

In the biomedically driven *clinical-ethics approach,* decisions about reporting individual biomonitoring results rest with scientists and medical experts and are based on whether the risk relationship between exposure and health effects is understood (Shalowitz and Miller 2005). If this relationship is known, the clinical action level of exposure, or "the level at which biomarker results will be of concern,"

TABLE 13.1 Frameworks for communicating biomonitoring results

Framework	Orientation	Right-to-know emphasis	Communication strategy	Protocol development
Clinical ethics	Biomedical	Weak	Individual results communicated if exposures reach clinical action levels, or if relationships between exposure and health outcome are understood.	Protocols developed primarily by scientific and medical experts. Participant confidentiality is paramount. No opportunities exist for participants to exchange results.
Community-based participatory research	Prevention	Strong, while also protecting participants' right *not* to know their results	Encourages communication of aggregate and individual results to participants, with emphasis on explaining scientific uncertainties and addressing concerns about community stigmatization. Participants' right to know is explained at the point of study recruitment and consent.	Protocols developed jointly by scientific and community partners. Confidentiality of participants is important, although some studies may offer opportunities for participants to share results if they wish. Protocols seek to balance community right to know with individual right to know.
Citizen-science data judo	Advocacy	Strong	Encourages reporting of aggregate and individual results to study participants to support precautionary individual action, communications, and policy change.	Protocols developed by scientific experts affiliated with advocacy organizations, sometimes in consultation with study participants. Participants encouraged to share results with each other and to speak publicly about their results.

should be determined prior to the start of the study (Deck and Kosatsky 1999). If the results fall below this level, individual data are generally not reported to participants.

The clinical ethics model gives more weight to the expert researcher's role in avoiding possible harm to study participants from reporting uncertain information and less weight to the study participants' ability to process complex and uncertain scientific information and respond autonomously. The decision to withhold clinically insignificant data may preclude precautionary action by participants in cases where even a low level of exposure to a contaminant may affect health, as with lead or mercury. Moreover, possible beneficial actions are usually seen as limited to medical or public health interventions based on regulatory guidelines or a legal mandate (such as screening children for lead exposure). These regulatory benchmarks are sometimes legally or scientifically contested.

In practice, the clinical ethics framework overlooks the significant evolution of clinical communications in recent decades. Individuals have become more proactive in directing their own health care: for example, many people monitor their own blood pressure and cholesterol, even when the results fall below a clinical action criterion (Bury 2004; Shalowitz and Miller 2005). In addition, withholding individual data may preclude action in the future, when links between exposure and health outcomes may be better understood. As one academic research scientist interviewed stated, individual results "are part of their medical history, so potentially in a few years that might be useful information."

For the majority of chemicals tested in biomonitoring studies, no health effects are conclusively linked to individual low-level exposure. In consequence, this clinical framework is likely to lead researchers to report only aggregate data. Nevertheless, our interviews with three medical doctors who conduct biomonitoring research suggest a potential shift in the clinical ethics framework. They saw certain advantages in engaging participants openly about biomonitoring results and their uncertainties to ensure productive clinical interactions.

Although health-based benchmarks are not available for most of the chemicals tested in humans, population-surveillance biomonitoring programs conducted over the past several years provide useful comparison data for reporting individual biomonitoring results. Indeed, scientists involved in an epidemiological cohort study of the developmental effects of pesticide exposures explained that the research team began by reporting only aggregate biomonitoring results but subsequently reported individual results because they could be compared to the national average levels provided by the CDC's biomonitoring information (CDC 2005). Although these comparisons are useful, they often do not help to elucidate exposure pathways and sources, nor do they relate exposures to levels associated with health effects.

In *community-based participatory research,* decisions about individual results communication are shared equally between scientists and the study community. This approach assumes that the reporting of individual and aggregate scientific study results can empower communities and individuals to act (Bishop 1994) and can restructure unequal and discriminatory power relationships (Wallerstein and Duran 2003). The sharing of knowledge (such as biomonitoring results) between researchers and participants is seen to have implications beyond the relevance of the knowledge to individual health (Foucault 1980). Therefore, CBPR encourages disseminating as much information as possible to study participants and posits that the participants from whose homes or bodies the original samples were taken have primary ownership of collected data (Bishop 1994).

An article on reporting pesticide exposure results to farmworker families in North Carolina echoes this approach, stating that "communicating risk to affected individuals should be an integral part of any community-based project. It is ethical to return information to the owner of that information" (Quandt et al. 2004, 642). In this study, the main question was not whether to report individual results, but how. According to this CBPR framework, even information about exposure to a substance whose health effects are unknown can have some benefits to participants, such as enabling them to take action to reduce personal exposures. The North Carolina study emphasizes community involvement in the development of protocols to address the interests and concerns of study participants: "In terms of the ambiguity, [the participants] thought it was important that the scientists present *la verdad* (the truth). If this meant telling women that it was not possible to know the level of danger represented by the findings, they would prefer to know that rather than to have the scientists give them a simpler but incomplete answer" (Quandt et al. 2004, 641).

Thus the CBPR approach to reporting data seeks not only to communicate health information but also to address disparities in access to knowledge that traditionally characterize "lay-expert" relationships (Sullivan et al. 2001). The CBPR approach must be strategic, however, as this framework raises potential conflicts between community versus individual right to know: the broad dissemination of biomonitoring results can adversely affect communities under study, even if the rights and confidentiality of individual participants are protected. Communities exposed to toxic contaminants with significant health risks may be stigmatized. Individuals associated with an "at risk" population may be denied jobs or health or life insurance. Collectively, a community perceived as contaminated may be passed over for programs or benefits, experience stereotyping that affects the quality of health care, suffer a decline in real-estate values, or face financial liability for remediation (Weijer 1999). For example, as early news broke of elevated PCB levels in the community of Broughton Island in northern Canada, and before the contamination was understood to extend throughout the circumpolar region, Broughton Islanders were shunned as the "PCB people." This stigma damaged the livelihood of the fishing community (Colborn, Dumanoski, and Myers 1996).

These pitfalls of biomonitoring studies can be addressed if researchers develop protocols and communication strategies in partnership with study communities

(Cone 2005; Brody et al. 2007a). This process requires a collective understanding about who represents the interests of study communities and how their issues can be effectively deliberated and incorporated into the protocol.

Citizen-science data judo, or "advocacy biomonitoring," is a strategy in which study design and communication of individual results are shaped primarily by policy goals (in this case, to improve chemical regulation). This framework assumes that personalized information about chemical body burdens can broaden public support for toxics-use reduction policies and motivate individuals to pursue both activism and personal exposure reduction. Environmental advocacy groups and communities marshal their own scientific resources and expertise to conduct research, and report-back strategies are specifically designed to advance regulatory and policy change (Morello-Frosch et al. 2005b). Our interviews with scientists who conducted biomonitoring studies for environmental organizations, as well as the individuals who participated, support this framework.

Although the goals of the data judo approach overlap with those of the CBPR framework, there are some important differences. CBPR is primarily research driven and aims to use report-back strategies to break down power and knowledge disparities between scientists and communities; the data judo approach is advocacy driven and seeks to mobilize constituencies by increasing public awareness about a specific regulatory issue or policy initiative. In recent years, body burden studies spearheaded by environmental organizations have proliferated. Three milestone activist studies were conducted by the Environmental Working Group (EWG). The first study, known as the Body Burden Study, recruited nine volunteers, most of whom were prominent environmental advocates, to have their blood and urine tested for the presence of 210 chemicals commonly found in consumer products and industrial pollution streams (Environmental Working Group 2003a). An average of 91 industrial compounds, pollutants, and other chemicals were found in the blood and urine of the study participants, with a total of 167 chemicals found in the entire group. The report on this study appears on the EWG website: viewers can click on a thumbnail photo of each study participant to see what contaminants are in that person's body.

The second EWG study examined the presence of a category of brominated flame retardants (PBDEs) in the breast milk of twenty first-time mothers in the United States (Environmental Working Group 2003b). This study found an average level of bromine-based chemicals in breast milk that was seventy-five times the average found in recent European studies (Norén and Meironyté 2000; Strandman, Koistinen, and Vartiainen 2000). Milk from two study participants contained the highest levels of fire-retardant chemicals ever reported in the United States, and several of the mothers had among the highest levels of these chemicals yet detected worldwide.

The third study examined the presence of chemicals commonly used in cosmetics and body-care products marketed to teenage girls. The study detected sixteen chemicals from four chemical families—phthalates, triclosan, parabens, and musks—in blood and urine samples from twenty participants between the ages of 14 and 19. Many of these chemicals are linked to potential health effects, including cancer and hormone disruption (Environmental Working Group 2008).

Advocacy biomonitoring has made human exposures to chemicals a prominent media and policy issue and has led to a proliferation of studies by other environmental and media organizations, including Commonweal, the World Wildlife Federation, Greenpeace, Environmental Defence (Canada), the Sightline Institute, National Geographic, and the *Oakland Tribune* in California (Body Burden Work Group and Commonweal Biomonitoring Resource Center 2007; World Wildlife Federation 2004; Greenpeace International 2005; Environmental Defence 2005; Sightline Institute 2004; Duncan 2006; Fischer 2005). It highlights the failure of environmental regulations and policies, such as the Toxic Substances Control Act (TSCA), to protect the public from exposures to ubiquitous contaminants, few of which have been tested to assess their health effects. As a result of extensive public outreach by both scientists and study participants, advocacy biomonitoring has garnered substantial regulatory attention and legitimized public concern about the presence of these chemicals in consumer products and elsewhere (Iles 2007). With few exceptions, these advocacy studies report data to study participants individually and also provide participants opportunities to talk publicly about their results. For example, EWG provides online personal biographies of consenting study participants in their body-burden and breast-milk studies (Environmental Working Group 2003a, 2003b, 2005). Many of these biographies emphasize participants' efforts to lead healthy lifestyles and point out that they did not work directly with chemicals in their jobs or live near major pollution sources.

Nearly all participants in advocacy biomonitoring studies savored the opportunity to share their results with other study participants to better contextualize and understand them and find opportunities for exposure reduction. As one participant noted: "The important thing, I think, to me, was understanding my results in the context of other people's results. So that while each of us got our results individually . . . it was only sort of when most of us [study participants] agreed to be in a conference call together to talk about it that I sort of began to understand what my own results meant, and how I felt about it in the context of other people's reactions. . . . And so it was very important to me that as a group we agreed to share our results. Not that we now know exactly what it means, but it was interesting to note that the biggest fish eaters had the highest levels of mercury."

Advocacy biomonitoring explicitly challenges traditional institutional review board (IRB) protocols for protecting participant confidentiality by giving study participants opportunities to discuss their results publicly, with the media, and with each other. IRB guidelines for biomedical studies have typically been developed to protect individuals in more controlled studies, such as clinical trials and lab experiments. Many IRBs have allowed aggregate reporting of study results while restricting or strongly discouraging the conveying of individual information. For example, some academic IRBs require passive individual report-back protocols that require participants to explicitly request their results. Although IRB concern about participant confidentiality is warranted, protocols that require greater initiative on the part of study participants to acquire their results ignore the fact that many individuals want to know their own results in order to take action to reduce exposures. Participants may also want to share their results with other study participants or through their own networks, communities, and public forums. As one scientist from an advocacy organization argued: "I think part of the challenge for all of the biomonitoring studies that are going on, including ours, is that you want to do it by the book, so that you write up an IRB [protocol] like any other study with human subjects, but in a way, doing it by the book is exactly what this is not about." Some advocacy biomonitoring studies have encouraged IRBs to examine how traditional standards of confidentiality may impose problematic restrictions on individual results communication.

Central Issues in Reporting Exposure Data to Individuals and Communities

Our analysis of the three approaches to biomonitoring results communication also elucidated some general guidelines for reporting exposure data to study participants.

Providing Adequate Background Information.   Several scientists and participants recommended comparing individual data with aggregate study results. Such comparisons are useful for putting the information into a familiar context. As Quandt and colleagues found, "presenting individual exposure data with reference to actual community data, rather than more abstract population-level reference data, engages community members' interest" (Quandt et al. 2004, 642). The use of comparisons is also recognized in the risk communication literature as important when the values being communicated appear small or when risks are unfamiliar to the involved community (Williams 2004). Body burden studies can fit both of these criteria: chemicals are often detected in seemingly low concentrations, and they may involve chemicals unfamiliar to the general population.

Another system for reporting individual data is to compare them with data from other published studies, such as the CDC reports (CDC 1999, 2003, 2005), when such studies exist. There can, however, be some confusion about what such a comparison implies. For example, one researcher indicated that when pesticide exposure results were reported to individuals, it was critical to ensure that any comparisons to general population levels from the CDC report were not misinterpreted as safety benchmarks. The exposure distribution for the population may be understood as a norm (Deck and Kosatsky 1999; Quandt et al. 2004). This misconception can have two negative effects on the participants' understanding of their risk. First, it can lead to a false sense of security among participants who have exposure levels at or below a community average; second, it can lead to unnecessary concern among those with higher exposure levels than the study average, regardless of the fact that the entire cohort might have exposures that are significantly below levels that indicate cause for concern. One scientist we interviewed, who directed an exposure study on brominated flame retardants, reported that two study participants had extremely high levels of PBDEs in their tissue samples. This caused at least one participant to be concerned, although currently there are no human health studies to indicate whether her results posed health risks for her or her child: "The participant who had the second-highest result was really pretty blown away by it. She had done the study expecting that she would be one of the more healthy, safe, you know, protected. . . . It's really an unfortunate part about enrolling [participants] in studies and giving them results about contaminant levels in their bodies when you don't have an even distribution or a way that would kind of predict or prepare them for where they might be in that distribution. and she took it really hard. . . . [T]he rest of the . . . [participants] felt lucky and felt protected."

The pitfalls of comparing individual data to study or population averages should not, however discourage the dissemination of this information. Instead, care should be taken to ensure that study participants understand that population averages should not be considered safety benchmarks. Whenever possible, information about comparison measures in other populations should be coupled with an explanation of the potential health implications of these levels and appropriate regulatory benchmarks.

Contention among Researchers about Reporting Protocols.   Our interviews revealed that the process for developing report-back protocols varies widely in both academic and advocacy biomonitoring studies. Some researchers develop protocols with little community input, whereas others solicit input from the study community, scientific colleagues not directly involved in the study, and social scientists. Most interviewees acknowledged the importance of involving community representatives in decisions about reporting results. They felt that it should be the community's decision whether individuals receive their own data, especially in situations when studies included participants whose illness might be linked to a substance or site under study. Nevertheless, for academic research involving community-academic collaborations, this view must contend with the fact that all entities receiving federal funding for research must operate in accordance with federally prescribed IRB procedures; this makes IRBs the final arbiters of whether to approve individual-level notification of study participants.

The academic scientists we interviewed reported wide variations in the willingness of their institutions' IRBs to grapple with the bureaucratic and logistical challenges of reviewing and approving individual reporting for biomonitoring studies. In addition, some described a lack of consensus among study collaborators, including academic scientists and members of community advisory panels. The disagreements show that even when there is a commitment to the right to know and community-based research, deciding how to implement those principles may not be simple. For example, physicians on an advisory board for one biomonitoring study tended to discourage individual report-back because of concerns that patients might have health-related questions linked to their study results that most doctors could not realistically answer. Conversely, community advocates and some industry representatives tended to favor releasing individual results to study participants, viewing this as a right-to-know issue.

Factors Affecting How Results Are Reported.   Most scientists described a system of individual and aggregate reporting that involved a combination of written materials and conversations with experts, either over the phone or in person. Some used a form of passive reporting, whereby study participants could contact researchers if they wanted to receive their personal results confidentially. This system gave participants the opportunity to opt out of receiving their information. Another researcher stressed the need to offer counseling or to give participants the name of someone to contact later to discuss new health issues or concerns. One scientist discussed the need to remain extremely flexible and available to participants, as one-third of the participants who did not initially opt to call in for results expressed interest in getting their results during a follow-up survey a few weeks later. This experience suggests that passive (opt-in) reporting may not be sufficient for providing results to participants.

The report-back process offers the potential to use aggregate and individual information to develop ways to reduce chemical exposures. Indeed, participants in two pesticide-exposure studies reported that receiving information about how to remove pesticides from the home and how to prevent future contamination was the most important part of the process. The support of public health interventions directly related to study results helps scientists ensure that the information provided to participants helps them take action to promote their health and well-being (Altman et al. 2008). One scientist brought up the importance of reporting individual study results in combination with specific measures that participants could take: "The most important component of that for us was not only giving the information but giving information about what the [participants] could do. So that reporting back is always linked to action, so that they are not getting the information without having any idea of what they can do about it."

In one pesticide exposure study of women, the health workers explained actions that all women could take to prevent pesticides from entering their homes and getting picked up by children, including closing windows during crop spraying and having farmworkers change their clothes before entering the home. In addition, brochures were provided, with information in Spanish, explaining that pesticide residues can be invisible and advising storing and washing work clothes separately (Deck and Kosatsky 1999; Quandt et al. 2004). Other biomonitoring studies of persistent organic pollutants that accumulate in the food chain have suggested that participants might choose to reduce their consumption of animal products or decrease the presence of contaminants in household dust by switching to less toxic consumer products.

However, scientists are often forced to balance the potential health benefits of such measures against the disruption and cost of an intervention (Cone 2005; Brody et al. 2007a). This is especially true if the effectiveness of the intervention has not been assessed. For example, one scientist leading a study on brominated flame retardants indicated that he would explain to participants how to reduce levels of animal fat in their diet, citing other health benefits associated with this action. But he also indicated that he would refrain from advising participants to take costly or inconvenient action to minimize the presence of PBDEs in household dust: "Right now my gut feeling would be not to tell people you should throw away all your furniture and buy all new furniture. That seems kind of extreme, right?"

Some biomonitoring results raise conflicts with an existing practice known to have a health benefit. Studies of contaminants in breast milk, for example, have been controversial because of concerns that the results might discourage breastfeeding, despite its known health benefits. A recent survey suggests that learning about the presence of chemicals in their breast milk may lead breastfeeding mothers to wean infants earlier than they had intended (Geraghty et al. 2008), although the survey was hypothetical, and the study did not measure whether reporting monitoring results actually changed the duration of breastfeeding.

In response to this debate, a recent article proposed a model informed-consent protocol for breast-milk biomonitoring studies that includes advice that "breastfeeding is almost always considered to be the best form of nutrition for a baby, and that the fact that the study is being carried out should in no way be taken as implying anything to the contrary" (Bates et al. 2002, 1873). All three scientists we interviewed who were involved in breast-milk studies reported that they encouraged participants to breastfeed. Additional empirical investigation of mothers' responses in breast-milk studies that encourage breastfeeding could inform the design of future monitoring efforts.

Debates over "risk messaging," or how to communicate about possible health risks revealed through biomonitoring research, are most difficult when health implications warrant exposure reduction but effective interventions are impossible, unjust, or likely to produce more deleterious consequences. In the 1980s and early 1990s, communication of biomonitoring results among Arctic Inuit communities called into question the consumption of large marine mammals, a traditional food source. Although the tissues of these mammals contain potentially dangerous levels of bioaccumulating contaminants, hunting and consuming them are practices essential to the subsistence and cultural survival of the community. Viable alternative food sources are few: commercially produced foods pose their own, arguably more dire health consequences in the form of malnutrition, obesity, cardiovascular disease, and diabetes (Furgal et al. 2003; Cone 2005).

Increasingly, messages encourage consumption of particular species with lower contaminant levels or specific cuts of flesh. Yet mounting evidence of the reproductive, immunological, and developmental effects of these persistent contaminants leave many communities and scientists in an uncertain situation (Cone 2005). Scientists and community members involved in these studies support the community's right to know; however, exposure reduction strategies are extremely difficult to employ. Reducing pollutant levels in marine mammals requires international political action and a long time horizon (Inuit Tapiriit Kanatami 1995; Furgal et al. 2003).

Addressing Varying Levels of Literacy.   Biomonitoring studies involve populations with varying levels of literacy (Boston Consensus Conference 2006; Nelson et al. 2008). In some cases, as with the Environmental Working Group's breast-milk study, participants are drawn from populations of environmental activists with high levels of environmental health literacy. One academic scientist we interviewed who was conducting breast-milk biomonitoring noted that participants came from two distinct groups: one that was upper middle class with a postgraduate level of education, and another that was working class, with a high-school or lower level of education. The latter group was far less inclined to request their biomonitoring results. However, participants who are members of marginalized groups with low levels of scientific literacy may still be eager to learn their results: they may prefer to have materials read to them and be shown diagrams, graphs, and pictures to help them interpret data (Quandt et al. 2004).

Another scientist involved in a cohort study on pesticides in low-income urban women and children provided further evidence that populations of low literacy are interested in receiving their individual results: "Yeah, the research workers have been getting the same questions that they've been getting for years now, you know, when are we going to get our individual results for our kids? You know, when are we going to know about pesticides? When are we going to know the results from our [monitoring]?"

Conveying complex results to populations with low levels of scientific literacy requires carefully crafting reports so that participants are engaged and able to understand the material presented to them. It is also necessary to communicate with members of the community during the creation of these materials to ensure that the information is relevant to their life experiences. If these measures are undertaken, our interviews suggest that populations with lower levels of scientific literacy are as interested in receiving their individual data as are more highly educated groups. Ultimately, participants can make a clear, deliberate choice regarding their right to know or not to know.

IRB Requirements and Standards of Confidentiality.   IRBs' focus on protecting the rights and confidentiality of individuals may lead them to discourage individual reporting. The scientists we interviewed faced a range of responses from IRBs to their proposed report-back protocols. One researcher was able to convince IRB members to reconsider their opposition to individual reporting by demonstrating that community representatives on the study's advisory board supported it. Another IRB limited researchers to calling participants and referring to them by their individual code number, rather than their names, in order to protect confidentiality.

By contrast, studies conducted by environmental advocacy organizations gave participants numerous opportunities to discuss their individual results with each other. In one study we examined, conference calls were held for all participants before and after results were disseminated, and group members were encouraged to share their personal responses to receiving their results. This process enabled them to share thoughts regarding pollutant sources and ways to reduce exposures. Such an approach encourages a reevaluation of traditional protocols aimed at protecting participant confidentiality and suggests new ways for researchers to enhance the participatory nature of disseminating and interpreting biomonitoring results. An IRB's duty to protect confidentiality ensures that personal information is not released without a participant's explicit and informed consent. Nevertheless, as with any health information, individuals should be free to share their own personal information with others.

DISCUSSION

Biomonitoring provides new ways of detecting and understanding the health implications of chemical trespass in people's bodies. It raises new ethical challenges that require democratizing the research enterprise to allow study participants to play a larger role in interpreting, disseminating, and acting on study results.

A consensus has yet to emerge on the ethics of reporting individual data on environmental exposures when the relationship between exposures and health outcomes is not established (Keune, Morrens, and Loots 2008). Indeed, some environmental health advocates and scientists who generally support the notion of the community right to know remain wary of individual reporting of data when the clinical implications are uncertain. Nevertheless, participatory research models are spilling over into the environmental health arena, compelling more scientists and advocacy organizations to consider whether and how to provide individual-level biomonitoring information (Quandt et al. 2004; Brody et al. 2007a). The literature and our interviews with scientists and study participants, although not unequivocal, indicate a trend in favor of including report-back strategies in the recruitment and consent process for research studies. The ethical issues of reporting exposure-monitoring results necessitate addressing the rights of study participants to information before, during, and after studies so that they can make informed decisions and be empowered to take action.

Perhaps the most important issue to emerge from our interviews is the need to set expectations for any exposure assessment or biomonitoring study *before* commencing data collection and setting up reporting protocols. It is important to clarify the inherent uncertainties and limitations of interpreting the data and its implications for community and individual health. If health implications are unknown, individual report-back may still provide an impetus for people to take action that could reduce their exposure. This information can also provide participants with opportunities to act collectively to use their results to support broader biomonitoring efforts. In time, these may enable researchers and participants to more fully understand population variability in exposures and propose interventions that promote protective regulation and toxics-use reduction.

CONCLUSION

Much of the new biomonitoring work involves informing individuals of their chemical exposures. The individual report-back approaches discussed here represent a departure from traditional models of reporting aggregate study results only in academic settings, such as professional meetings and peer-reviewed publications. Of note is the increased effort among scientists to report chemical exposures whose clinical significance is not fully known. Guidance is needed on the ethical responsibilities associated with communicating individual and community-level data. This guidance cannot come solely from the established arbiters of clinical and research practice or from government health officials but must also be shaped by the communities engaged in research efforts.

NOTE

Originally published as Rachel Morello-Frosch, Julia Green Brody, Phil Brown, Rebecca Gasior Altman, Ruthann A. Rudel, and Carla Pérez, "Toxic Ignorance and the Right-to-Know: Assessing Strategies for Biomonitoring Results Communication in a Survey of Scientists and Study Participants," *Environmental Health* 8, no. 6 (2009).

14

IRB Challenges in Community-Based Participatory Research on Human Exposure to Environmental Toxics

A Case Study

Phil Brown, Rachel Morello-Frosch, Julia Green Brody, Rebecca Gasior Altman,
Ruthann A. Rudel, Laura Senier, Carla Pérez, and Ruth Simpson

In 1979 the Belmont Report established principles for the use of human subjects in scientific research (National Institutes of Health 1979). Developed partly in response to the Tuskegee syphilis study (the infamous forty-year study of deliberate nontreatment of syphilis), the Belmont Report identified three basic principles governing the ethical use of human research subjects, including their informed consent. The first principle, respect for persons, stressed that an individual's decision to become a research participant must be voluntary, and it called for special protection for those who lacked the capacity to make such a decision themselves. The second principle, beneficence, called on researchers to do no harm or at least to maximize the benefits of their research while minimizing the risk to the subject. Finally, the principle of justice required careful attention to the fair distribution of risks and benefits, calling on researchers to select subjects only "for reasons directly related to the problem being studied" and to vigilantly avoid the selection of subjects for "their easy availability, their compromised position, or their manipulability." Justice also required that those who bear the risks of research should, whenever possible, be among the first to benefit from its insight.

The implementation of these principles fell to institutional review boards (IRBs), oversight groups within research organizations that are charged with ensuring that studies protect individual participants through confidentiality, informed consent, and oversight. But although IRBs have been the traditional enforcers of the Belmont principles, the same principles form the basis of community-based participatory research (CBPR), a method that has become increasingly important in the work of environmental justice and environmental public health activists who are engaging more directly in scientific research design and the collection and analysis of individual data (Shepard et al. 2002; McCormick, Brown, and Zaves-toski 2003; Morello-Frosch et al. 2005b; Brody et al. 2007a). CBPR focuses on problems that affect whole communities—environmental toxins, for example—and thus is different from most biomedical research, which takes the individual as its primary subject. In CBPR projects, researchers work closely with community members and community-based organizations to develop appropriate research agendas, conduct analyses, and disseminate results and information. This merging of community interests and community action reflects another distinct quality of CBPR: its commitment to advocacy for the public good and to providing open access to information.

CBPR takes "respect for persons" to a new level: not only do research subjects participate voluntarily, but they also participate *actively* in research design, data collection, analysis, implementation, and dissemination. This inclusion reflects CBPR's commitment to the principles of beneficence and justice, as the active involvement and scrutiny of subjects encourages the fair assessment and distribution of the research's risks and benefits. Further, the practice of giving research subjects the choice of having full access to research results helps ensure that they have sufficient information to make informed decisions during and after the study and is thus consistent with the Belmont Report's emphasis on informed consent. In CBPR, research subjects are transformed into research participants.

Ironically, however, IRB review of CBPR projects frequently results in unintended violations of the very principles they share. This conflict is due in part to implicit assumptions embedded in the Belmont Report that were adopted by IRBs but that contradict other CBPR principles. For example, IRBs, following Belmont, assume that the research participant is an individual, whereas CBPR sees research participants as both individuals and a community of individuals (Deeds et al. 2008). This difference has profound implications for confidentiality, the dissemination of information, and the assessment of risks and benefits. Similarly, CBPR's inclusion of laypeople, community-based organizations, and other entities in the carrying out of the research means that university IRBs must consider whether and how to extend their jurisdiction. These differences and the general unfamiliarity of many IRBs with the CBPR approach can result in obstacles and delays and hence can reduce the benefit of the research for the participants and even cause them harm, if their access to information that could inform their own decisions about their future health and welfare is restricted or delayed. A third difficulty arises when communities request that scientists study environmental problems and work with scientific collaborators to design and fund a project, but the IRBs either delay approval or decline to oversee the project.

The increasing use of CBPR in the work of environmental justice and environmental public health activists makes it particularly important that all those involved work toward defining IRB oversight procedures that will advance CBPR projects instead of inadvertently hindering them. We draw on our own experiences to demonstrate the various problems that can arise during institutional review and show how those problems undermine rather than support the spirit of the Belmont Report. We supplement our accounts with reports from other researchers engaged in CBPR projects, and we use these experiences to identify the causes of these problems and propose solutions. We conclude by recommending an alternative approach to informed consent and ethical review that will empower communities and social-change organizations to participate fully in both the scientific process and the protection of human research subjects.

METHODS

Our research collaborative involves a partnership between three institutions: Brown University, Silent Spring Institute (a nonprofit environmental health research organization based in Massachusetts), and Communities for a Better Environment (CBE; a California environmental justice organization that combines organizing, advocacy, litigation, and research). Our project entails sampling household air and dust in three study sites: Richmond and Bolinas in California, and Cape Cod in Massachusetts. We also conducted human biomonitoring on Cape Cod. In response to community concerns about environmental justice and environmental links to breast cancer, we tested for endocrine-disrupting compounds and additional pollutants from industry and transportation corridors near the Richmond site. The project reports individual results to study participants who choose to receive them and disseminates aggregate results through community meetings, peer-reviewed publications, and media outreach.

Brown University's IRB was initially reluctant to oversee the researchers in the community partner organizations but ultimately facilitated an effective oversight strategy that ensured human subjects protection for the entire collaborative. Hence our experience serves as a model for others and adds weight to a changing research protection paradigm that understands and values community-based participatory research.

We also report the experiences of twelve colleagues collaborating on CBPR projects at other institutions. We selected these colleagues from the list of current projects funded by the National Institute of Environmental Health Sciences Environmental Justice Program. Because we were, at the time, only seeking information to guide our own IRB request, we were not subject to human-subjects protection oversight for these consultations. Therefore we report on lessons learned without direct reference to the researchers or their institutions. While preparing for a research proposal to study these IRB issues in greater depth, we spoke with four additional researchers involved in biomonitoring and household exposure studies.

In addition, we draw data from a workshop we led at the NIEHS Environmental Justice Program grantees conference in Talkeetna, AK, in September 2005 and a workshop on community review boards led by West Harlem Environmental Action (WE ACT) at the NIEHS Environmental Justice Program grantees conference in Boston in December 2007. Uncited material is taken from our interviews, conversations, and observations.

RESULTS: CBPR EXPERIENCES WITH IRB REVIEW

CBPR researchers have joined a growing group of scholars concerned that the institutional review process has become too formulaic and inflexible. Designed for overseeing biomedical and behavioral research, the process is often inappropriate to the methods, challenges and objectives of studies in other disciplines. Social scientists, for example, have criticized the application of stringent informed-consent procedures for low-risk, nonintrusive interview research, such as interviewing public officials who are legally obliged to reply to citizens' queries (Bosk and DeVries 2004).

But CBPR researchers face unique challenges in the review process. The differing assumptions that CBPR researchers and IRBs bring to the process are most apparent in IRBs' opposition to two particular CBPR practices: layperson participation in the research process and the reporting of individual results to study participants. The involvement of laypeople and community-based organizations in CBPR research means that some of those involved in conducting research are outside the conventional jurisdiction of institutional IRBs. And the CBPR practice of report-back, and especially the philosophy of openness that informs it, challenges IRB assumptions about who owns the data produced in human-subjects research, when and whether those data should be made available to members of an affected community, and the nature and duration of the researcher-subject relationship.

IRB Oversight of Community-Based Organizations

Unlike conventional research, in which the researcher maintains total control over the research and research subjects, CBPR is collaborative, inviting community members and community-based organizations to work alongside the professional researchers studying that community. Laypeople help define the research agenda, form research questions, carry out the study, and disseminate results and information to the community and other relevant parties, such as public health practitioners and social service agencies (Israel et al. 1998; Shepard et al. 2002). CBPR thus blurs the traditional roles of researcher and subject and takes seriously the contributions that members of the affected community can bring to the project.

The active involvement of laypersons in CBPR research expresses the Belmont principle of "respect for persons," intended to protect research participants from being objectified and dehumanized. By encouraging this involvement, CBPR greatly reduces the chances that they will be objectified in the first place. As participants in the design and implementation of the research plan, members of the affected community have a level of informed consent far deeper than typically occurs in conventional research; and scientific and medical experts work alongside laypeople, rather than treating them simply as objects of study.

Facilitating collaboration and communication among scientists, medical professionals, and laypeople has its own challenges, but often the biggest hurdle for CBPR researchers is introducing IRBs to the idea. We and our colleagues have found that IRBs are uneasy when community-based organizations (CBOs) serve as formal partners in a research initiative. The main problem is jurisdictional: university IRBs are reluctant to take responsibility for human-subjects protection when projects involve organizations outside the university. That discomfort is sometimes magnified by the routine activities of the CBO. For example, a CBO's process of seeking feedback from its constituency—evaluating whether a presentation has successfully reached its target audience, for example—could appear to an academic IRB as human-subjects research requiring review. This judgment could appear to the CBO as an unwelcome intrusion into its internal affairs. (Exceptions for such routine activities already exist in federal regulations and could be a basis for exempting CBO educational evaluations, but IRBs are not always aware of this.) IRBs may be particularly disturbed when a CBO openly merges research and activism, thus challenging traditional academic norms. Concerned by the close coexistence of research and common CBO activities such as outreach, IRBs may attempt to influence activities that many CBOs believe should be under their own control.

Many of these problems were apparent when we sought human-subjects review from Brown University's IRB for a project that involved two CBOs: Silent Spring Institute and Communities for a Better Environment. Silent Spring Institute was the principal investigator for several reasons. The institute originated the study of large numbers of diverse analytes in homes. It remains the foremost research organization in this field and was the only partner on the team with the capacity to design and implement methods of exposure assessment. It also originated the idea of studying participants' report-back experiences. Moreover, NIEHS had encouraged CBPR project teams to promote leadership by CBO partners. The IRB initially doubted its own capacity to oversee and hold accountable organizations that were not legal entities of the university. But in fact, this IRB, like many others, routinely has oversight of research conducted in other countries by locally hired researchers. Of primary concern was the possibility that some CBO activities might violate federal standards and jeopardize federally funded research activities and the reputation of the university as a whole.

From our standpoint, the concerns about jurisdiction were unfounded. The Department of Health and Human Services Policy for the Protection of Human Subjects makes clear that CBOs can be reprimanded directly by the HHS Office for Human Research Protection (OHRP) for violations of federal regulations for the protection of human subjects (revised in 2005). Brown's IRB could have contacted the OHRP directly with any concern about a CBO partner's ability to conduct research or protect human subjects in federally funded research. All CBOs conducting research are required to obtain and periodically update an OHRP assurance of compliance with human-subjects protection guidelines and must report any suspension or termination of research by an IRB.

To allay IRB concerns, we demonstrated that our community partners were experienced in scientific research and well versed in human-subjects protection protocols. Silent Spring Institute has a long track record of obtaining state IRB approval for environmental health research supported by state, federal, and private funds. Communities for a Better Environment is a long-established organization whose research using secondary data (such as oil refinery emissions, for example) was well known to academic institutions and government agencies. Moreover, individual CBE staff members had experience working for universities and health providers conducting human-subjects research. In addition, staff from both Silent Spring and CBE completed human-subjects protection training through the National Institute of Health's online certification training and exam.

Despite these credentials, the Brown University IRB remained reluctant. Deciding that NIH certification was insufficient, it required that staff from both organizations also take the Collaborative Institutional Training Initiative (CITI) online course and exam. Focusing on issues related to clinical and behavioral research, the CITI training program does not address the human-subjects issues unique to CBPR projects. Thus CBO staff received training on research scenarios that were largely irrelevant to their own projects. In addition, the training module assumed familiarity with online electronic systems, experience with multiple-choice tests, and strong English literacy—all potentially disruptive to an environmental justice project, for example, if it is staffed by people who speak English as a second language or have little or no experience navigating web-based programs. The five or six hours required to complete the training added to the frustration of already overextended CBO staff. At the NIEHS Environmental Justice grantees conferences and other events, our colleagues described similar problems.

Ideally, we would have turned to NIEHS for help in getting community partners through the university IRB process. Unfortunately, although NIEHS promotes CBPR research, it does not offer guidance to IRBs for reviewing academic and community partnerships. In consequence, researchers and IRB staff members were on their own to resolve unique and sometimes conflicting institutional concerns. We developed procedures making Brown University faculty partners responsible for protecting study participants in interviews, collection of human and household samples, and record keeping. These faculty members agreed to make quarterly visits to Communities for a Better Environment and Silent Spring to check record-keeping and data-storage protocols and reported to the IRB on the collaborative's adherence to approved study protocols.

In the end, the IRB agreed to provide oversight for our research collaborative, initially for only eighteen months of a four-year project, but eventually for the full duration of the project. Although we were pleased to have obtained approval, the many problems caused substantial delays in initiating and conducting the project.

Who Gets to Know? CBPR and IRB Conflicts over the Dissemination of Information

IRBs frequently clash with CBPR researchers over their methods of disseminating information and results. IRBs are accustomed to overseeing conventional research projects, in which study participants often are not informed of personal results that lack regulatory or clinical significance. The CBPR practice of having study participants work alongside researchers confounds assumptions about who should control and have access to the resulting data.

In CBPR, the subjects' right to have access to the results of research derives from a source more fundamental than their own participation in the research effort. CBPR posits that the participants from whom the samples are taken have primary ownership of collected data (Bishop 1994). From this perspective, it would be inappropriate and unjust to deny people full access to information that came from their own bodies, homes, and communities, through their willing participation.

IRBs frequently express concerns that disseminating uncertain data may harm human subjects. For example, a participant might be psychologically harmed by receiving results if their clinical significance is unknown or if no valid options exist to address the potential health risks they reveal (Shalowitz and Miller 2005). Indeed, the National Bioethics Advisory Commission (1999) issued guidelines directing researchers to report biological markers of contamination or disease only when health implications are significant and recourse is available. These discussions may not, however, have adequately considered the distinction between communications related to genetic biomarkers, which are not modifiable, and chemical exposures, many of which are modifiable. When these clinical guidelines are applied to research about chemical exposure measures, people are left unaware of the presence in their own bodies of foreign substances known to be harmful from animal studies and sometimes from in vitro and in vivo human studies. From the perspective of CBPR, such guidelines are an affront to individuals' and communities' rights to know, and by extension a tarnish on the scientific process.

In CBPR, respect for persons thus requires and reinforces a commitment to report-back, an ethical practice that encourages the dissemination of individual and aggregate results to study participants who want them. This openness is valued in CBPR because it democratizes knowledge production and helps restructure unequal power relationships (Wallerstein and Duran 2003), especially the disparities in access to knowledge that have traditionally characterized relationships between laypeople and professional researchers (Sullivan et al. 2001). CBPR also assumes that the sharing of knowledge between researchers and participants empowers communities and individuals to use scientific evidence to advocate for their own interests (Bishop 1994). Report-back thus upholds the principle of beneficence by maximizing the benefits of the research project for participants, both by giving them access to information crucial for their health and well-being and by empowering them to act on their own behalf (Brody et al. 2007a). From a beneficence perspective, even information about an exposure for which a corresponding risk relationship is not available can have some benefits to participants, such as enabling them to reduce personal exposures. The sharing of aggregate data can also make communities aware of a problem in their midst and give them both the motivation and the evidence they need to take action. Our project has expended considerable effort on reporting data to individual participants and to community gatherings in order to advance general knowledge, build local capacity for community improvement, and encourage policy shifts in government and corporate practice (Brody et al. 2009; Morello-Frosch et al. 2009a).

As we and our colleagues discovered, the voluntary sharing of information in CBPR may be foreign to IRB conceptions of confidentiality. For example, in the Body Burden study (a joint project of the Environmental Working Group, Mt. Sinai School of Medicine, and Commonweal) researchers discovered 167 pollutants (of 210 for which they tested) in the blood and urine of nine volunteers, with an average of 56 carcinogens in each person's samples. Aggregate study results appeared in *Public Health Reports* (Thornton, McCally, and Houlihan 2002), but study participants voluntarily placed their individual data on the internet, with photos and personal biographies to accompany the contaminant data (Environmental Working Group 2003a). Voluntary though it was, the website would have been perceived by most IRBs as a violation of confidentiality.

Similarly, IRBs were frequently bothered by the extended interactions between researchers and participants that are typical of CBPR. For example, community residents' requests for information to reduce exposure, and our own sense of responsibility, led us to build into our project an intervention phase for reducing household toxics use. We also distributed information sheets to participants about nontoxic alternatives and environmental organizations. We saw our actions as akin to health care workers providing treatment and prevention advice in medical screening.

The enduring, proactive, and flexible relationship between researchers and study participants is crucial to CBPR but can be troublesome to IRBs. For example, some academic IRBs require "passive" reporting protocols that restrict researchers from asking participants if they want to receive and discuss their own results. Instead, researchers may only inform study participants that they can contact researchers should they wish to receive individual results in the future. IRBs may feel obliged to review each phase of the relationship and any and all communications between researcher and participant before the research can proceed. Such requirements can delay research, prevent study participants from getting information necessary for their health and well-being, and threaten collaborations between researchers and members of the affected community.

Such delays and disruptions occurred in the Cape Cod project. Because many study participants were initially identified through the Massachusetts Cancer Registry, the Massachusetts Department of Public Health's Research and Data Access Review (RaDAR) Committee had jurisdiction over the project. Any subsequent work with these participants (such as developing protocols to inform them of their individual household sampling and biomonitoring results) had to be cleared by the RaDAR Committee. Unfortunately, that review process took many months, and the committee and others within the Massachusetts DPH lodged a number of objections to the CBPR project. One delay occurred when Cape Cod homes with high levels of chemicals were retested to get more detailed measurements that might determine sources of contamination and point to possible remediation strategies. The DPH Bureau of Environmental Health Assessment initially asked to review the letters that went to every one of these households, raising the possibility of protracted negotiation about the scientific interpretation of each individual's finding. Finally, after a meeting with Silent Spring Institute and Brown University researchers, they approved a prototype letter that would be tailored by the research team for each recipient.

The DPH action was a prime example of IRB review threatening the very principles it hopes to uphold—in this case the principles of beneficence and justice. Recurring delays from lengthy reviews, on top of funding cuts, kept study participants from getting their results in a timely fashion and jeopardized relations between the research team and participants, thus threatening good CBPR practice. Women who had provided human tissue and household dust and air samples for the study were understandably disconcerted by the delay in receiving their results. Fortunately, Silent Spring Institute's respected status in the community and its skillful handling of the situation, which enabled participants to stay informed on the progress of the research, helped maintain the participants' trust and goodwill.

IRB resistance to ongoing interactions between researchers and study participants was also manifest in its resistance to storing samples after the main research was accomplished, when traditionally samples have been destroyed.

Exposure-assessment research is a rapidly evolving field in which analytical methods and knowledge are constantly improving. Stored samples provide an opportunity to reanalyze data as research methods become better and more cost-effective. For example, a study on a possible link between breast cancer and DDT exposure, published in 2007, reanalyzed blood samples that had been donated between 1959 and 1967 for a child health and development study. The results showed that women exposed to the highest levels of DDT before midadolescence had a fivefold increase in breast cancer risk (Cohn et al. 2007). Because many women heavily exposed to DDT in childhood are still under fifty, we may see startling effects in the coming decades. Had those samples been destroyed, the potential loss to public health would have been monumental.

In one instance during the Cape Cod project, the DPH threatened to require the destruction of environmental and biological samples immediately after the first laboratory chemical analyses were completed, even though study participants had given permission for samples and data to be retained for ten years for further analysis. The DPH requirement would have undermined one of the critical goals of the research project: to identify sources of endocrine-disrupting compounds in homes. New assays might be developed in the future to detect additional EDCs, and if samples were destroyed, researchers would miss the opportunity to analyze them. After much negotiation, the RaDAR Committee required the research team to get new consent from study participants in order to continue storing their samples at the research laboratory.

The Cape Cod case demonstrated that maintaining such samples can become crucial for reasons unforeseeable at the time of IRB review. During the research, the study team unexpectedly found breakdown products of a banned flame retardant. Had the samples been destroyed, researchers would have been unable to retest the samples to confirm the source of the residues. When research participants want their own samples destroyed, their wishes should, of course, be respected, but when they have consented to sample and data storage, IRB requirements to destroy biological specimens can in fact contravene the Belmont principles to maximize research benefits for study participants. Because the last few years have seen a dramatic increase in knowledge about flame retardants, especially PBDEs, these samples have retroactively become a part of front-line public health research (Hites 2004; Blum 2007; Zota et al. 2008).

Despite significant obstacles and delays related to IRB review, our research progressed. We moved the Massachusetts RaDAR Committee on several critical issues through continual pressure by academic partners, Silent Spring Institute, supporters from the Massachusetts Breast Cancer Coalition, pro bono legal representation, and state legislators. The Brown University IRB found the experience valuable, too, and they invited us to give a presentation at a statewide research conference they organized in 2007.

Educating the IRB about the CBPR Process

While attempting to shepherd CBPR projects through the IRB process, we and our colleagues at other institutions employed a range of strategies with varying degrees of success. For example, to help the Cape Cod project through institutional review at Brown University, we prepared extensive memos to our university IRB that laid out the history and practices of CBPR, bolstered by extensive in-person and e-mail dialogue with IRB staff. We demonstrated precedent by showing that other researchers at prominent institutions had carried out this kind of collaborative work while observing sound ethical practices, and that another institutional review board had approved such multipartner collaborative research.

One researcher we consulted suggested researching IRB members' familiarity with CBPR. Others have remarked that because IRBs need to be educated about CPBR, researchers often find themselves in advocacy roles with IRB members. At one state university in the western United States, one faculty member invited the IRB and human subjects administration to an all-day CBPR workshop to improve overall understanding of the principles of CBPR and to establish regular communication between researchers and IRBs.

Despite the many obstacles to collaborative projects, some academic IRBs understand the unique circumstances of CBPR work and go out of their way to facilitate it. Still, in our consultations with other CBPR researchers, we learned of only one other case in which the IRB of a major research university agreed to be the IRB of record for a CBO partner in a CBPR project.

STRATEGIES FOR NAVIGATING THE IRB PROCESS

The problems that arise in IRB review of CBPR projects stem from the different assumptions and objectives of diverse parties. An effective solution requires effort by all involved. Based on our experience, we suggest the following guiding principles for advancing multipartner CBPR projects through the IRB process.

What CBPR Researchers and CBO Partners Can Do

Take Time to Educate the IRB.   Helping IRBs learn about the objectives and approach of CBPR research proved very useful in the review process. IRB members may be unfamiliar with CBPR and might benefit from presentations on the history of the work, its basic principles, the funding agencies that support it, the scientific and community benefits, and the unique ethical considerations it raises. Getting to know the IRB members in advance of the review process can help researchers assess the extent of education about CBPR that may be necessary.

Make Sure Academic IRBs Know Community Partners.   Academic research-ers should try to connect community partners with IRB staff to demonstrate the community's involvement in the research process and the importance of their perspective on human-subjects protection to the project's success. One approach is to invite community partners to meetings with the IRB. Research partners can include this "community consent" in the IRB application. If the IRB lacks the familiarity, experience, or the skills necessary for assessing the ethical issues posed by a CBPR research project, an outside expert can be brought in to educate the board and encourage members to think critically about the research proposal (Pritchard 2002).

What IRBs and Funding Institutions Can Do

Keep Abreast of CBPR and Other Cutting-Edge Research Approaches.   Just as IRB officials keep up with the literature on conventional human-subjects research, they need to keep current on the CBPR literature. Rather than wait until they are approached for approval of a CBPR project, IRBs should prepare themselves in advance for that encounter. Attending meetings and conferences where CBPR is broadly discussed (e.g. the meetings of the Community-Campus Partnerships for Health, International Society for Environmental Epidemiology, and International Society for Exposure Analysis) or inviting CBPR experts to share their experi-ences would help IRBs better understand CBPR approaches.

Develop a Procedure for the Review of CBPR Projects.   Routinizing IRB review of CBPR would keep new applicants from having to reinvent the wheel and would increase the viability of CBPR projects. The procedure could be developed incre-mentally as successful projects provide models for others. Alternatively, federal funding agencies could develop guidelines. For example, NIEHS could contract out the development of a protocol to a research institution that deals with ongoing CBPR issues (such as Campus-Community Partnerships for Health, a nonprofit organization that has created partnerships between 1,500 communities and cam-puses). The resulting guidelines could be posted on relevant websites and form the basis for training sessions.

Provide Clear Guidance and Tools for Navigating IRB Issues Unique to Academic and Community Collaboratives.   Funding institutions, especially the National Institutes of Health (NIH) and the National Science Foundation (NSF), should offer human-subjects training specific to CBPR research and should sensitize universities to the importance of supporting community groups. University IRBs should be aware that community organizations may operate on different time-lines, and that the intense and lengthy university IRB reporting process can create difficulties for them. This is particularly true when the community partner is the principal investigator—responsible for ensuring timely progress of the research, but dependent on a university IRB that has a slow review process. Researchers doing grant-funded community-based research should include ample time for IRB review in their grant proposals.

Funding agencies should encourage academic IRBs to provide oversight to both academic and community partners to avoid unnecessary delays and expenses in protocol reviews. They may want to promote consortium-based approval, whereby one institution's IRB is accepted by others in the consortium (Silent Spring Institute has an agreement of this type with Boston University, a partner in some of its other projects; indemnification may be necessary so that universities do not bear responsibility for the actions of community partners). Funding agencies should ensure that all community partners in the projects they sponsor will have the resources necessary to complete the IRB process and comply with reporting requirements. In addition, funding agencies could help communicate to IRBs that community groups should not have to expend their own resources to navigate the review process. Addressing these issues can help all IRB processes and offer improved protection to individuals and communities. Funding institutions could use grant announcements and descriptions to give clear guidance about the IRB issues that CBPR partners are likely to face. Another possible resource is the Applied Research Ethics National Association, an organization that provides resources and information about ethical and procedural issues of campus IRBs (Strand et al. 2003).

Regulate Any Conflicts of Interest IRBs May Bring to the Review Process.   IRB members, like those on the Massachusetts DPH RaDAR Committee, should not review human-subjects protection for a project when they might have a vested interest in the outcome (because of its implications for public health agency action, for example). Creating an independent IRB for such situations would protect human subjects while avoiding conflicts of interest that could hinder the progress of a worthy study. That IRBs may have their own conflicts of interest is a legitimate concern. A recent survey of 893 IRB members at 100 academic institutions found that 36 percent of IRB members had had at least one relationship with industry in the previous year, of which only two-thirds had been disclosed to the IRB. Of those who reported conflicts, nearly one-third had participated in the reviews anyway (Campbell et al. 2006). Of course, some have argued that conflicts of interest are widespread even among independent IRBs (Forster 2002), so further action may be needed.

Reassess How IRBs Oversee Situations in which Participants Desire Access to and Disclosure of Their Own Study Results.   In some cases, ensuring participants' access to their study data necessitates continued interaction between researchers and participants, a process that IRBs may be reluctant to allow and are poorly designed to manage. Iterative rounds of approval for ongoing communication with study participants result in delays that undermine researchers' relationships with participants. Although IRB concerns about confidentiality are warranted, they may disregard the fact that individuals often want access to their own data in order to take individual or collective action to reduce their exposures. They may also want to share their personal results with other study participants and have the power to disseminate their results through their own networks and broader public forums. Restricting individual report-back could push confidentiality protections to collide with the principle of beneficence. Thus, CBPR challenges IRBs to reassess the seemingly contradictory elements of the Belmont Report principles and to develop alternatives that do not require choosing one principle over another.

Working with Community and Tribal IRBs

Academic IRBs are not the only forums in which community benefits of the research may be assessed. Some communities have convened their own review boards to assess collectively whether proposed research is justified and benefits the community (Quigley 2006). For example, the Navajo Nation maintains its own IRB to protect its people from research that would not directly help them (Sharp and Foster 2002). The Indian Health Service adds respect for communities to the Belmont principles and expects proposals to discuss whether there are tribal consultants who could be involved, whether the project entails community capacity building that would benefit the tribe, whether researchers understand community research priorities, and whether researchers will provide regular and timely community consultations (Romero 2003). Similarly, the citizens' organization that oversees research on residential exposures from the Fernald, OH, nuclear weapons plant permits researchers access to its records only when the researchers can demonstrate a concrete benefit for the community, regardless of academic IRB approval (Gerhardstein and Brown 2005).

Researchers involved in community-based participatory research are increasingly seeking community review boards that emphasize community protections alongside traditional IRB responsibilities (Gilbert 2006). While tribal IRBs have the power of regular IRBs, other community review boards do not yet meet the requirements for oversight of federally funded research. Factors such as geographic dispersion, political disorganization, and the lack of authority to review research protocols can impede the formation of such boards. In consequence, an additional IRB is required to provide formal guarantees. Academic IRBs reviewing research proposals on behalf of such communities need to understand their form and organization, their needs and vulnerabilities, and their existing governance and communication structures for disseminating research (Weijer 1999).

Community representation in the review process would be helpful not only to those engaged in community-based research but also to those engaged in individual research who may not have considered the effects of their research on communities. NIH rules were clarified in 1998 to ensure that IRBs have "knowledge of the local research context," but although they require that one member of the IRB must be from outside the institution, direct community representation is not required (National Institutes of Health 1998). Community representatives on academic IRBs usually come from large, well-established organizations rather than grassroots groups, and such organizations do not usually reflect the demographic composition of the communities under study (Taylor 2003). Two 2001 reports from the Office of Human Subjects Research of NIH and the National Bioethics Advisory Commission have pointed to the need to expand community involvement in research beyond mere representation on IRBs (Dickert and Sugarman 2005), but most pressure for deep community involvement stems from activist groups (Strand et al. 2003).

RECOMMENDATIONS FOR FUTURE RESEARCH

Health and social science researchers should study a large sample of scientists working in human exposure and related areas to gather more detailed information on IRB challenges. It is important to learn whether and how IRBs may have changed their procedures in response to pressure for individual report-back and community-level protection, and whether and how researchers may have changed their beliefs about or methods for the reporting of individual data. Extensive interviews with IRB staff and academic members should supplement interviews with researchers. Future research should study how participants experience the process of informed consent in biomonitoring and household exposure studies, the degree to which they desire detailed information and supplementary information used for reducing exposure, and the ways they use their personal data to explain exposure, understand disease causation, and seek regulatory and other changes.

CONCLUSION

Resolving IRB challenges is not solely a matter of revising study requirements. Rather, it is part of a larger process by which CBOs and their academic supporters reframe the entire research enterprise and empower community organizations to protect individual subjects and communities (whether those communities are defined by geography, class, ethnicity, or other distinctions). Such changes pose fundamental challenges to researcher-participant relationships, academic and community interaction, and the people's right to know about chemicals and toxins in their environments, homes, and bodies.

The spirit of community and openness that informs CBPR has special significance for environmental justice. Communities facing environmental justice issues have understandable concerns about the power, objectives, and decision-making processes of government and scientific agencies. Further, the stress and complexities of an environmental hazard can cause divisions within a community even in the face of a shared problem. CBPR's emphasis on report-back is crucial for establishing a productive working relationship between community members and outside researchers by promoting the interest of the former over the research objectives of the latter. In addition, encouraging lay participation in collaborative research can help overcome divisions and motivate a community to take the action necessary to achieve environmental justice. In short, the very practices that disturb many IRBs are exactly those that make CBPR so valuable for environmental justice issues. It is thus all the more crucial that the review process be revised in a way that will improve CBPR rather than hinder it.

Despite the challenges of the IRB experience, research partners can use this process as a way to explore issues of collaboration, privacy and confidentiality, relations with government agencies, and organizational workloads. As we negotiated the bureaucracies and researched and prepared this chapter, we were pleased by the complexities we uncovered, the improvements in our own collaborative work, and the new networks with which we connected.

NOTE

Originally published as Phil Brown, Rachel Morello-Frosch, Julia Green Brody, Rebecca Gasior Altman, Ruthann A. Rudel, Laura Senier, Carla Pérez, and Ruth Simpson, "Institutional Review Board Challenges in Community-Based Participatory Research on Human Exposure to Environmental Toxins," *Environmental Health* 9 (2010): 39.

15

Conclusion

Phil Brown, Rachel Morello-Frosch, and Stephen Zavestoski

For more than a decade the Contested Illnesses Research Group (CIRG) has combined policy-rooted fieldwork with scientific inquiry to build a multilayered research program. We have created an ethnographic fieldwork approach with roots in public sociology that has community-engaged research as its primary orientation. CIRG is part of a larger network of academics and activists that has created synergies to advance the health social movements that we study.

We believe the methodological and theoretical approaches discussed in this book provide new ways of understanding contested-illness struggles within the broader field of health social movements, particularly those movements focused on environmental health. Since our initial examination of disputes over environmental factors in asthma, breast cancer, and Gulf War illnesses, we have expanded our research to many new areas in a burgeoning environmental health movement. Over time, we have observed dramatic shifts in the science base and the policy implications that follow.

BUILDING AND SHARING THEORY

CIRG has invested significant effort in discussing, reflecting on, and revising our theory (see chapter 2), which bridges the multiple disciplines and content areas of our work. Seeking feedback from colleagues in related fields has enabled us to advance our theoretical framework for health social movements, which has been widely adopted by others (Cooper, Kirton, and Schrecker 2007; Annetts et al. 2009; Keirns 2009). Our community partners are also interested in how the theoretical framework facilitates understanding of the ways health social movements emerge, evolve, and connect with each other as they work to reshape scientific fact-making in medicine and public health and to transform policy.

BUILDING A NEW SET OF TECHNIQUES
AND METHODS

The field analysis and policy ethnography tools described in chapter 4 help us locate a health social movement in historical, socioeconomic, political, and institutional contexts. Using a multisited field analysis elucidates how social movements develop and evolve in response to political opportunities, challenges, scientific discovery and shifting movement dynamics. They operate in multifaceted social and institutional worlds, which include diverse strategic allies and coalition partners in academia, government, and the private sector who may have conflicting perspectives. Our field analysis approach has also allowed our social movement partners to reflect on their background, legacy, and cross-organizational and cross-movement connections, which has helped them to build broader alliances and more diverse constituencies (e.g., linking environmental justice and breast cancer advocacy). These links in turn have made our partners' work more attractive to government funding agencies and foundations and enabled them to advance their advocacy and scientific work in innovative ways. Thus our methods have not only been helpful to our research but have also boosted the organizational capacity of our activist partners.

We have also assessed the effectiveness and evolution of CBPR projects aimed at advancing community environmental health, studying how environmental health movement organizations have simultaneously contested science while conducting scientific work in order to influence policy and regulation or transform dominant theories of disease causation. Policy ethnography has also enabled us to seize policy opportunities when they present themselves. For example, as described in chapter 12, our community outreach with the Environmental Neighborhood Awareness Committee of Tiverton (ENACT) enabled CIRG to work with Rhode Island legislators to pass a bill that makes home equity loans available to homeowners living in contaminated areas so that they can maintain their property as they await cleanup. Similarly, community-based research with the Southern California Environmental Justice Collaborative (chapter 5) contributed to the tightening of emissions regulations for industrial facilities in Southern California. This work illustrates how CBPR can advance the concrete policy objectives of advocacy partners (Minkler et al. 2008). And our work with the Northern California Household Exposure study, in collaboration with Silent Spring Institute and Communities for a Better Environment, helped to stall the expansion of major refinery operations in Richmond, California (chapter 9). These specific policy outcomes highlight how academic research teams can conduct scholarly work that has specific policy advocacy objectives and achieves practical goals. At its inception, CIRG did not foresee its direct involvement in policy debates, although the group's recent work has sought to influence policy as well as to make contributions in environmental health science, social science and social theory. Merging research with policy aims is consistent with recent directions in public sociology that encourage academic engagement with policy goals as part of main-stream scholarship (Burawoy 2005).

MERGING COMMUNITY-BASED PARTICIPATORY RESEARCH WITH COMMUNITY OUTREACH

CBPR and community-engaged activities are not tools for research teams to gain access to marginalized communities but rather are central to research partner-ships that build enduring community capacity. A unique component of our team's work is the combination of CBPR with community-engaged outreach. As we note in chapter 4, community-engaged outreach and service are not collabora-tive CBPR but are still designed to give voice and aid to communities. Our project linking breast cancer advocacy and environmental justice, described in chapter 8, is emblematic of our commitment to CBPR, while the Superfund Research Program's community outreach core work (chapter 12) is representative of our community-engaged outreach initiatives. Having community-based organiza-tions as funded partners in the community outreach core of SRP promotes a form of academic and community partnership similar to that found in CBPR. We fol-low the leads and needs of community partners, we bring university resources to them, and we learn from each other in ways that advance our research and organizational goals.

The ideas and sensibilities of CBPR can also be applied to other forms of community-engaged outreach. For example, our outreach work with ENACT is not driven exclusively by research aims but is also designed to assist that con-taminated community through policy, education, and remediation. Our project design allows ample time to evaluate these activities with our community partner. Further, the outreach partnership is intended to build capacity for ENACT's indi-vidual members and the group as a whole. Merging CBPR with concrete outreach activities in collaboration with community advocates enables CIRG to better inte-grate the political, policy, methodological, and theoretical elements of our work.

IMPLICATIONS OF INTERDISCIPLINARITY

CIRG continually reaffirms the need for rigorous methodological training, whether in environmental health sciences or the social sciences. We work to com-bine disciplinary expertise and skill sets, and we mix qualitative and quantitative analysis to achieve synergies that advance theory and research methods in the social and environmental-health sciences. This integration of disciplines gives our research group the flexibility and nimbleness to take on a wide range of issues. For example, we can take on a project that requires expertise in exposure assessment, environmental epidemiology, ethical communication of results to study participants and affected communities, engagement with advocates and policy makers, and the dissemination of research findings to academic colleagues, the media, and the broader public. The quantitative skills allow us to produce high-quality exposure assessment results; the qualitative skills provide rich community context, a more complete picture of the field (e.g., a history of pollution, neighborhood structure, and economic and industrial legacies) and a method for evaluating the effectiveness of projects.

Our interdisciplinarity also helps us reach broad audiences: academic colleagues as well as community-based organizations, policy makers, and regulators. It has promoted the value and scientific contributions of such work for tenure and promotion at universities and with major funding agencies such as the National Science Foundation and the National Institute of Environmental Health Sciences. Our approach has also encouraged university volunteer centers to expand their work to include much more interaction between students and community groups. Most important, the interdisciplinary orientation of CIRG suggests how faculty can effectively train undergraduate and graduate students for community-engaged research within health social movements.

The expanding field of health social movements and contested illnesses requires interdisciplinary collaboration, and the results of our work suggest that this form of community-engaged scholarship is becoming increasingly important. Much of our work has been disseminated in widely read academic journals in several fields, as well as through more mainstream outlets, such as *Scientific American*. Moreover, as environmental health challenges become more complex, disciplinary boundaries must be crossed to address them. Funding agencies have begun to encourage the formation of interdisciplinary teams. We believe that this trend has been an important factor in our ability to secure financial support from diverse funders, such as the National Institutes of Health, the National Science Foundation, the Robert Wood Johnson Foundation, the Ford Foundation, the California Endowment, and the California Wellness Foundation. Our strong track record also suggests that undergraduate and graduate students can forge successful research careers using interdisciplinary and community-based participatory methods.

The success of engaged research must also be transferred to the classroom. We have developed courses in which we can impart our advocacy-based scientific approach to a more general audience of graduate and undergraduate students, thereby enlarging the pool of students who can contribute to our research and outreach work. Our courses allow students to experience a style of community-engaged work that is both challenging and rewarding. For example, faculty members at Brown University developed a seminar in environmental justice that includes service-learning placements with environmental health and justice organizations, allowing students to learn firsthand about the principles, practices, and obligations involved in community-based participatory research. We have been able to make this a rewarding experience for both the students and the community partner organizations because we have worked to maintain collaborative relationships with community groups. Similarly, we developed a research ethics seminar that scrutinizes the ethical concerns involved in community-based environmental health research. We have also shared with other faculty members and graduate students the lessons we have learned about how to make service learning and community-engaged research and outreach successful. By speaking in small workshops and in public and university forums, we have been able to disseminate our strategies for community-engaged, interdisciplinary research and teaching.

EVALUATION AND REFLEXIVITY

Evaluation and reflection are very important to us—for nurturing our partnerships, helping with theoretical development, examining ethical quandaries and obligations about what data to report and how to report it, assessing advances in policy making, and applying our work to improve public health. One of the biggest challenges is finding the time and resources to do all this well. In our breast cancer advocacy and environmental justice project, all participants met periodically to reflect on the benefits that we derived, individually and collectively, from the collaboration. That regular reflection and self-assessment helped us measure progress and identify challenges.

As CBPR becomes more popular, there is a danger that the approach may be watered down, co-opted, or carried out inappropriately. Continuing evaluation, especially critical self-assessment, is needed to ensure that the work meets the goals and aspirations of community and academic partners. Other CBPR scholars have contributed to a growing body of literature that analyzes the policy effects of CBPR strategies. Minkler and colleagues presented ten case studies that offer a procedural and methodological framework for evaluating the effectiveness of CBPR (Minkler et al. 2008): its criteria include meeting policy goals as well as the capacity-building needs of community partners.

FUTURE DIRECTIONS

As this volume documents, our approach to the study of contested illnesses has spanned a range of issues and the activities of multiple actors in diverse social settings. But our work could still expand in many directions. The rise of a food justice movement, although it is not solely focused on health, is ripe for policy ethnography, because the scientific knowledge base that links our food system to human disease is complex and hotly contested, and because (like the dominant epidemiological paradigm) the industrial food-production system is dominated by powerful industry, media, and government stakeholders. Its critics, who call for more sustainable and healthier food production, lay the blame for hunger and certain chronic diseases on its inherent structural inequalities. They will therefore find themselves in conflict with deeply vested interests as they push for policy change. For example, sustainable food-system advocates often point to the high rates of obesity in the United States as evidence of the harm being done by government subsidization of corn-based ingredients, which are used to make highly processed foods with little nutritional value. But a growing body of research suggests that at least part of the pattern of obesity may be due to exposure to endocrine-disrupting chemicals, especially during the perinatal phase of development (Heindel 2003). Future research will need to parse the complexities of a contested illness (or contested health condition, such as obesity) in which a suspected environmental exposure, instead of leading directly to disease, leads to a physical condition associated with a wide range of negative health outcomes.

Our work could also expand geographically. Our research has been mainly limited to contested illness in the United States (though our group is beginning to examine examples in developing nations, as with Stephen Zavestoski's [2009] work on Bhopal), and most other research has similarly been focused on either the United States or Europe. Of particular interest would be illness contestation in developing countries, where science infrastructure, existing laws, and cultures of collective action vary greatly. Research on patterns of illness contestation can expand our knowledge of a diversity of contested forms (Dauvergne 2005). Inasmuch as Western scientific, medical, and humanitarian organizations lead the charge against emerging health threats in the developing world, in the case of pollution-related disease, more emphasis is needed on underlying causes. For example, at a recent conference on breast cancer in the developing world, only one of the six sessions addressed the causes of rising rates of breast cancer in developing countries, whereas numerous sessions were devoted to treatment and screening. This pattern suggests that the developing world is institutionalizing some of the same norms that in the developed world have led to biases toward genetic and lifestyle explanations of disease at the expense of attention to environmental causes. Further research on the social forces that shape the scientific agenda in the developing world might have the potential to challenge these individualized and biomedicalized ways of framing health issues.

Comparative research on health social movements in different countries could further develop theoretical frameworks that explain the formation and contestation of scientific knowledge and collective action. For example, climate change is likely to result in widespread contestation about emerging diseases and the disparate effects of adaptation and mitigation strategies. Illness will result not just from hotter, wetter, drier, or colder climates, but also from adaptations that introduce new technologies and the wider application of existing technologies. These may include heavier applications of pesticides and water-treatment chemicals and heavier reliance on genetically modified organisms in agriculture. Similarly, market-based strategies to reduce greenhouse gas emissions might concentrate toxic copollutants in communities that disproportionately host heavily polluting facilities, thus worsening local air quality and associated health effects (Shonkoff et al. 2009). Already we are witnessing ways in which community advocates and scientists have come together to identify the potential effects of climate change and shape social responses to them (Morello-Frosch et al. 2009b).

The CIRG has sought to expand the field of health social movements by studying how lay people and experts make sense of illness and recovery and how they engage in collective action when illness is perceived as a social problem instead of a personal one. This volume documents not only several case studies of contested illnesses but also the methodological and ethical challenges of biomonitoring research—an approach that is rapidly becoming a commonly employed means of documenting the presence and extent of chemicals in our bodies. Our research has enabled us to forge strong ties with academic colleagues and diverse community partners. Here we have sought to share our project experiences and the tools we use to combine research, policy advocacy, public education, and community capacity-building. We hope that our contributions will motivate others to pursue similar work.

Contested Illnesses Research Group's Nuts and Bolts and Lessons Learned

Laura Senier, Rebecca Gasior Altman,
Rachel Morello-Frosch, and Phil Brown

The Contested Illnesses Research Group (CIRG) was established in 1999 at Brown University with funding from the Robert Wood Johnson Foundation and the National Science Foundation. The original project studied contestation over environmental factors that might contribute to asthma, breast cancer, and Gulf War illnesses. Today, with new funding, new faces, and new research areas, CIRG meets for weekly discussions, bringing together faculty, postdoctoral fellows, and graduate and undergraduate students from sociology, anthropology, ethnic studies, community health, and science studies. Often our alumni join in. We host visits from outside scholars and collaborate with scholars at other institutions (including the group's own recent graduates and scientists at Silent Spring Institute, Boston University, and the University of California, Berkeley). We also work with environmental health and justice groups that do community organizing and policy work (such as Communities for a Better Environment in Oakland, CA).

We do not merely study citizen-science alliances but actively participate in them. We work to ensure that the alliances we engage in benefit the communities we study, as well as advancing our own theoretical formulations. Like many scholars before us, we have found that the best way to learn is by doing. Over the past eleven years, by doing, we have learned many lessons. For the benefit of researchers who want to pursue similar work, here are seven of them.

Lesson 1
Today's Research Participant Is Tomorrow's Research Partner

Policy ethnography often leads to collaboration with groups that were initially the focus of our research. More recently, our work on contested environmental illnesses and citizen-science alliances has segued into participation in novel research collaborations among environmental health and justice activists, environmental scientists, and social scientists.

In 1999, the contested illness project included Silent Spring Institute as a research site to examine disputes over environmental causation of breast cancer. Over time, our relationship grew into a productive and ground-breaking research partnership. In 2004, we expanded this partnership, joining with Silent Spring Institute and Communities for a Better Environment to conduct a project linking breast cancer advocacy with environmental justice activism. The project conducted personal exposure assessments of hormonally active pollutants found in home environments from consumer products, industrial emissions, and transportation sources. Researchers collaborated with community members on the design and implementation of the study and on reporting our findings back to participants and the community. Community activists were trained to collect air and dust samples to assess indoor and outdoor levels of pollutants, especially endocrine disruptors, which have been linked to breast cancer, reproductive and neurological anomalies, and other health outcomes. This project led us to further work focusing on the ethical issues associated with the practice of reporting environmental study results to individual study participants.

Lesson 2
Fortune Favors the Researcher Who Has Cultivated Community Relationships

Serendipity can provide opportunities for the application of existing resources and infrastructure to advance intellectual and policy goals, but a "directed serendipity" such as we have experienced arises from the cultivation of relationships with community partners. For example, through a research project with the Massachusetts Committee on Occupational Safety and Health (MassCOSH) on labor unions and environmental activism, CIRG learned about a new collaboration between MassCOSH and the Boston Urban Asthma Coalition, and we were able to devote graduate student research time to study this project. As related in chapter 10, we helped MassCOSH and its partners evaluate their campaign to introduce environmentally friendly cleaning products into a public school system. This work led not only to a program evaluation that we wrote for MassCOSH but also to a peer-reviewed journal article. While serendipity could be seen as the most proximate cause of our involvement in the Green Cleaners Project, we were able to pursue the project because we had previously invested in relationships with the people and organizations involved.

Lesson 3
Share the Data with Participants

Documenting the policy ethnography process for participants helps to create and reinforce connections between scholars and activists and to disseminate important information to concerned audiences. The household exposure studies on Cape Cod and in Northern California illustrate how important it is to share data with participants and the communities in which they live. In earlier projects, we shared our findings with the organizations that we studied, which led to further conversations, which in turn deepened our relationship and created further opportunities for collaboration.

Our team's strategies for individual reporting of personal exposure information have been influential in other locales, ranging from academic research to government-run biomonitoring projects that monitor pollutants in human bodies. We believe that participants have the right to have access to data that was gathered from them and their community, should they choose to receive it. This access democratizes the scientific process, and the data may help participants make informed decisions about whether and how to take action.

Lesson 4
Share Methods with Other Researchers

We hope that the burgeoning network of scholars involved with policy ethnography will not only produce work that will advocate for communities burdened by environmental injustice but also will help to improve, refine, and expand the methodological sophistication of policy ethnography tools. Many of our articles detail the collaborative nature of our work on community-based participatory research and community-engaged activities, and we have also sought to disseminate our philosophy and experiences in other ways. For example, we designed a colloquium series on public sociology and community-based participatory research for the Brown Sociology department, which was well attended and fostered thought-provoking conversations in and beyond the department.

The Contested Illnesses Research Group offers unique opportunities to students, allowing them to explore both the theoretical and applied elements of environmental health and social movement scholarship. Students have had opportunities for authorship on journal articles and book chapters as well as projects and reports used by our community-based partner organizations and grant applications. Students have organized several of the outreach initiatives outlined above, including work with the Toxics Action Center, a grassroots support group based in Boston, MA, with regional offices in every New England state, and with community groups served by the Brown Superfund Research Program Outreach activities.

Lesson 5
Engaging Community Organizations in the Scientific Process
Will Lead to Even More Community-Directed Research

Scientific capacity-building can enable organizations to launch their own data-collection initiatives that inform community organizing and policy advocacy strategies. On a local level, Communities for a Better Environment chose to continue the scientific work in Richmond by conducting their own survey to assess community perceptions of environmental health and neighborhood stressors. Our team assisted CBE in writing a successful Avon Foundation grant to fund work on this community survey. We also assisted in developing the questionnaire, field methods, and techniques for data analysis. Not only did this endeavor provide valuable health data, but it also allowed CBE to use the survey to advance its organizing efforts in several Richmond neighborhoods and to make productive links with other community organizations in the area.

Lesson 6
Policy Ethnography Has Practical Impact

Our work has been effective in assessing the policy, legal, and regulatory effects of community-based participatory research. Under the auspices of a new National Science Foundation grant, we are now exploring the implications of biomonitoring in the three arenas where it is typically conducted and debated: national-level population surveillance; state-based biomonitoring studies; and place- or community-based studies that investigate local environmental problems. Engaging with researchers and activists in these arenas has augmented our expertise in designing ethical report-back approaches and made our project more visible to the growing community of people doing biomonitoring and household exposure studies. For example, one member of our team has been invited to participate in planning new biomonitoring projects with the California Biomonitoring Program. Our partners at Silent Spring Institute were invited to present our approach to reporting back individual exposure data at the grantees' conference of NIEHS's Breast Cancer and the Environment Research Centers and to a special workgroup of the Centers for Disease Control and Prevention.

Our findings in the household air and dust monitoring project uncovered very high rates of flame retardants, especially PBDEs, in human body fluids in Cape Cod, and then in air and dust in California, most likely because of that state's stringent but misinformed furniture flammability standards. This finding led us to develop additional research on flame retardants. It also promoted new collaborations between our team and scientists who are trying to change California policy, prevent federal policy from adopting similarly dangerous flammability standards, and prevent the adoption of international protocols that would add billions of pounds of flame retardants to electronic devices.

Another practical outgrowth of our policy ethnography work on health social movements has been a research focus on coalitions among activist groups concerned about health and the environment, particularly between the labor and environmental movements. Although recent history suggests an adversarial relationship between labor unions and environmental groups, a longer history points to a mutually supportive relationship between unionists and others concerned with the health effects of chemical exposures. Our own work has shown that when so-called blue-green coalitions form around a shared health concern, they more easily bridge their ideological divides to form viable coalitions.

Lesson 7
Build Community Capacity to Sustain Research
and Outreach Activities

One of the reasons CIRG has been able to cultivate long-term partnerships for both research and outreach is that we have worked for years to build the capacity of community organizations, allowing them to establish sustainable organizational structures that enhance the effectiveness of our research initiatives as well as their advocacy and organizing efforts. We started our work with community-based organizations in Rhode Island as early as 2003 but quickly formulated a goal of creating a statewide network of community groups that would cooperate on campaigns for environmental health and social justice. In 2007, the Environmental Justice League of Rhode Island (EJLRI) was launched, with grant support from the US Environmental Protection Agency and ten participating community groups. The CIRG helped to promote the EJLRI in three specific ways: first, by helping community groups connect to one another; second, by connecting the emerging statewide network of community groups to similar advocacy networks elsewhere; and third, by providing concrete and tangible university resources.

Long before beginning our work in Rhode Island, the CIRG team had a relationship with Toxics Action Center, a nonprofit agency based in Boston that has supported more than five hundred organizations across northern New England in fighting environmental pollution. In 2003–4, one of our master's degree students interviewed activists who received support from TAC in order to learn more about the pressures and difficulties faced by first-time activists (Altman 2004). This work brought the CIRG team in touch with community groups in Rhode Island working on environmental campaigns. Although our Rhode Island neighbors knew of TAC, we believed that they would benefit from a local forum where they could seek leadership-development support and technical assistance, and we began working to help TAC establish a presence in Rhode Island. The CIRG team helped TAC obtain foundation support from the Cox Charitable Trust and developed leadership-training and capacity-building workshops to train and sustain grassroots leaders in what can often be protracted campaigns.

Communities throughout Rhode Island are fighting lead poisoning, high rates of childhood asthma, substandard housing in subsidized housing developments, inappropriate siting of public schools on contaminated land, and toxic waste regulation, reduction, and cleanup. To help these communities connect with one another, CIRG began organizing workshops under the name of the Providence Environmental Justice Education Forum (PEJEF) in 2004. We used grant support from an NIH-funded project, the Collaborative Initiative for Research Ethics in Environmental Health, to hold quarterly meetings at which groups could meet one another, share stories, and cooperate on common problems and challenges. For example, two communities in southern Rhode Island were fighting air and water pollution caused by a local textile and dye firm. These community groups collaborated to form teams of volunteers known as bucket brigades to capture air-quality data in support of their case. They were able to negotiate a settlement with the corporate polluter that included equipment upgrades to reduce the amount of pollution emissions and funds for a comprehensive health assessment of the surrounding community.

These community groups reached out to their neighbors in Tiverton, RI, where more than one hundred property owners learned that their homes were built on contaminated fill. The PEJEF meetings thus became one means through which community groups could learn about other, similar problems in the state, sometimes sharing strategies and tactics but at other times simply offering their neighbors support and encouragement.

Because these campaigns are often so long and often so highly technical, community partners need specialized advice and technical assistance from other sources. We brought organizers from two Boston-based environmental advocacy groups—TAC and Alternatives for Community and Environment—to Rhode Island for strategy and training sessions. They offered advice on specific campaigns and also spoke about the resources and vision needed to build a long-range and sustainable organizational form. We also connected the PEJEF with the Connecticut Coalition for Environmental Justice, another emerging, regionally based environmental justice group. Finally, we connected the Rhode Island coalition to antitoxics groups on the national scene, including the Center for Health, Environment, and Justice (CHEJ). We invited Lois Gibbs, whose activism in Love Canal, NY, made her one of the founders of the environmental health movement, to Rhode Island to speak to activists who were fighting pollution in residential communities as well as to those who were campaigning against the construction of public elementary and secondary schools on or near contaminated land. We connected CHEJ to attorneys at Rhode Island Legal Services (RILS) and some Brown University students, who conducted a thorough analysis of state laws concerning school siting and found that twenty states, including Rhode Island, have no laws of any kind prohibiting construction of schools on or near contaminated land. In these various ways, the CIRG has helped connect the growing coalition of Rhode Island–based environmental justice groups to regional and national networks and contributed to the dialogue about how contamination is affecting communities across the country.

Whenever possible, CIRG supported the emerging statewide network by providing specific, concrete resources, including skill-building opportunities as well as personnel and financial support. For example, we ran workshops for PEJEF members on communicating with the media and writing grants. Two of our member groups subsequently received grants from the EPA's Healthy Communities Program. We also assigned graduate and undergraduate students to service-learning projects in these communities. They analyzed government and scientific reports, designed websites, wrote and translated pamphlets, organized fund-raising walkathons, and coached middle schoolers in public speaking. We also recruited students to work with communities through the community outreach core of Brown's Superfund Research Program grant and through the Swearer Center for Public Service.

We provided financial support to communities through several different mechanisms. Community-based organizations are often named as partners in our grant applications, so that they receive funds to hire and retain staff, secure office space, and support operating budgets. Our grants also budget for public meetings and community outreach so that we can reach a more general public audience. And we have helped our community partners when they have written their own applications for independent grant funding. We assisted the EJLRI in its first grant application to the US EPA Community Action for Renewed Environment (CARE) program, from which the group was awarded a $100,000 grant. We also helped the EJLRI obtain a special grant from the national program office of the Superfund Research Program. Together these grants provided salary support for two staff members and a graduate student research assistant.

Conclusion

We believe that outreach activities are most likely to be effective when developed in response to the needs and interests of community groups. We have been able to tap into a diverse range of groups and networks and to demonstrate the importance of environmental health and environmental justice as organizing frames. While the work of our own group has been organized around the serious theoretical and empirical investigation of various aspects of environmental health and health social movements, we have been conscious of the need to connect these theories with practice, often providing concrete support to help our community partners in their campaigns.

Additional appendixes are available at www.ucpress.edu/go/contestedillnesses.

All appendixes, as well as other information on our current research, are also available at the Contested Illnesses Research Group web site, www.brown.edu/Research/Contested_Illnesses_Research_Project/resources.htm.

REFERENCES

Abdel-Rahman, A., Shetty, A., and Abou-Donia, M. 2002. "Disruption of the Blood-Brain Barrier and Neuronal Cell Death in Cingulate Cortex, Dentate Gyrus, Thalamus, and Hypothalamus in a Rat Model of Gulf-War Syndrome." *Neurobiology of Disease* 10: 306–26.

Akinbami, L. J., and Moorman, J. E. 2011. *Asthma Prevalence, Health Care Use and Mortality: United States, 2005–2009.* National Health Statistics Report. Atlanta, GA: Centers for Disease Control and Prevention. January 12, www.cdc.gov/nchs/data/nhsr/nhsr032.pdf.

Aldinger, C. 2000. "Study Links Agent Orange, Diabetes." *New York Times,* March 29.

Altman, R. G. 2004. "Biographical Disruption and Local Anti-toxics Activism." MA thesis, Brown University.

——— 2008. "Chemical Body Burden and Place-Based Struggles for Environmental Health and Justice." PhD diss., Brown University.

Altman, R., Morello-Frosch, R., Brody, J., Rudel, R., Brown, P., and Averick, M. 2008. "Pollution Comes Home and Gets Personal: Women's Experience of Household Chemical Exposure." *Journal of Health and Social Behavior* 49 (4): 417–35.

Amdur, M. 1996. "Animal Toxicology." In *Particles in Our Air: Concentrations and Health Effects,* ed R. W. J. Spengler, 85–122. Cambridge, MA: Harvard University Press.

American Cancer Society. 2007. *Breast Cancer Facts and Figures 2007–2008.* Atlanta, GA: American Cancer Society.

American Conference of Governmental Industrial Hygienists. 2005. *TLVs and BEIs Based on the Documentation of the Threshold Limit Values and Biological Exposure Indices.* Cincinnati, OH: American Conference of Governmental Industrial Hygienists.

American Lung Association. 2004. *Children and Asthma in America.* New York: American Lung Association.

Anderson, A. 1997. *Media and the Environment.* New Brunswick, NJ: Rutgers University Press.

Anderson, S. 2000. "The School That Wasn't: Politics and Pollution in LA." *Nation,* June.

Anderton, D. 1996. "Methodological Issues in the Spatiotemporal Analysis of Environmental Equity." *Social Science Quarterly* 77: 508–15.

Annetts, J., Law, A., McNeish, W., and Mooney, G. 2009. *Understanding Social Welfare Movements.* Bristol, UK: Policy Press.

Arcury, T. A., Quandt, S. A., and McCauley, L. 2000. "Farmworkers and Pesticides: Community-Based Research." *Environmental Health Perspectives* 108 (8): 787–92.

Arendt, M. 2008. "Communicating Human Biomonitoring Results to Ensure Policy Coherence with Public Health Recommendations: Analysing Breastmilk whilst Protecting, Promoting and Supporting Breastfeeding." *Environmental Health* 7 (Supp. 1): S6.

ASA (American Sociological Association). 2005. *Public Sociology and the Roots of Sociology: Re-establishing Our Connections to the Public.* American Sociological Assocation Task Force on Institutionalizing Public Sociologies, http://pubsoc.wisc.edu/page.php?3, accessed December 4, 2009.

Aschengrau, A., Ozonoff, D., Coogan, P., Vezina, R., Heeren, T., and Zhang, Y. 1996. "Cancer Risk and Residential Proximity to Cranberry Cultivation in Massachusetts." *American Journal of Public Health* 86 (9): 1289–96.

Auyero, J., and Swistun, D. 2007. "Confused Because Exposed: Towards an Ethnography of Environmental Suffering." *Ethnography* 8 (2): 123–44.

Azaroff, Lenore S., Hoa Mai Nguyen, Tuan Do, Rebecca Gore, and Marcy Goldstein-Gelb. 2011. "Results of a Community-University Partnership to Reduce Deadly Hazards in Hardwood Floor Finishing." *Journal of Community Health* (January): 1–11. http://dx.doi.org/10.1007/s10900–011–9357–7, accessed April 26, 2011.

Baker, D. 2007. "Oil Facilities Are Getting Refined." *San Francisco Chronicle,* January 5.

Balshem, M. 1993. *Cancer in the Community: Class and Medical Authority.* Washington, DC: Smithsonian Institution Press.

Banaszak-Holl, J., Levitsky, S., and Zald, M., eds. 2010. *Social Movements and the Development of Health Institutions.* New York: Oxford University Press.

Baquet, C., Mishra, S., Commiskey, P., Ellison, G., and DeShields, M. 2008. "Breast Cancer Epidemiology in Blacks and Whites: Disparities in Incidence, Mortality, Survival Rates and Histology." *Journal of the National Medical Association* 100 (5): 480–88.

Barraza-Villarreal, A., Sunyer, J., Hernandez-Cadena, L., Escamilla-Nuñez, M. C., Sienra-Monge, J. J., Ramírez-Aguilar, M., Cortez-Lugo, et al. 2008. "Air Pollution, Airway Inflammation, and Lung Function in a Cohort Study of Mexico City Schoolchildren." *Environmental Health Perspectives* 116 (6): 832–38.

Bates, M. N., Selevan, S. G., Ellerbee, S. M., and Gartner, L. M. 2002. "Reporting Needs for Studies of Environmental Chemicals in Human Milk." *Journal of Toxicology and Environmental Health A* 65: 1867–79.

Beamish, T. D. 2002. *Silent Spill: The Organization of an Industrial Crisis.* Cambridge, MA: MIT Press.

Beasley, R., Crane, J., Lai, C. K., and Pearce, N. 2000. "Prevalence and Etiology of Asthma." *Journal of Allergy and Clinical Immunology* 105 (2, pt. 2): S466–S472.

Beck, U. 1992. *Risk Society: Towards a New Modernity.* London: Sage.

Becker, H. 1967. "Whose Side Are We On?" *Social Problems* 14: 239–47.

Bener, A., Abdulrazzaq, Y., Debuse, P., and Abdin, A. 1994. "Asthma and Wheezing as the Cause of School Absence." *Journal of Asthma* 31 (2): 93–98.

Benford, R. D., and Snow, D. A. 2000. "Framing Processes and Social Movements: An Overview and Assessment." *Annual Review of Sociology* 26 (1): 611.

Berman, D. 1981. "Grassroots Coalitions in Health and Safety: The COSH Groups." *Labor Studies Journal* 6 (Spring): 104–13.

Bernstein, J., Saunder, T., Bernstein, D., and Bernstein, I. 1994. "A Combined Respiratory and Cutaneous Hypersensitivity Syndrome Induced by Work Exposure to Quaternary Amines." *Journal of Allergy and Clinical Immunology* 94 (2, pt. 1): 257–59.

Best, J., Ed. 1989. *Images of Issues: Typifying Contemporary Social Problems.* New York: Aldine.

Bhatia, R., Brenner, B., Salgado, B., Shumasunder, B., and Prakash, S. 2005. "Biomonitoring: What Communities Must Know." *Race, Poverty and Environment* 11: 56.

Bird, C. E., Conrad, P., and Fremont, A., eds. 2000. *Handbook of Medical Sociology.* Upper Saddle River, NJ: Prentice-Hall.

Bishop, R. 1994. "Initiating Empowering Research?" *New Zealand Journal of Educational Studies* 29 (1): 175–88.

Bloom, B., Cohen, R., Vickerie, J., and Wondimu, E. 2003. "Summary Health Statistics for US Children: National Health Interview Survey, 2001." *Vital Health Statistics* 10: 1–54.

Bloor, M. 1988. "Notes on Member Validation." In *Contemporary Field Methods,* ed. R. Emerson, 156–72. Prospect Heights, IL: Waveland Press.

Blum, A. 2007. "The Fire Retardant Dilemma." *Science* 318 (5848): 194b–195.

Blum, E. D. 2008. *Love Canal Revisited: Race, Class, and Gender in Environmental Activism.* Lawrence: University of Kansas Press.

Blume, H. 2000. "No Vacancy: The School District's Space Crunch Is Much Worse Than You Know." *LA Weekly,* June 7.

Body Burden Work Group and Commonweal Biomonitoring Resource Center. 2007. "Is It in Us? Toxic Trespass, Regulatory Failure, and Opportunities for Action." http://isitinus.org/project.php, accessed November 8, 2007.

Bosk, C., and DeVries, R. 2004. "Bureaucracies of Mass Deception: Institutional Review Boards and the Ethics of Ethnographic Research." *Annals of the American Academy of Political and Social Science* 595: 249–63.

Boston Consensus Conference. 2006. *Measuring Chemicals in People: What Would You Say? A Boston Consensus Conference on Biomonitoring.* www.biomonitoring06.org, accessed June 16, 2007.

Boston Urban Asthma Coalition. 2006. "The BUAC Mission." www.buac.org/about_us.html, accessed August 31, 2006.

Boswell-Penc, M. 2006. *Tainted Milk: Breastmilk, Feminisms, and the Politics of Environmental Degradation.* Albany: State University of New York Press.

Bourdieu, P. 1984. *Distinction: A Social Critique of the Judgment of Taste.* Cambridge, MA: Harvard University Press.

Bourgeault, I. L., DeVries, R., and Dingwall, R., eds. 2010. *The Sage Handbook of Qualitative Methods in Health Research.* Thousand Oaks, CA: Sage.

Brenner, B. A. 2000. "Sister Support: Women Create a Breast Cancer Movement." *Breast Cancer: Society Shapes an Epidemic*, ed. A. S. Kasper and Susan J. Ferguson, 325–54. New York: St. Martin's Press.

———. 2003. "BCA Withdraws Support for Breast-Milk Biomonitoring Program." *Breast Cancer Action Newsletter 75*.

Brody, J. G., Vorhees, D. J., Melly, S. J., Swedis, S. R., Drivas, P. J., and Rudel, R. A. 2003. "Environmental Pollutants and Breast Cancer." *Environmental Health Perspectives* 111 (8): 1007–19.

Brody, J. G., Morello-Frosch, R., Brown, P., Rudel, R. A., Altman, R. G., Frye, M., Osimo, C. A., Pérez, C., and Seryak, L. M. 2007a. "Improving Disclosure and Consent: Is It Safe? New Ethics for Reporting Personal Exposures to Environmental Chemicals." *American Journal of Public Health* 97 (9): 1547–54.

Brody, J. G., Moysich, K. P., Humblet, O., Attfield, K. R., Beehler, G. B., and Rudel, R. A. 2007b. "Environmental Pollutants and Breast Cancer: Epidemiologic Studies." *Cancer* 109 (S12): 2667–2711.

Brody, J. G., Morello-Frosch, R., Zota, A., Brown, P., Perez, C., and Rudel, R. A. 2009. "Linking Exposure Assessment Science with Policy Objectives for Environmental Justice and Breast Cancer Advocacy: The Northern California Household Exposure Study." *American Journal of Public Health* 99 Supp. 3: S600–S609.

Brown, M. L., Kessler, L. G., and Reuter, F. G. 1990. "Is the Supply of Mammography Machines Outstripping Need and Demand?" *Annals of Internal Medicine* 113: 547–52.

Brown, P. 2007. *Toxic Exposures: Contested Illnesses and the Environmental Health Movement*. New York: Columbia University Press.

Brown, P., and Mikkelsen, E. J. 1997 [1990]. *No Safe Place: Toxic Waste, Leukemia, and Community Action.* Berkeley: University of California Press.

Brown, P., Zavestoski, S., McCormick, S., Mandelbaum, J., and Luebke, T. 2001a. "Print Media Coverage of Environmental Causation of Breast Cancer." *Sociology of Health and Illness* 23: 747–75.

Brown, P., Zavestoski, S., McCormick, S., Mandelbaum, J., Luebke, T., and Linder, M. 2001b. "A Gulf of Difference: Disputes over Gulf War–Related Illnesses." *Journal of Health and Social Behavior* 42: 235–57.

Brown, P., Zavestoski, S., Mayer, B., McCormick, S., and Webster, P. 2002. "Policy Issues in Environmental Health Disputes." *Annals of the American Academy of Political and Social Science* 584: 175–202.

Brown, P., Zavestoski, S., Luebke, T., Mandelbaum, J., McCormick, S., and Mayer, B. 2003. "The Health Politics of Asthma: Environmental Justice and Collective Illness Experience in the United States." *Social Science and Medicine* 57: 453–64.

Brown, P., Zavestoski, S., McCormick, S., Mayer, B., Morello-Frosch, R., and Altman, R. G. 2004. "Embodied Health Movements: Uncharted Territory in Social Movement Research." *Sociology of Health and Illness* 26 (1): 1–31.

Brown, P., Zavestoski, S., McCormick, S., Mayer, B., Morello-Frosch, R., Altman, R. G., and Senier, L. 2006. "'A Lab of Our Own': Environmental Causation of Breast Cancer and Challenges to the Dominant Epidemiological Paradigm." *Science, Technology, and Human Values* 31: 499–536.

Bullard, R. D. 1990. *Dumping in Dixie: Race, Class, and Environmental Quality.* Boulder, CO: Westview Press.

———. 1994. "Overcoming Racism in Environmental Decision-Making." *Environment* 36 (4): 10–44.

———, ed. 1993. *Confronting Environmental Racism: Voices from the Grassroots.* Boston: South End Press.

Bullard, R. D. and Johnson, G. S. 1997. *Just Transportation: Dismantling Race and Class Barriers to Mobility.* Gabriola Island, BC: New Society Publishers.

Burawoy, M. 2000. "Reaching for the Global." In *Global Ethnography: Forces, Connections, and Imaginations,* by M. Burawoy, J. A. Blum, S. George, Z. Gille, M. Thayer, T. Gowan, L. Haney, M. Klawiter, S. H. Lopez, and S. O'Riain. Berkeley: University of California Press.

———. 2005. "2004 Presidential Address: For Public Sociology." *American Sociological Review* 70: 4–28.

Bury, M. 2004. "Researching Patient-Professional Interactions." *Journal of Health Services Research and Policy* 9 (Supp. 1): 48–54.

Caldwell, J., Woodruff, T., Morello-Frosch, R., and Axelrad, D. 1998. "Application of Health Information to Hazardous Air Pollutants Modeled in EPA's Cumulative Exposure Project." *Toxicology and Industrial Health* 14 (3): 429–54.

Cal-EPA (California Environmental Protection Agency). 2004. "Environmental Justice Action Plan." www.calepa.ca.gov/EnvJustice/ActionPlan/, accessed August 6, 2008.

Cal-EPA Advisory Committee on Environmental Justice. 2003. "Recommendations of the California Environmental Protection Agency (Cal/EPA) Advisory Committee on Environmental Justice to the Cal/EPA Interagency Working Group on Environmental Justice, Final Report." www.calepa.ca.gov/EnvJustice/Documents/2003/FinalReport.pdf, accessed February 20, 2003.

California. Senate. 2006. California Environmental Contaminant Biomonitoring Program. *SB 1379.* Sacramento: OSP.

Campbell, E. G., Weissman, J. S., Vogeli, C., Clarridge, B. R., Abrahama, M., Marder, J. E., and Koski, G. 2006. "Financial Relationships between Institutional Review Boards and Industry." *New England Journal of Medicine* 355: 2321–29.

CARB. 2005. "Air Quality and Land Use Handbook: A Community Health Perspective." www.arb.ca.gov/ch/handbook.pdf, accessed June 5, 2009.

Carpenter, D. 2008. "Environmental Contaminants as Risk Factors for Developing Diabetes." *Review of Environmental Health* 23 (1): 59–74.

Carson, R. 1962. *Silent Spring.* New York: Houghton Mifflin.

Casamayou, M. H. 2001. *The Politics of Breast Cancer.* Washington, DC: Georgetown University Press.

Casper, M. J., ed. 2003. *Synthetic Planet: Chemical Politics and the Hazards of Modern Life.* New York: Routledge.

Casper, M. J., and Moore, L. J. 2009. *Missing Bodies: The Politics of Visibility.* New York: New York University Press.

Caufield, C. 1990. *Multiple Exposures: Chronicles of the Radiation Age.* Chicago: University of Chicago Press.

CDC (Centers for Disease Control and Prevention). 1999. *First National Report on Human Exposure to Environmental Chemicals.* Atlanta, GA: National Center for Environmental Health.

————. 2003. *Second National Report on Human Exposure to Environmental Chemicals.* Atlanta, GA: National Center for Environmental Health.

————. 2005. *Third National Report on Human Exposure to Environmental Chemicals.* Atlanta, GA: National Center for Environmental Health.

————. 2010. *Fourth National Report on Human Exposure to Environmental Chemicals,* available at www.cdc.gov/exposurereport/pdf/FourthReport.pdf, accessed June 13, 2010.

CDMRP (Congressionally Directed Medical Research Program, Department of Defense). 2010. "Funding History." http://cdmrp.army.mil/about/fundinghistory.shtml, accessed May 2010.

Cecchine, G., Golomb, B., Hilborne, L., Spektor, D., and Anthony, C. 2000. *A Review of the Scientific Literature as It Pertains to Gulf War Illnesses,* vol. 8, *Pesticides.* Washington, DC: RAND.

Center, R. 2000. *Poverty, Ethnicity, and Pediatric Asthma in Rhode Island.* Providence, RI: Center for Environmental Studies, Brown University.

Center for Health, Environment, and Justice. 2002. *Creating Safe Learning Zones: The ABCs of Healthy Schools.* Falls Church, VA: Center for Health, Environment, and Justice.

Charles, C., and DeMaio, S. 1993. "Lay Participation in Health Care Decision-Making: A Conceptual Framework." *Journal of Health Politics, Policy, and Law* 18: 881–904.

Charmaz, K. 1991. *Good Days, Bad Days: The Self in Chronic Illness and Time.* New Brunswick, NJ: Rutgers University Press.

Checker, M. 2005. *Polluted Promises : Environmental Racism and the Search for Justice in a Southern Town.* New York: New York University Press.

Chess, C., and Purcell, K. 1999. "Public Participation and the Environment: Do We Know What Works?" *Environmental Science and Technology* 33 (16): 2685–92.

Chevron Corporation. 2009a. "Chevron: What We Do; The Refining Process." www.chevron.com/products/sitelets/richmond/about/what_we_do.aspx, accessed January 17, 2009.

————. 2009b. "Chevron: About the Refinery." www.chevron.com/products/sitelets/richmond/about/, accessed February 6, 2009.

Chrousos, G., and Gold, P. 1992. "The Concepts of Stress and Stress System Disorders: Overview of Physical and Behavioral Homeostasis." *Journal of the American Medical Association* 267: 1244–52.

Clark, N., Brown, R., Parker, E., Robins, T., Remick, D., Philbert, M., Keeler, G., and Israel, B. 1999. "Childhood Asthma." *Environmental Health Perspectives* 107 (Supp. 3): 421–29.

Clarke, A. 2001. "Negotiating New Relationships Again and Again: U.S. Women's Health Movements and (Bio)Medicine." Annual meeting of the Society for the Social Study of Science, Cambridge, MA, November.

————.2005. *Situational Analysis: Grounded Theory after the Postmodern Turn.* Thousand Oaks, CA: Sage.

Clarke, L. 1989. *Acceptable Risk? Making Decisions in a Toxic Environment.* Berkeley: University of California Press.

Clawson, D. 2003. *The Next Upsurge: Labor and the New Social Movements*. Ithaca, NY: Cornell University Press.

Cohen, L., and Legion, V. 2000. "Urban Asthma and Community Health Workers." Annual meeting of the American Public Health Association, Boston, November.

Cohn, B., Wolff, M., Cirillo, P., and Sholtz, R. 2007. "DDT and Breast Cancer in Young Women: New Data on the Significance of Age at Exposure." *Environmental Health Perspectives* 115: 1406–14.

Colborn, T., Dumanoski, D., and Myers, J. P. 1996. *Our Stolen Future: Are We Threatening Our Fertility, Intelligence, and Survival?* New York: Dutton.

Collaborative on Health and the Environment. 2009. "Battle Scars: Findings from the Federal Report on Gulf War Veterans' Illness," webinar, April 6, www.healthandenviron ment.org/partnership_calls/5837, accessed August 2010.

Collins, H. 1996. "In Praise of Futile Gestures: How Scientific Is the Sociology of Scientific Knowledge?" *Social Studies of Science* 26: 229–44.

Communities for a Better Environment. n.d. *Communities for a Better Environment: Environmental Health and Justice for California's Urban Communities*. www.cbecal.org, accessed May 12, 2004.

Cone, M. 2005. *Silent Snow*. New York: Grove Press.

Cooper, A. F., Kirton, J. J., and Schrecker, T. 2007. *Governing Global Health: Challenge, Response, Innovation*. Aldershot, UK: Ashgate.

Corburn, J. 2005. *Street Science: Community Knowledge and Environmental Health Justice*. Cambridge, MA: MIT Press.

———. 2007. "Returning to Our Roots: American Urban Planning and Public Health in the 21st Century." *Urban Affairs Review* 42: 688–713.

Couch, S. R., and Kroll-Smith, J. S. 1985. "The Chronic Technological Disaster: Toward a Social Scientific Perspective." *Social Science Quarterly* 66: 564–75.

———. 1994. "Environmental Controversies, Interactional Resources, and Rural Communities: Siting versus Exposure Disputes." *Rural Sociology* 59: 25–44.

———, eds. 1991. *Communities at Risk: Collective Responses to Technological Hazards*. New York: Peter Lang.

Cox, S. M., and McKellin, W. 1999. "'There's This Thing in Our Family': Predictive Testing and the Construction of Risk for Huntington's Disease." *Sociology of Health and Illness* 21 (5): 622–46.

Crom, W. 1994. "Pharmacokinetics in the Child." *Environmental Health Perspectives* 102 (Supp. 11): 111–17.

Croteau, D., and Hicks, L. 2003. "Coalition Framing and the Challenge of a Consonant Frame Pyramid: The Case of a Collaborative Response to Homelessness." *Social Problems* 50 (2): 251–72.

Dauvergne, P. 2005. "Cancer and Global Environmental Politics: Proposing a New Research Agenda." *Global Environmental Politics* 5 (3): 6–13.

Davis, D. L., and Bradlow, H. L. 1995. "Can Environmental Estrogens Cause Breast Cancer?" *Scientific American* 273 (4): 144–49.

Davis, D. L., and Webster, P. 2002. "The Social Context of Science: Cancer and the Environment." *Annals of the American Academy of Political and Social Science* 584: 13.

Davis, M. 2000. "Gulf War Illnesses and Recognizing New Diseases." In Institute of Medicine, *Gulf War and Health*, vol. 1, *Depleted Uranium, Sarin, Pyridostigmine Bromide, and Vaccines.* Washington, DC: National Academy Press.

Deahl, M. 2005. "Smoke, Mirrors, and Gulf War Illness." *Lancet* 365 (9460): 635–38.

Deapen, D., Liu, L., Perkins, C., Bernstein, L., and Ross, R. 2002. "Rapidly Rising Breast Cancer Incidence Rates among Asian-American Women." *International Journal of Cancer* 99 (5): 747–50.

DeCaprio, A. 1997. "Biomarkers: Coming of Age for Environmental Health and Risk Assessment." *Environmental Science and Technology* 31: 1837–48.

Deck, W., and Kosatsky, T. 1999. "Communicating Their Individual Results to Participants in an Environmental Exposure Study: Insights from Clinical Ethics." *Environmental Research* 80 (2, pt. 2): S223–S229.

Deeds, B. G., Castillo, M., Beason, Z., Cunningham, S. D., Ellen, J. M., and Peralta, L. 2008. "An HIV Prevention Protocol Reviewed at 15 National Sites: How Do Ethics Committees Protect Communities?" *Journal of Empirical Research on Human Research Ethics* 3 (2): 77–86.

Defense Science Board Task Force on Persian Gulf War Health Effects. 1994. *Report of the Defense Science Board Task Force on Persian Gulf War Health Effects.* Washington, DC: Office of the Under Secretary of Defense for Acquisition and Technology, www.gulflink .osd.mil/dsbrpt, accessed May 13, 2009.

Della Porta, D., and Diani, M. 1999. *Social Movements: An Introduction.* Oxford: Blackwell Publishing.

Destounis, S. V., DiNitto, P., Logan-Young, W., Bonaccio, E., Zuley, M. L., and Willison, K. M. 2004. "Can Computer-Aided Detection with Double Reading of Screening Mammograms Help Decrease the False-Negative Rate?" *Radiology* 232: 578–84.

Dickersin, K., Braun, L., Mead, M., Millikan, R., Wu, A. M., Pietenpol, J., Troyan, S., Anderson, B., and Visco, F. 2001. "Development and Implementation of a Science Training Course for Breast Cancer Activists: Project LEAD (Leadership, Education and Advocacy Development)." *Health Expectations* 4 (4): 213–20.

Dickert, N., and Sugarman, J. 2005. "Ethical Goals of Community Consultation in Research." *American Journal of Public Health* 95: 1123–27.

Diette, G., Markson, L., Skinner, E., Nguyen, T., Algatt-Bergstrom, P., and Wu, A. 2000. "Nocturnal Asthma in Children Affects School Attendance, School Performance, and Parents' Work Attendance." *Archives of Pediatrics and Adolescent Medicine* 154 (9): 923–29.

DiMaggio, P. J., and Powell, W. W. 1983. "The Iron Cage Revisited: Institutional Isomorphism and Collective Rationality in Organizational Fields." *American Sociological Review* 47: 147–60.

Dingwall et al. 2010 (see ch. 3, p. 87, query C)

Dockery, D. 2000. "Fine Particulate Air Pollution: Smoke and Mirrors of the '90s or Hazard of the New Millennium?" Annual meeting of the American Public Health Association, Boston, November.

Dockery, D., Pope, C. A. 3rd, Xu, X., Spengler, J., Ware, J., Ray, M., Ferris, B., and Speitzer, F. 1993. "An Association between Air Pollution and Mortality in Six U.S. Cities." *New England Journal of Medicine* 329 (24): 1753–59.

Dorgan, J. F., Brock, J. W., Rothman, N., Needham, L. L., Miller, R., Stephenson, H. E., Schussler, N., and Taylor, P. R. 1999. "Serum Organochlorine Pesticides and PCBs and Breast Cancer Risk: Results from a Prospective Analysis (USA)." *Cancer Causes and Control* 10 (1): 1–11.

Downs, A. 1972. "Up and Down with Ecology: The 'Issue-Attention Cycle.'" *Public Interest* 28: 38–51.

Doyle, J. 2004. *Trespass against Us: Dow Chemical and the Toxic Century.* Monroe, ME: Common Courage Press/Environmental Health Fund.

Duncan, D. E. 2006. "Toxic People: The Pollution Within." *National Geographic,* October 2006, www.nationalgeographic.com/ngm/0610/feature4/, accessed October 30, 2006.

Edelstein, M. 2004 [1988]. *Contaminated Communities: The Social and Psychological Impacts of Residential Toxic Exposure.* Boulder, CO: Westview Press.

Ehrenreich, B. 2009. "We Need a New Women's Health Movement." *Los Angeles Times,* December 2.

Emmet, E. A., Zhang, H., Shofer, F. S., Rodway, N., Desai, C., Freeman, D., and Hufford, M. 2009. "Development and Successful Application of a 'Community-First' Communication Model for Community-Based Environmental Health Research." *Journal of Occupational and Environmental Medicine* 51 (2): 146–56.

Engel, C. C., Liu, X., Clymer, R., Miller, R. F., Sjoberg, T., and Shapiro, J. R. 2000. "Rehabilitative Care of War-Related Health Concerns." *Journal of Occupational and Environmental Medicine* 42: 385–90.

Engler, R. 1992. *Fighting for the Right-to-Act in New Jersey.* Trenton, NJ: New Jersey Right-to-Know and Act Coalition.

Environmental Defence. 2005. "Toxic Nation: A Report on Pollution in Canadians." www.environmentaldefence.ca/toxicnation/resources/publications.htm, accessed November 2007.

Environmental Working Group. 2003a. *Body Burden: The Pollution in People.* Oakland, CA: Environmental Working Group, www.ewg.org/reports/bodyburden1, accessed May 2011.

———. 2003b. *Mother's Milk.* Oakland, CA: Environmental Working Group, www.ewg.org/reports/mothersmilk, accessed May 2011.

———. 2005. *Body Burden: The Pollution in Newborns.* Oakland, CA: Environmental Working Group, www.ewg.org/reports/bodyburden2, accessed May 2011.

———. 2008. *Teen Girls' Body Burden of Hormone-Altering Cosmetics Chemicals.* www.ewg.org/book/export/html/26953, accessed January 25, 2009.

Epstein, S. 1996. *Impure Science: AIDS, Activism, and the Politics of Knowledge.* Berkeley: University of California Press.

Erikson, K. 1976. *Everything in Its Path: Destruction of Community in the Buffalo Creek Flood.* New York: Simon & Schuster.

———. 1994. *A New Species of Trouble: Explorations in Disaster, Trauma, and Community.* New York: W. W. Norton.

Estabrook, T. 2006. *Labor-Environmental Coalitions: Lessons from a Louisiana Petrochemical Region.* New York: Baywood Publishing.

Evans, N. 2006. *The State of the Evidence: What Is the Connection between Breast Cancer and the Environment?* San Francisco, CA: Breast Cancer Fund.

Executive Order 13045. 1997. *Protection of Children from Environmental Health Risks and Safety Risks.*

Felix, H. C. 2007. "The Rise of the Community-Based Participatory Research Initiative at the National Institute for Environmental Health Sciences: An Historical Analysis Using the Policy Streams Model." *Progress in Community Health Partnerships: Research, Education, and Action* 1: 31–39.

Ferguson, S. J., and A. S. Kasper. 2000. "Living with Breast Cancer." In *Breast Cancer: Society Shapes an Epidemic,* by A. S. Kasper and S. J. Ferguson, 5–22. New York: St. Martin's Press.

First National People of Color Environmental Leadership Summit. 1991. "Washington Office of Environmental Justice." www.ejnet.org/ej/principles.html, accessed January 31, 2007.

Fischer, D. 2005. "What's in You?" *Oakland Tribune,* March 10.

Fischer, F. 2000. *Citizens, Experts, and the Environment: The Politics of Local Knowledge.* Durham, NC: Duke University Press.

Fishman, J. 2000. "Assessing Breast Cancer: Risk, Science and Environmental Activism in An 'At Risk' Community." In *Ideologies of Breast Cancer: Feminist Perspectives,* ed. Lana Potts, 181–204. New York: St. Martin's Press.

Fitzpatrick, K., and LaGory, M. 2000. *Unhealthy Places: The Ecology of Risk in the Urban Landscape.* New York: Routledge.

Foreman, C. 1998. "The Promise and Peril of Environmental Justice." Washington, DC: Brookings Institution.

Forster, D. 2002. "Independent Institutional Review Boards." *Seton Hall Law Review* 32: 513–23.

Foskett, J., Karran, A., and LaFia, C. 2000. "Breast Cancer in Popular Women's Magazines from 1913 to 1996." In *Breast Cancer: Society Shapes an Epidemic,* ed. A. Kasper and S. Ferguson, 302–24. New York: Palgrave.

Foucault, M. 1980. *Power/Knowledge: Selected Interviews and Other Writings, 1972–1977.* New York: Pantheon Books.

Fowler, M., Davenport, M., and Garg, R. 1992. "School Functioning of US Children with Asthma." *Pediatrics* 90 (6): 939–44.

Fowler W. J., Jr., and Walberg, H. J. 1991. "School Size, Characteristics, and Outcomes." *Educational Evaluation and Policy Analysis* 13 (2): 189–202.

Freudenburg, W. R. 1993. "Risk and Recreancy: Weber, the Division of Labor, and the Rationality of Risk Perceptions." *Social Forces* 71: 909–32.

Frickel, S. 2004. *Chemical Consequences: Environmental Mutagens, Scientist Activism, and the Rise of Genetic Toxicology.* New Brunswick, NJ: Rutgers University Press.

Frickel, S., and Gross, N. 2005. "A General Theory of Scientific/Intellectual Movements." *American Sociological Review* 70: 204–32.

Frickel, S., and Vincent, M. B. 2007. "Hurricane Katrina, Contamination, and the Unintended Organization of Ignorance." *Technology in Society* 29: 181–88.

Friedman, A., Kaufer, D., Shemer, J., Hendler, I., Soreq, H., and Tur-Kaspa, I. 1996. "Pyridostigmine Brain Penetration under Stress Enhances Neuronal Excitability and Induces Early Immediate Transcriptional Response." *Nature Medicine* 2 (12): 1382–85.

Friedman, M. S., Powell, K. E., Hutwagner, L., Graham, L. M., and Teague, W. G. 2001. "Impact of Changes in Transportation and Commuting Behaviors during the 1996 Summer Olympic Games in Atlanta on Air Quality and Childhood Asthma." *Journal of the American Medical Association* 285 (7): 897–905.

Friedrich, M. 2000. "Poor Children Subject to 'Environmental Injustice.'" *Journal of the American Medical Association* 283 (23) 3057–58.

Fukuda, K., Nisenbaum, R., Stewart, G., Thompson, W. W., Robin, L., Washko, R. M., Noah, D. L., et al. 1998. "Chronic Multisymptom Illness Affecting Air Force Veterans of the Gulf War." *Journal of the American Medical Association* 280: 981–88.

Furgal, C., Kalhok, S., Loring, E., and Smith, S. 2003. *Knowledge in Action: Canadian Arctic Contaminants Assessment Report, II*. Ottawa, ON: Ministry of Indian Affairs and Northern Development.

Gamson, W. 1990. *The Strategy of Social Protest*. Homewood, IL: Dorsey Press.

Gamson, W., Fireman, B., and Rytina, S. 1982. *Encounters with Unjust Authority*. Homewood, IL: Dorsey Press.

Geiser, K. 2001. *Materials Matter: Toward a Sustainable Materials Policy*. Cambridge, MA: MIT Press.

Geraghty, S., Khoury, J., Morrow, A., and Lanphear, B. 2008. "Reporting Individual Test Results of Environmental Chemicals in Breastmilk: Potential for Premature Weaning." *Breastfeeding Medicine* 3 (4): 207–13.

Gerhards, J., and Rucht, D. 1992. "Mesomobilization: Organizing and Framing in Two Protest Campaigns in West Germany." *American Journal of Sociology* 98: 555–95.

Gerhardstein, B., and Brown, P. 2005. "The Benefits of Community Medical Monitoring At Nuclear Weapons Production Sites: Lessons from Fernald." *Environmental Law Reporter* 35: 10530–38.

Gieryn, T. F. 1983. "Boundary-Work and the Demarcation of Science from Non-science: Strains and Interests in Professional Ideologies of Scientists." *American Sociological Review* 48 (6): 781–95.

———. 1999. *Cultural Boundaries of Science: Credibility on the Line*. Chicago: University of Chicago Press.

Gilbert, S. G. 2006. "Supplementing the Traditional Institutional Review Board with an Environmental Health and Community Review Board." *Environmental Health Perspectives* 114: 1626–9.

Gille, Z., and O'Riain, S. 2002. "Global Ethnography." *Annual Review of Sociology* 28 (1): 271–95.

Gilliland, F., McConnell, R., Peters, J., and Gong, H. 1999. "A Theoretical Basis for Investigating Ambient Air Pollution and Children's Respiratory Health." *Environmental Health Perspectives* 107 (Supp. 3): 403–7.

Ginns, S., and Gatrell, A. 1996. "Respiratory Health Effects of Industrial Air Pollution: A Study in East Lancashire, UK." *Journal of Epidemiology and Community Health* 50 (6): 631–35.

Godleski, J. 2000. "Mechanisms of Particulate Air Pollution Health Effects." Annual meeting of the American Public Health Association, Boston, November.

Goffman, E. 1974. *Frame Analysis: An Essay on the Organization of Experience.* New York: Harper Colophon.

Gold, D., Rotnitzky, A., Damokosh, A., Ware, J., Speizer, F., Ferris, B., and Dockery, D. 1993. "Race and Gender Differences in Respiratory Illness Prevalence and Their Relationship to Environmental Exposures in Children 7 to 14 Years of Age." *American Review of Respiratory Disease* 148: 10–18.

Gold, D., and Wright, R. 2005. "Population Disparities in Asthma." *Annual Review of Public Health* 26: 89–113.

Goldstein, B. D. 2005. "Advances in Risk Assessment and Communication." *Annual Review of Public Health* 26: 141–63.

Golomb, B. A. 2008. "Acetylcholinesterase Inhibitors and Gulf War illnesses." *Proceedings of the National Academy of Sciences* 105: 4295–4300.

Gomzi, M., and Saric, M. 1997. "Respiratory Impairment among Children Living in the Vicinity of a Fertilizer Plant." *International Archives of Occupational and Environmental Health* 70 (5): 314–20.

Goodman, D. C., Stukel, T. A., and Chang, C. 1998. "Trends in Pediatric Asthma Hospitalization Rates: Regional and Socioeconomic Differences." *Pediatrics* 101 (2): 208–13.

Goodwin, J., Jasper, J. M., and Polletta, F., eds. 2001. *Passionate Politics: Emotions and Social Movements.* Chicago: University of Chicago Press.

Gottlieb, R. 2001. *Environmentalism Unbound: Exploring New Pathways for Change.* Cambridge, MA: MIT Press.

———. 2005 [1993]. *Forcing the Spring: The Transformation of the American Environmental Movement.* 2nd ed. Washington, DC: Island Press.

Gould, K. A., Lewis, T., and Roberts, J. T. 2004. "Blue-Green Coalitions: Constraints and Possibilities in the Post 9-11 Political Environment." *Journal of World-Systems Research* 10 (1): 91–116.

Grandjean, P., and Landrigan, P. J. 2006. "Developmental Neurotoxicity of Industrial Chemicals." *Lancet* 368: 2167–78.

Gray, G. C., and Kang, H. K. 2006. "Healthcare Utilization and Mortality among Veterans of the Gulf War." *Philosophical Transactions of the Royal Society London, Biological Sciences* 361: 553–69.

Gray, G. C., Knoke, J. D., Berg, S. W., Wignall, F. S., and Barrett-Connor, E. 1998. "Counterpoint: Responding to Suppositions and Misunderstandings." *American Journal of Epidemiology* 148: 328–33.

Gray, G. C., Gackstetter, G. D., Kang, H. K., Graham, J. T., and Scott, K. C. 2004. "After More Than 10 Years of Gulf War Veteran Medical Evaluations, What Have We Learned?" *American Journal of Preventive Medicine* 26 (5): 443–52.

Greenbaum, D. 2000. "Interface of Science with Policy." Annual meeting of the American Public Health Association, Boston, November.

Greene, A., Morello-Frosch, R., and Shenassa, E. D. 2006. "Inadequate Prenatal Care and Elevated Blood Lead Levels among Children Born in Providence, Rhode Island: A Population-Based Study." *Public Health Reports* 121: 729–36.

Greenhouse, L. 2000. "E.P.A.'s Authority on Air Rules Wins Supreme Court's Backing." *New York Times,* February 28.

Greenpeace International. 2005. *A Present for Life: Hazardous Chemicals in Umbilical Cord Blood.* www.greenpeace.org/eu-unit/press-centre/reports/a-present-for-life, accessed November 2, 2007.

Groch, S. 1994. "Oppositional Consciousness: Its Manifestation and Development; The Case of People with Disabilities." *Sociological Inquiry* 64: 369–95.

Guo, Y., Lin, Y., Sung, F., Huang, S., Ko, Y., Lai, J., Su, H., Shaw, C., Lin, R., and Dockery, D. 1999. "Climate, Traffic-Related Air Pollutants, and Asthma Prevalence in Middle-School Children in Taiwan." *Environmental Health Perspectives* 107 (12). 1001–6.

Gurney, James G., Fritz, Melissa S., Ness, Kirsten K., Sievers, Phillip, Newschaffer, Craig J., and Shapiro, Elsa G. 2003. "Analysis of Prevalence Trends of Autism Spectrum Disorder in Minnesota." *Archives of Pediatric and Adolescent Medicine* 157: 622–27.

Güttes, S., Failing, K., Neumann, K., Kleinstein, J., Georgii, S., and Brunn, H. 1998. "Chlororganic Pesticides and Polychlorinated Biphenyls in Breast Tissue of Women with Benign and Malignant Breast Disease." *Archives of Environmental Contamination and Toxicology* 35 (1): 140–47.

Guzelian, P. S., Henry, C. J., and Olin, S. S. 1992. *Similarities and Differences between Children and Adults: Implications for Risk Assessment.* Washington, DC: ILSI Press/International Life Sciences Institute.

Haas, P. 1992. "Introduction: Epistemic Communities and International Policy Coordination." *International Organization: Knowledge, Power, and International Policy Coordination* 46: 1–35.

Haley, R., Kurt, T., and Hom, J. 1997. "Is There a Gulf War Syndrome? Searching for Syndromes by Factor Analysis of Symptoms." *Journal of the American Medical Association* 277: 215–22.

Hammersley, M., and Atkinson, P. 1995. *Ethnography: Principles in Practice.* New York: Routledge.

Hardin, R. 2001. "Conceptions and explanations of Trust." In *Trust in Society,* ed. K. S. Cook, 3–39. New York: Russell Sage Foundation.

Harley, N., Foulkes, E., Hilborne, L., Hudson, A., and Anthony, C. R. 1999. *A Review of the Scientific Literature as It Pertains to Gulf War Illness,* vol. 7, *Depleted Uranium.* Santa Monica, CA: RAND.

Harr, J. 1996. *A Civil Action.* New York: Vintage Books.

Harris, J. S. 1983. "Toxic Waste Uproar: A Community History." *Journal of Public Health Policy* 4 (2): 181–201.

Heaton, K., Palumbo, C., Proctor, S., Killiany, R., DA: Y.-T., and White, R. 2007. "Quantitative Magnetic Resonance Brain Imaging in U.S. Army Veterans of the 1991 Gulf War Potentially Exposed to Sarin and Cyclosarin." *Neurotoxicology* 28 (4): 761–69.

Heindel, J. J. 2003. "Endocrine Disruptors and the Obesity Epidemic." *Toxicological Sciences* 76: 247–49.

Hernandez, J. 1999. "Is Belmont High School's Legacy Racist Environmental Standards?" *Planning Report* 13 (3), www.ablinc.net/trp, accessed April 10, 2002.

Hess, D. J. 2002. "Technology-Oriented Social Movements and the Problem of Globalization." Unpublished paper.

Hilborne, L., and Golomb, B. 2001. *A Review of the Scientific Literature as It Pertains to Gulf War Illnesses,* vol. 1, *Infectious Diseases.* Santa Monica, CA: RAND.

Hilgartner, S., and Bosk, C. 1988. "The Rise and Fall of Social Problems: A Public Arenas Model." *American Journal of Sociology* 94 (1): 53–78.

Hites, R. 2004. "Polybrominated Diphenyl Ethers in the Environment and in People: A Meta-analysis of Concentrations." *Environmental Science and Technology* 38 (4): 945–56.

Holguin, F. 2008. "Traffic, Outdoor Air Pollution, and Asthma." *Immunology and Allergy Clinics of North America* 28 (3): 577–88.

Hooper, K., and She, J. 2003. "Lessons from the Polybrominated Diphenyl Ethers (PBDEs): Precautionary Principle, Primary Prevention, and the Value of Community-Based Body-Burden Monitoring Using Breast Milk." *Environmental Health Perspectives* 111: 109–14.

Høyer, A. P., Jørgensen, T., Brock, J. W., and Grandjean, P. 2000. "Organochlorine Exposure and Breast Cancer Survival." *Journal of Clinical Epidemiology* 53 (3): 323–30.

Hunter, D. J., and Kelsey, K. T. 1993. "Pesticide Residues and Breast Cancer: The Harvest of a Silent Spring?" Editorial. *Journal of the National Cancer Institute* 85: 598–99.

Hunter, D. J., Hankinson, S. E., Laden, F., Colditz, G. A., Manson, J. A. E., Willett, W. C., Speizer, F. E., and Wolff, M. S. 1997. "Plasma Organochlorine Levels and the Risk of Breast Cancer." *New England Journal of Medicine* 337 (18): 1253–58.

Hyams, K. C., Wignall, F. S., and Roswell, R. 1996. "War Syndromes and Their Evaluation: From the US Civil War to the Persian Gulf War." *Annals of Internal Medicine* 125 (5): 398–405.

Iles, A. 2007. "Identifying Environmental Health Risks in Consumer Products: Non-governmental Organizations and Civic Epistemologies." *Public Understanding of Science* 16: 371–91.

Institute of Medicine. 1994. *Veterans and Agent Orange: Health Effects of Herbicides Used in Vietnam.* Washington, DC: National Academy Press.

———. 1999. *Toward Environmental Justice: Research, Education, and Health Policy Needs.* Washington, DC: Committee on Environmental Justice, Health Sciences Policy Program, Health Sciences Section, Institute of Medicine.

———. 2000. *Gulf War and Health,* vol. 1, *Depleted Uranium, Sarin, Pyridostigmine Bromide, and Vaccines.* Washington, DC: National Academy Press.

Inuit Tapiriit Kanatami. 1995. *Communicating about Contaminants in Country Foods: The Experience of Aboriginal Communities.* Ottawa, ON:, Inuit Tapiriit Kanatami.

Iowa Persian Gulf Study Group. 1997. "Self-Reported Illness and Health Status among Gulf War Veterans." *Journal of the American Medical Association* 277: 238–45.

Irwin, A., and Wynne, B., eds. 1996. *Misunderstanding Science? Public Reconstruction of Science and Technology.* Cambridge: Cambridge University Press.

Israel, B. A., Schulz, A., Parker, E. A., and Becker, A. B. 1998. "Review of Community-Based Research: Assessing Partnership Approaches to Improve Public Health." *Annual Review of Public Health* 19 (1): 173–202.

Jackson, R. 2007. "Environment Meets Health, Again." *Science* 315: 1337.

Jackson, R., Locke, P., Pirkle, J., Thompson, F., and Sussman, D. 2002. "Will Biomonitoring Change the Way We Regulate Toxic Chemicals?" *Journal of Law, Medicine and Ethics* 30 (3): 177–83.

Jan, Tracy. 2004. "Environmental Report Details City School Ills." *Boston Globe,* November 19.

Jasanoff, S. 1987. "Contested Boundaries in Policy-Relevant Science." *Social Studies of Science* 17: 195–230.

———. 1990. *The Fifth Branch: Science Advisers as Policymakers.* Cambridge, MA: Harvard University Press.

———, ed. 2004. *States of Knowledge: The Co-production of Science and Social Order.* New York: Routledge.

———. 2005. *Designs on Nature.* Princeton, NJ: Princeton University Press.

Jedrychowski, W., and Flak, E. 1998. "Separate and Combined Effects of the Outdoor and Indoor Air Quality on Chronic Respiratory Symptoms Adjusted for Allergy among Preadolescent Children." *International Journal of Occupational Medicine and Environmental Health* 11 (1): 19–35.

Jenkins, R., Kopits, E., and Simpson, D. 2006. *Measuring the Social Benefits of EPA Land Cleanup and Reuse Programs.* Washington, DC: National Center for Environmental Economics, Environmental Protection Agency.

Johnston, H. 1995. "A Methodology for Frame Analysis: From Discourse to Cognitive Schemata." In *Social Movements and Culture,* ed. H. J. a. B. Klandermans, 217–45. Minneapolis: University of Minnesota Press.

Jones, A. W., Hutchinson, R. N., Van Dyke, N., Gates, L., and Companion, M. 2001. "Coalition Form and Mobilization Effectiveness in Local Social Movements." *Sociological Spectrum* 21 (2): 207–31.

Jones, C. 2008. "Richmond Council OKs Chevron Refinery Plan." *San Francisco Chronicle,* July 18.

Jonsen, A. R. 1991. "Ethical Considerations and Responsibilities when Communicating Health Risk Information." *Journal of Clinical Epidemiology* 44 (Supp. I): 69S–72S.

Kang, H., and Bullman, T. 2001. "Mortality among US Veterans of the Persian Gulf War: 7-year Follow-up." *American Journal of Epidemiology* 154: 399–405.

Kant, A. K., Schatzkin, A., Graubard, B. I., and Schairer, C. 2000. "A Prospective Study of Diet Quality and Mortality in Women." *Journal of the American Medical Association* 283 (16): 2109–15.

Kaplan, L. 1997. "The Hanford Education Action League: An Informed Citizenry and Radiation Health Effects." *International Journal of Contemporary Sociology* 34: 255–66.

Kaplan, S., and Morris, J. 2000. "Kids at Risk." *US News and World Report* 128 (24): 47–53.

Kazis, R., and Grossman, R. L. 1990. *Fear at Work: Job Blackmail, Labor, and the Environment.* New York: Pilgrim Press.

Keck, M., and Sikkink, K. 1998. "Transnational Advocacy Networks in the Movement Society." In *The Social Movement Society,* ed. D. Meyer and S. Tarrow, 217–38. Lanham, MD: Rowman & Littlefield.

Keeler, J. R., Hurst, C. G., and Dunn, M. A. 1991. "Pyridostigmine Used as a Nerve Agent Pretreatment under Wartime Conditions." *Journal of the American Medical Association* 266 (5): 693–95.

Keirns, C. C. 2009. "Asthma Mitigation Strategies: Professional, Charitable, and Community Coalitions." *American Journal of Preventive Medicine* 37 (6S1): S244–S250.

Keune, H., Morrens, B., and Loots, I. 2008. "Risk Communication and Human Biomonitoring: Which Practical Lessons from the Belgian Experience Are of Use for the EU Perspective?" *Environmental Health* 7 (Supp. 1): S1–11.

Kiecolt-Glaser, J. K., McGuire, L., Robles, T. F., and Glaser, R. 2002. "Psychoneuroimmunology and Psychosomatic Medicine: Back to the Future." *Psychosomatic Medicine* 64 (1): 15–28.

Klawiter, M. 1999. "Racing for the Cure, Walking Women, and Toxic Touring: Mapping Cultures of Action within the Bay Area Terrain of Breast Cancer." *Social Problems:* 104–26.

———. 2001. "Breast Cancer Activism in the U.S.: Diverse Perspectives." Annual meeting of the Society for the Social Study of Science, Cambridge, MA, November.

Knorr, R. S., Condon, S. K., Dwyer, F. M., and Hoffman, D. F. 2004. "Tracking Pediatric Asthma: The Massachusetts Experience Using School Health Records." *Environmental Health Perspectives* 112: 1424–27.

Knorr-Cetina, K. 1999. *Epistemic Cultures: How the Sciences Make Knowledge.* Cambridge, MA: Harvard University Press.

Kolata, G. 1996. "No Rise Found in Death Rates after Gulf War." *New York Times,* November 14.

———. 2002." Epidemic That Wasn't." *New York Times,* August 29

Kopans, D. 1991. "The Positive Predictive Value of Mammography." *American Journal of Roentgenology* 153: 521–26.

Koretz, Daniel. 1997. "Indicators of Educational Achievement." In *Indicators of Children's Well-Being,* ed. R. M. Hauser, B. V. Brown, and W. R. Prosser, 208–34. New York: Russell Foundation.

Kraft, M., and Scheberle, D. 1995. "Environmental Justice and the Allocation of Risk: The Case of Lead and Public Health." *Policy Studies Journal* 23 (1): 113–22.

Kriebel, D., Tickner, J., Epstein, P., Lemons, J., Levins, R., Loechler, E., Quinn, M., Rudel, R., Schettler, T., and Stoto, M. 2001. "The Precautionary Principle in Environmental Health Science." *Environmental Health Perspectives* 109 (9): 871–76.

Krieger, J. K., Takaro, T. K., Allen, C., Song, L., Weaver, M., Chai, S., and Dickey, P. 2002. "The Seattle-King County Healthy Homes Project: Implementation of a Comprehensive Approach to Improving Indoor Environmental Quality for Low-Income Children with Asthma." *Environmental Health Perspectives* 110 (Supp. 2): 311–22.

Krimsky, S. 1999. *Hormonal Chaos: The Scientific and Social Origins of the Environmental Endocrine Hypothesis.* Baltimore, MD: John Hopkins University Press.

———. 2000. *Hormonal Chaos: The Scientific and Social Origins of the Environmental Endocrine Hypothesis.* Baltimore, MD: Johns Hopkins University Press.

Krimsky, S., and Plough, A. 1988. *Environmental Hazards: Communicating Risks as a Social Process.* Dover, MA: Auburn House.

Kroll-Smith, J. S., and Couch, S. 1990. *The Real Disaster Is Above Ground: A Mine Fire and Social Conflict.* Lexington: University Press of Kentucky.

———. 1991. "What Is a Disaster? An Ecological-Symbolic Approach to Resolving the Definitional Debate." *International Journal of Mass Emergencies and Disasters* 9: 355–66.

Kroll-Smith, S., and Floyd, H. H. 1997. *Bodies in Protest: Environmental Illness and the Struggle over Medical Knowledge.* New York: New York University Press.

Kroll-Smith, S., Brown, P., and Gunter, V., eds. 2000. *Illness and the Environment: A Reader in Contested Medicine*. New York: New York University Press.

Krueger, A. 1999. "Experimental Estimates of Educational Production Functions." *Quarterly Journal of Economics* 114 (2): 497–532.

Kubal, T. J. 1998. "The Presentation of Political Self: Cultural Resonance and the Construction of Collective Action Frames." *Sociological Quarterly* 39 (4): 539.

Kuehn, R. R. 1996. "The Environmental Justice Implications of Quantitative Risk Assessment." *University of Illinois Law Review* 1996 (1): 103–72.

Landrigan, P. 1997. "Illness in Gulf War Veterans: Causes and Consequences." *Journal of the American Medical Association* 277: 259–61.

Landrigan, P., and Goldman, L. R. 2011. "Children's Vulnerability to Toxic Chemicals: A Challenge and Opportunity to Strengthen Health and Environmental Policy." *Health Affairs* 30: 842–50.

Landrigan, P., Claudio, L., Markowitz, S., Berkowitz, G., Brenner, B., Romero, H., Wetmur, J., et al. 1999. "Pesticides and Inner-City Children: Exposures, Risks and Prevention." *Environmental Health Perspectives* 107 (Supp. 3): 431–37.

Landrigan, P., Schechter, C. B., Lipton, J M., Fahs, M C., and Schwartz, J. 2002. "Environmental Pollutants and Disease in American Children: Estimates of Morbidity, Mortality, and Costs for Lead Poisoning, Asthma, Cancer, and Developmental Disabilities." *Environmental Health Perspectives* 110: 721–28.

Latin, H. 1988. "Good Science, Bad Regulation, and Toxic Risk Assessment." *Yale Journal on Regulation* 5 (1): 89–148.

Latour, B., and Woolgar, S. 1987. *Science in Action: How to Follow Scientists and Engineers through Society*. Cambridge, MA: Harvard University Press.

Lawton, J. 2003. "Lay Experiences of Health and Illness: Past Research and Future Agendas." *Sociology of Health and Illness* 25 (3): 23–40.

Lee, C. 2002. "Environmental Justice: Building a Unified Vision of Health and Environment." *Environmental Health Perspectives* 110 (Supp. 2): 141–44.

Leikauf, G., Line, S., Albert, R., Baxter, C., Bernstein, D., and Buncher, C. 1995. "Evaluation of a Possible Association of Urban Air Toxics and Asthma." *Environmental Health Perspectives* 103 (Supplement 6): 253–71.

Lerner, S. 2005. *Diamond: A Struggle for Environmental Justice in Louisiana's Chemical Corridor*. Cambridge, MA: MIT Press.

Levine, A. 1982. *Love Canal: Science, Politics and People*. New York: Rowman & Littlefield.

Lichtenstein, P., Holm, N., Verkasalo, P. K., Iliadou, A., Kaprio, J., Koskenvuo, M., Pukkala, E., Skytthe, A., and Hemminki, K. 2000. "Environmental and Heritable Factors in the Causation of Cancer: Analyses of Cohorts of Twins from Sweden, Denmark, and Finland." *New England Journal of Medicine* 343: 78–85.

Lichterman, P. 1995. "Piecing Together Multicultural Community: Cultural Differences in Community Building among Grass-Roots Environmentalists." *Social Problems* 42 (4): 513–34.

Lindem, K., Heeren, T., and White, R., et al. 2003. "Neuropsychological Performance in Gulf War Era Veterans: Traumatic Stress Symptomatology and Exposure to Chemical-Biological Warfare Agents." *Journal of Psychopathology and Behavioral Assessment* 25: 105–19.

Lioy, P. J., Freeman, N. C. G., and Millette, J. 2002. "Dust: A Metric for Use in Residential and Building Exposure Assessment and Source Characterization." *Environmental Health Perspectives* 110 (10): 969–83.

Liu, L., Poon, R., Chen, L., Frescura, A.-M., Montuschi, P., Ciabattoni, G., Wheeler, A., and Dales, R. 2009. "Acute Effects of Air Pollution on Pulmonary Function, Airway Inflammation, and Oxidative Stress in Asthmatic Children." *Environmental Health Perspectives* 117 (4): 668–74.

Lofland, J., and Lofland, L. H. 1995. *Analyzing Social Settings*. Belmont, CA: Wadsworth.

MacIntyre, S., Ellaway, A., and Cummins, S. 2002. "Place Effects on Health: How Can We Conceptualize, Operationalize and Measure Them?" *Social Science and Medicine* 55 (1): 125–39.

MacKendrick, N. 2007. "Contaminants, the Human Body, and the Framing of Risk: A Study of Canadian News Coverage, 1986–2006." Annual meeting of the American Sociological Association, Montreal, August.

Mannino, D., Homa, D., and Pertowski, C. 1998. "Surveillance for Asthma: United States, 1960–1995." *Mortality and Morbidity Weekly Report* 47 (SS-1): 1–28.

Mannino, D., Homa, D. M., Akinbami, L. J., Moorman, J. E., Gwynn, C., and Redd, S. C. 2002. "Surveillance for Asthma: United States, 1980–1999." *Mortality and Morbidity Weekly Report Surveillance Summaries* 51 (1): 1–13.

Mansbridge, J., and Morris, A. D. 2001. *Oppositional Consciousness: The Subjective Roots of Social Protest*. Chicago: University of Chicago Press.

Marcus, G. E. 1995. "Ethnography in/of the World System: The Emergence of Multi-sited Ethnography." *Annual Review of Anthropology* 24: 95–118.

Markowitz, G., and Rosner, D. 2002. *Deceit and Denial: The Deadly Politics of Industrial Pollution*. Berkeley: University of California Press.

Marshall, C. 2005. "New Emission Rule for Bay Area Refineries." *New York Times*, July 15.

Martin, B. 1996. "Sticking a Needle into Science: The Case of Polio Vaccines and the Origin of AIDS." *Social Studies of Science* 26: 245–76.

Martin, J. L. 2003. "What is Field Analysis?" *American Journal of Sociology* 109: 1–49.

Mayer, B. 2008. *Blue-Green Coalitions: Fighting for Safe Workplaces and Healthy Communities*. Ithaca, NY: Cornell University Press.

Mayer, B., and Brown, P. 2005. "Constructing a Coalition Frame in a Cross-Movement Coalition: New Jersey's Labor-Environmental Alliance." Annual meeting of the American Sociological Association, Philadelphia. August.

Mayer, B., Brown, P., and Linder, M. 2002. "Moving Further Upstream: From Toxics Reduction to the Precautionary Principle." *Public Health Reports* 117: 574–86.

Mayer, B., Brown, P., and Senier, L. 2008. "Health, Labor, and the Environment." Annual meeting of the American Sociological Association, Boston, August.

McAdam, D. 1982. *Political Process and the Development of Black Insurgency, 1930–1970*. Chicago: University of Chicago Press.

McAdam, D., McCarthy, J., and Zald, M. N. 1996. *Comparative Perspectives on Social Movements: Opportunities, Mobilizing Structures, and Framing*. Cambridge: Cambridge University Press.

McAdam, D., Tarrow, S., and Tilly, C. 2001. *Dynamics of Contention*. New York: Cambridge University Press.

McCammon, H. J., and Campbell, K. E. 2002. "Allies on the Road to Victory: Coalition Formation between the Suffragists and the Women's Christian Temperance Union." *Mobilization* 7: 231–51.

McConnell, R., Berhane, K., Gilliland, F., London, S. J., Islam, T., Gauderman, W. J., Avol, E., Margolis, H. G., and Peters, J. M. 2002. "Asthma in Exercising Children Exposed to Ozone: A Cohort Study." *Lancet* 359 (9304): 386–91.

McCormick, S. 2009. *No Family History: The Environmental Links to Breast Cancer.* Lanham, MD: Rowman & Littlefield.

McCormick, S., and Baralt, L. 2006. "The Breast Cancer Movement: Overlapping Success and Co-optation." Annual meeting of the Society for the Study of Social Problems, Montreal, August.

McCormick, S., Brown, P., and Zavestoski, S. 2003. "The Personal is Scientific, The Scientific is Political: The Public Paradigm of the Environmental Breast Cancer Movement." *Sociological Forum* 18: 545–76.

McCormick, S., Brody, J., Brown, P., and Polk, R. 2004. "Lay Involvement in Breast Cancer Research." *International Journal of Health Services* 34: 625–46.

McKelvey, W., Brody, J. G., Aschengrau, A., and Swartz, C. H. 2003. "Association between Residence on Cape Cod, Massachusetts, and Breast Cancer." *Annals of Epidemiology* 14 (2): 89–94.

Mechanic, D., and Meyer, S. 2000. "Concepts of Trust among Patients with Serious Illness." *Social Science and Medicine* 51: 657–68.

Mendell, M., and Heath, G. 2005. "Do Indoor Air Pollutants and Thermal Conditions in Schools Influence Student Performance? A Critical Review of the Literature." *Indoor Air* 15 (1): 27–52.

Metcalf, S. W., and Orloff, K. G. 2004. "Biomarkers of Exposure in Community Settings." *Journal of Toxicology and Environmental Health A* 67: 715–26.

Metropolitan Forum Project. 1999. *What If? New Schools, Better Neighborhoods, More Livable Communities.* Los Angeles, CA: Metropolitan Forum Project.

Meyer, D. S., and Corrigal-Brown, C. 2005. "Coalitions and Political Context: U.S. Movements against Wars in Iraq." *Mobilization* 10 (3): 327–46.

Meyer, D. S., and Whittier, N. 1994. "Social Movement Spillover." *Social Problems* 41: 277–98.

Miller, B. 2000. "Media Art and Activism." In *Reclaiming the Politics of Health: Environmental Debate in a Toxic Culture,* ed. R. Hofrichter, 313–25. Cambridge, MA: MIT Press.

Mills, C. Wright. 1959. *The Sociological Imagination.* New York: Oxford University Press.

Minchin, T. J. 2003. *Forging a Common Bond: Labor and Environmental Activism during the BASF Lockout.* Gainesville: University of Florida Press.

Minkler, M. 2000. "Participatory Action Research and Healthy Communities." *Public Health Reportsorts* 115: 191–97.

Minkler, M., and Wallerstein, N., eds. 2003. *Community-Based Participatory Research for Health.* San Francisco: Jossey-Bass.

Minkler, M., Vasquez, V. B., Chang, C., and Miller, J. 2008. *Promoting Health Public Policy through Community-Based Participatory Research: Ten Case Studies.* Oakland, CA: PolicyLink.

Minkoff, D. C. 1997. "The Sequencing of Social Movements." *American Sociological Review* 62 (5): 779–99.

Mix, T., and Cable, S. 2006. "Condescension and Cross-Class Coalitions: Working Class Activists' Perspectives on the Role of Social Status." *Sociological Focus* 39: 99–114.

Moore, K. 1999. "Political Protest and Institutional Change: The Anti-Vietnam War Movement and American Science." In *How Social Movements Matter*, ed. M. Giugni, D. McAdam, and C. Tilly, 313–25. Minneapolis: University of Minnesota Press.

———. 2008. *Disrupting Science: Social Movements, American Scientists, and the Politics of the Military, 1945–1975*. Princeton, NJ: Princeton University Press.

Morello-Frosch, R. 1997. "The Politics of Reproductive Hazards in the Workplace: Class, Gender, and the History of Occupational Lead Exposure." *International Journal of Health Services* 27: 501–21.

———. 2002. "The Political Economy of Environmental Discrimination." *Environment and Planning C* 20: 477–96.

———. 2008. "Report to Richmond City Permitting Council on Proposed Changes in Refinery Operations." Unpublished document.

Morello-Frosch, R., and Shenassa, E. 2006. "The Environmental 'Riskscape' and Social Inequality: Implications for Explaining Maternal and Child Health Disparities." *Environmental Health Perspectives* 114 (8): 1150–53.

Morello-Frosch, R., Pastor, M., and Sadd, J. 2001. "Environmental Justice and Southern California's 'Riskscape': The Distribution of Air Toxics Exposures and Health Risks Among Diverse Communities." *Urban Affairs Review* 36 (4): 551–78.

———. 2002. "Integrating Environmental Justice and the Precautionary Principle in Research and Policy-Making: The Case of Ambient Air Toxics Exposures and Health Risks among School Children in Los Angeles." *Annals of the American Academy of Political and Social Science* 584: 47–68.

Morello-Frosch, R., Woodruff, T., Axelrad, D., and Caldwell, J. 2000. "Air Toxics and Health Risks in California: The Public Health Implications of Outdoor Concentrations." *Risk Analysis* 20 (2): 273–91.

Morello-Frosch, R., Pastor, M., Porras, C., and Sadd, J. 2005a. "Environmental Justice and Regional Inequality in Southern California: Implications for Future Research." *Community Research in Environmental Health: Studies in Science, Advocacy and Ethics*, ed. D. Brugge and H. P. Hynes, 205–18. Aldershot, UK: Ashgate.

Morello-Frosch, R., Pastor, M., Sadd, J., Porras, C., and Prichard, M. 2005b. "Citizens, Science, and Data Judo: Leveraging Community-Based Participatory Research to Build a Regional Collaborative for Environmental Justice in Southern California." In *Methods for Conducting Community-Based Participatory Research in Public Health*, ed. E. E. Barbara Israel, Amy Shultz, and Edith Parker, 371–92. San Francisco: Jossey-Bass.

Morello-Frosch, R., Zavestoski, S., Brown, P., Altman, R. G., McCormick, S., and Mayer, B. 2006. "Embodied Health Movements: Responses to a 'Scientized' World." In *The New Political Sociology of Science: Institutions, Networks, and Power*, ed. Kelly Moore and Scott Frickel, 244–71. Madison: University of Wisconsin Press.

Morello-Frosch, R., Brody, J. G., Brown, P., Altman, R. G., and Rudel, R. 2009a. "Toxic Ignorance and Right-To-Know in Biomonitoring Results Communication: A Survey of Scientists and Study Participants." *Environmental Health* 8 (6).

Morello-Frosch, R., Pastor, M., Sadd, J., and Shokoff, S. 2009b. *The Climate Gap: Inequalities in How Climate Change Hurts Americans and How to Close the Gap.* http://college.usc.edu/geography/ESPE/documents/The_Climate_Gap_Full_Report_FINAL.pdf.

Morgen, S. 2002. *Into Our Own Hands: The Women's Health Movement in the United States, 1969–1990.* New Brunswick, NJ: Rutgers University Press.

Morris, A. 1984. *The Origins of the Civil Rights Movement.* New York: Free Press.

Motosue, A., Petronella, S., Sullivan, J., Castillo, S., Garcia, T., Murillo, M., Calhoun, J., Chhickara, R., Bethel, D., and Ward J., Jr. 2009. "Lead Exposure Risk Is Associated with Asthma in a Low-Income Urban Hispanic Population: Results of the Communities Organized against Asthma and Lead (COAL) Project." *Journal of Allergy and Clinical Immunology* 123 (2): S20.

Mottl, T. 1980. "The Analysis of Counter-movements." *Social Problems* 27: 620–35.

Murphy, M. 2006. *Sick Building Syndrome and the Problem of Uncertainty: Environmental Politics, Technoscience, and Women Workers.* Durham, NC: Duke University Press.

Murphy, R. 1997. *Sociology and Nature: Social Action in Context.* Boulder, CO: Westview Press.

Myers, D. J., and Cress, D., eds. 2004. *Authority in Contention: Research in Social Movements, Conflict and Change.* Amsterdam: Elsevier.

Myhre, J. 2001. "Contemporary Breast Cancer Activism in the United States." Annual meeting of the Society for the Social Study of Science, Cambridge, MA, November.

National Academy of Sciences. 2006. *Human Biomonitoring for Environmental Chemicals.* Washington, DC: National Research Council, www.nap.edu/catalog/11700.html, accessed July 2, 2006.

National Bioethics Advisory Commission. 1999. *Research Involving Human Biological Materials: Ethical Issues and Policy Guidance.* Rockville, MD: National Bioethics Advisory Committee.

National Cancer Institute. 2010. "Long Island Breast Cancer Project." http://epi.grants.cancer.gov/LIBCSP/, accessed May 2010.

National Gulf War Resource Center. 2001. *Uncounted Casualties: America's Ailing Gulf War Veterans.* Topeka, KS: National Gulf War Resource Center.

National Institutes of Health. 1979. *The Belmont Report: Ethical Principles and Guidelines for the Protection of Human Subjects of Research.* Bethesda, MD: National Institutes of Health, Office of Human Subjects Research.

———. 1994. *The Persian Gulf Experience and Health.* Technology Assessment Workshop, Washington, DC.

———. 1998. *IRB Knowledge of Local Research Context.* Bethesda, MD: National Institutes of Health, Division of Human Subjects Protection.

NBCC (National Breast Cancer Coalition). 2008. *Annual Report.* Washington, DC: NBCC.

NCHS (National Center for Health Statistics). 2008a. *National Health and Nutrition Examination Survey Data, 2007–2008.* Hyattsville, MD: U.S. Department of Health and Human Services, Centers for Disease Control and Prevention.

————. 2008b. *Summary Health Statistics for U.S. Adults: National Health Interview Survey,* CDC. Atlanta, GA: Centers for Disease Control and Prevention.

Needham, L L.,Ozhaynak, H., Whyatt, R. M., Barr, D. B., Wang, R. Y., Haeher, L., et al. 2005. "Exposure Assessment in the National Children's Study: Introduction." *Environmental Health Perspectives* 113: 1076–82.

Nelkin, D. 1984. "Science and Technology Policy and the Democratic Process." In *Citizen Participation in Science and Policy,* ed. J. Peterson, 18–39. Amherst: University of Massachusetts Press.

————. 1995. *Selling Science: How the Press Covers Science and Technology.* New York: Freeman.

Nelson, J., Scammell, M. K., Altman, R. G., Webster, T. F., and Ozonoff, D. M. 2008. "A New Spin on Research Translation: The Boston Consensus Conference on Human Biomonitoring." *Environmental Health Perspectives* 117 (4): 495–99.

Newschaffer, C. J., Falb, M. D., and Gurney, J. G. 2005. "National Autism Prevalence Trends from United States Special Education Data." *Pediatrics* 115: 277–82.

New York Times. 2002. "Breast Cancer Mythology on Long Island." *New York Times,* August 31.

Norén, K., and Meironyté, D. 2000. "Certain Organochlorine and Organobromine Contaminates in Swedish Human Milk in Perspective of Past 20–30 years." *Chemosphere* 40: 1111–23.

Norgaard, K. 2006. "'We Don't Really Want to Know': The Social Experience of Global Warming; Dimensions of Denial and Environmental Justice." *Organization and Environment* 19 (3): 347–70.

Northwest Coalition for Alternatives to Pesticides. 2000. *Unthinkable Risk: How Children Are Exposed and Harmed When Pesticides Are Used at School.* Eugene, OR: Northwest Coalition for Alternatives to Pesticides.

NRC (National Research Council). 1993. *Pesticides in the Diets of Infants and Children.* Washington, DC: National Research Council.

Obach, B. 2004a. *Labor and the Environmental Movement: The Quest for Common Ground.* Cambridge, MA: MIT Press.

————. 2004b. "New Labor: Slowing the Treadmill of Production?" *Organization and Environment* 17 (3): 337–54.

Ochsner, M. L. 1992. "Worker and Community Right-to-Know: Case Studies in Policy Formation and Implementation." PhD diss., Columbia University.

O'Connell, V. 2003. "When a Child Has Cancer: Protecting Children from a Toxic World." In *Synthetic Planet: Chemical Politics and the Hazards of Modern Life,* ed. M. Casper, 111–29. New York: Routledge.

O'Fallon, L. R., Wolfle, G. M., Brown, D., Dearry, A., and Olden, K. 2003. "Strategies for Setting a National Research Agenda That Is Responsive to Community needs." *Environmental Health Perspectives* 111 (16): 1855–60.

Office of Behavioral and Social Sciences Research. 1999. *Qualitative Methods in Health Research: Opportunities and Considerations in Application and Review.* Bethesda, MD: National Institutes of Health.

Office of Environmental Health Hazard Assessment. 2009. *Cumulative Impacts and Precautionary Approaches Project.* http://oehha.ca.gov/ej/index.html, accessed June 5, 2009.

Omohundro, E. 2004. *Living in a Contaminated World: Community Structures, Environmental Risks, and Decision Frameworks.* Burlington, VT: Ashgate.

O'Neal, J. 2000. "For Generations Yet to Come: Junebug Productions' Environmental Justice Project." In *Reclaiming the Politics of Health: Environmental Debate in a Toxic Culture,* ed. R. Hofrichter, 301–11. Cambridge, MA: MIT Press.

Orfield, M. 1997. *Metropolitics: A Regional Agenda for Community and Stability.* Washington, DC: Brookings Institution.

O'Rourke, D., Connelly, L., and Koshland, C. P. 1996. "Industrial Ecology: A Critical Review." *International Journal of Environment and Pollution* 6: 89–112.

Ozonoff, D. M., and Boden, L. 1987. "Truth and Consequences: Health Agency Responses to Environmental Health Problems." *Science, Technology, and Human Values* 12 (3–4): 70–77.

Parkinson, A. 1996. *Casarett and Doull's Toxicology: The Basic Science of Poisons.* New York: McGraw-Hill.

Pastor, M. 2001. "Common Ground at Ground Zero? The New Economy and the New Organizing in Los Angeles." *Antipode* 33 (2): 260–89.

Pastor, M., Dreier, P., Lopez-Garza, M., and Grisby, E. 2000. *Regions That Work: How Cities and Suburbs Can Grow Together.* Minneapolis: University of Minnesota Press.

Pastor, M., Sadd, J., and Morello-Frosch, R. 2002a. "Reading, Writing and Toxics: Children's Health, Academic Performance and Environmental Justice in Los Angeles." Working paper, Center for Justice, Tolerance, and Community, University of California, Santa Cruz. January.

———. 2002b. "Who's Minding the Kids? Pollution, Public Schools, and Environmental Justice in Los Angeles." *Social Science Quarterly* 83 (1): 263–80.

Pausentbach, D., and Galbraith, D. 2006. "Biomonitoring: Is Body Burden Relevant to Public Health?" *Regulatory Toxicology and Pharmacology* 44: 249–61.

Pechter, E., Davis, L., Tumpowsky, C., Flattery, J., Harrison, R., Reinisch, F., Reily,M. J. et al. 2005. "Work-Related Asthma among Health Care Workers: Surveillance Data from California, Massachusetts, Michigan, and New Jersey, 1993–1997." *American Journal of Industrial Medicine* 47: 265–75.

Perera, F., Jedrychowski, W., Rauh, V., and Whyatt, R. M. 1999. "Molecular Epidemiological Research on the Effects of Environmental Pollutants on the Fetus." *Environmental Health Perspectives* 107 (Supp. 3): 451–60.

Pew Environmental Health Commission. 2000. *Attack Asthma.* Los Angeles: Pew Environmental Health Commission.

PGVCB-RWG (Persian Gulf Veterans Coordinating Board Research Working Group Members). 1999. *Annual Report to Congress: Federally Sponsored Research on Gulf War Veterans' Illnesses for 1999.* Washington, DC: Department of Veterans Affairs.

Picou, S. 1990. *Social Disruption and Psychological Stress in an Alaskan Fishing Community: The Impact of the Exxon Valdez Oil Spill.* Boulder: University of Colorado Natural Hazards Center.

Polletta, F., and Jasper, J. M. 2001. "Collective Identity and Social Movements." *Annual Review of Sociology* 27: 283–305.

Pope, C. A. 3rd. 1989. "Respiratory Disease Associated with Community Air Pollution and a Steel Mill, Utah Valley." *American Journal of Public Health* 79 (5): 623–28.

Powell, F., Pinto, L., Sullivan, K., Krengel, M., White, R., and Killiany, R. 2007. "MRI Reveals Evidence of Structural Brain Changes among Veterans Deployed in the First Gulf War." Meeting of the American Academy of Neurology, Boston, May.

Presidential Advisory Committee on Gulf War Veterans' Illnesses. 1996. *Final Report.* Washington, DC: US Government Printing Office.

Princen, T., Maniates, M., and Conca, K., eds. 2002. *Confronting Consumption.* Cambridge, MA: MIT Press.

Pritchard, I. A. 2002. "Travelers and Trolls: Practitioner Research and Institutional Review Boards." *Educational Researcher* 31 (3): 3–13.

Proctor, S. P., Heeren, T., White, R. F., Wolfe, J., Borgos, M. S., Davis, J. D., Pepper, L., et al. 1998. "Health Status of Persian Gulf War Veterans: Self-Reported Symptoms, Environmental Exposures and the Effect of Stress." *International Journal of Epidemiology* 27 (6): 1000–1010.

Prussel, D., and Tepperman, J. 2001. "Tackling Health Hazards at School." *Children's Advocate,* www.4children.org/news/901toxic.htm, aaccessed May 26, 2002.

———. 1996. *Environmentalism and Economic Justice: Two Chicano Studies in the Southwest.* Tucson: University of Arizona Press.

Purohit, A., Kopferschmitt-Kubler, M., Moreau, C., Popin, E., Blaumeiser, M., and Pauli, G. 2000. "Quaternary Ammonium Compounds and Occupational Asthma." *International Archives of Occupational and Environmental Health* 73 (6): 423–27.

Quandt, S. A., Doran, A. M., Rao, P., Hoppin, J. A., Snively, B. M., and Arcury, T. A. 2004. "Reporting Pesticide Assessment Results to Farmworker Families: Development, Implementation, and Evaluation of a Risk Communication Strategy." *Environmental Health Perspectives* 112 (5): 636–42.

Quigley, D. 2006. "A Review of Improved Ethical Practices in Environmental and Public Health Research: Case Examples from Native Communities." *Health Education and Behavior* 33: 130–47.

RAC (Research Advisory Committee on Gulf War Veterans' Illnesses). 2008. *Gulf War Illness and the Health of Gulf War Veterans.* Washington, DC: Department of Veterans Affairs.

Raffensperger, C., and Tickner, J., eds. 1999. *Protecting Public Health and the Environment: Implementing the Precautionary Principle.* Washington, DC: Island Press.

Rapp, R. 1999. *Testing Women, Testing the Fetus: The Social Impact of Amniocentesis in America.* New York: Routledge.

Ray, R. 1999. *Fields of Protest: Women's Movements in India.* Minneapolis: University of Minnesota Press.

Reeves, W. C., Fukuda, K., Nisenbaum, R., and Thompson, W. W. 1999. "Letters: Chronic Multisystem Illness among Gulf War Veterans." *Journal of the American Medical Association* 282: 327–29.

Reich, M. 1991. *Toxic Politics: Responding to Chemical Disasters.* Ithaca, NY: Cornell University Press.

Reiss, J. R., and Martin, A. R. 2000. *Breast Cancer 2000: An Update on the Facts, Figures and Issues.* San Francisco: Breast Cancer Fund.

Rettig, R. A. 1999. *Military Use of Drugs Not Yet Approved by the FDA for CW/BW Defense: Lessons from the Gulf War.* Santa Monica, CA: RAND.

Ritz, B., Yu, F., Fruin, S., Chapa, G., Shaw, G., and Harris, J. 2002. "Ambient Air Pollution and Risk of Birth Defects in Southern California." *American Journal of Epidemiology* 155 (1): 17–25.

Robbins, A. S., Brescianini, S., and Kelsey, J. L. 1997. "Regional Differences in Known Risk Factors and the Higher Incidence of Breast Cancer in San Francisco." *Journal of the National Cancer Institute* 89 (13): 960–65.

Roberts, J. T., and Toffolon-Weiss, M. 2001. *Chronicles from the Environmental Justice Front-line*. Cambridge: Cambridge University Press.

Robertson, A. 2000. "Embodying Risk, Embodying Political Rationality: Women's Accounts of Risks for Breast Cancer." *Risk and Society* 2 (2): 219–35.

Robnett, B. 1981. "African-American Women in the Civil Rights Movement, 1954–1965: Gender, Leadership, and Micromobilization." *American Journal of Sociology* 101 (6): 1661–93.

Romero, F. 2003. "The Fourth Basic Ethical Principle." Conference on Dialogues for Improving Research Ethics in Environmental and Public Health, Providence, RI, May.

Rose, F. 2000. *Coalitions across the Class Divide: Lessons from the Labor, Peace, and Environmental Movements*. Ithaca, NY: Cornell University Press.

Rosenbaum, A., Ligocki, M., and Wei, Y. 1999. *Modeling Cumulative Outdoor Concentrations of Hazardous Air Pollutants: Revised Final Report*. San Rafael, CA: Systems Applications International.

Rosenbaum, A., Axelrad, D. A., Woodruff, T. J., Wei, Y., Ligocki, M. P., and Cohen, J. P. 1999. "National Estimates of Outdoor Air Toxics Concentrations." *Journal of the Air and Waste Management Association* 49: 1138–52.

Rudel, R., Seryak, L., and Brody, J. G. 2008. "PCB-Containing Wood Floor Finish Is a Likely Source of Elevated PCBs in Residents' Blood, Household Air and Dust: A Case Study of Exposure." *Environmental Health* 7 (2).

Rudel, R. A., Geno, P., Sun, G., Yau, A., Spengler, J., Vallarino, J., and Brody, J. G. 2001. "Identification of Selected Hormonally Active Agents and Animal Mammary Carcinogens in Commercial and Residential Air and Dust Samples." *Journal of the Air and Waste Management Association* (51): 499–513.

Rudel, R. A., Camann, D. E., Spengler, J. D., Korn, L. R., and Brody, J. G. 2003. "Phthalates, Alkylphenols, Pesticides, Polybrominated Diphenyl Ethers, and Other Endocrine-Disrupting Compounds in Indoor Air and Dust." *Environmental Science and Technology* 37 (20): 4543–53.

Rudel, R. A., Attfield, K. R., Schifano, J., and Brody, J. G. 2007. "Chemicals Causing Mammary Gland Tumors in Animals Signal New Directions for Epidemiology, Chemicals Testing, and Risk Assessment for Breast Cancer Prevention." *Cancer* 109 (S12): 2635–66.

Rudestam, K. 2001. "The Important of Place: Asthmatic Children's Perceptions of Inside and Outside Environments." BA thesis, Brown University.

Ruzek, S. B. 1978. *The Women's Health Movement: Feminist Alternatives to Medical Control*. New York: Praeger.

Ruzek, S. B., Olesen, V. L., and Clarke, A. E., eds. 1997. *Women's Health: Complexities and Differences*. Columbus: Ohio State University Press.

Sadd, J., Pastor, M., Boer, T., and Snyder, L. 1999. "'Every Breath You Take': The Demographics of Toxic Air Releases in Southern California." *Economic Development Quarterly* 13 (2): 107–23.

Salzinger, L. 1991. "A Maid by Any Other Name: The Transformation of 'Dirty Work' by Central American Immigrants." In *Ethnography Unbound: Power and Resistance in the Modern Metropolis*, ed. M. Burawoy, 139–60. Berkeley: University of California Press.

Sarker, P. 2000. "Worried Locals Seek Blood Testing: Richmond Neighbors Fear Toxic Contaminants." *San Francisco Chronicle*, September 10.

Scammell, M. K., Ozonoff, D., Senier, L., Darrah, J., Brown, P., and Santos, S. 2009. "Tangible Evidence and Common Sense: Finding Meaning in a Community Health Study." *Social Science and Medicine* 68: 143–53.

Schettler, T., Solomon, G., Valenit, M., and Huddle, A. 1999. *Generations at Risk: Reproductive Health and the Environment*. Cambridge, MA: MIT Press.

Schettler, T., Stein, J., Reich, F., and Valenti, M. 2001. in *Harm's Way: Toxic Threats to Child Development*. Boston, MA: Greater Boston Physicians for Social Responsibility. Available online at www.igc.org/psr.

Schmitt, E. 1997. "Panel Criticizes Pentagon Inquiry on Gulf Illnesses." *New York Times*, January 8.

Schnaiberg, A., Watts, N., and Zimmermann, K. 1986. *Distributional Conflicts in Environmental-Resource Policy*. New York: St. Martin's Press.

Schulte, P. A. 1985. "The Epidemiologic Basis for the Notification of Subjects of Cohort Studies." *American Journal of Epidemiology* 121 (3): 351–61.

Schulte, P. A., and Singal, M. 1989. "Interpretation and Communication of the Results of Medical Field Investigations." *Journal of Occupational Medicine* 31 (7): 589–94.

———. 1996. "Ethical Issues in the Interaction with Subjects and Disclosure of Results." In *Ethics and Epidemiology*, ed. S. Coughlin and T. Beauchamp, 178–98. New York: Oxford University Press.

Schwartz, D. A., Sassaman, A. P., and Collman, G. W. 2006. "Environmental Health Sciences and the Community." *Environmental Health Perspectives* 114 (2): A80.

Schwartz, J., Gold, D., Dockery, D., Weiss, S., and Speizer, F. 1990. "Predictors of Asthma and Persistent Wheeze in a National Sample of Children in the United States: Association with Social Class, Perinatal Events and Race." *American Review of Respiratory Disease* 142: 555–62.

Schwartz, J., and Woodruff, T. 2008. *Shaping our Legacy: Reproductive Health and the Environment*. San Francisco: Program on Reproductive Health and the Environment, Department of Obstetrics, Gynecology, and Reproductive Sciences, University of California, San Francisco.

Schwarzman, M., and Wilson, M. 2009. "New Science for Chemicals Policy." *Science* 326: 1065–66.

Scott, D. N. 2009. "Confronting Chronic Pollution: A Socio-legal Analysis of Risk and Precaution." *Osgood Hall Law Journal* 46: 293–342.

Scott, P., Richards, E., and Brian, M. 1990. "Captives of Controversy: The Myth of the Neutral Social Researcher in Contemporary Scientific Controversies." *Science, Technology, and Human Values* 15: 474–94.

Scott, W. 1988. "Competing Paradigms in the Assessment of Latent Disorders: The Case of Agent Orange." *Social Problems* 35: 145–61.

Scott, W. R., and Meyer, J. W. 1992. "The Organization of Societal Sectors." In *Organizational Environments*, ed. J. W. Meyer and W. R. Scott, 129–53 Newbury Park, CA: Sage.

Sears, M. R. 1997. "Epidemiology of Childhood Asthma." *Lancet* 350 (9083): 1015–20.

Seifer, S. D., and Sisco, S. 2006. "Mining the Challenges of CBPR for Improvements in Urban Health." *Journal of Urban Health* 83 (6): 981–84.

Senier, L., Gasior Altman, R., Morello-Frosch, R., and Brown, P. 2006. "Research and Action for Environmental Health and Environmental Justice: A Report on the Brown University Contested Illnesses Research Group." *Critical Mass Bulletin* (Newsletter of the Collective Behavior and Social Movements section of the American Sociological Association), 3–6.

Sexton, K., and Adgate, J. 1999. "Looking at Environmental Justice from an Environmental Health Perspective." *Journal of Exposure Analysis and Environmental Epidemiology* 9 (1): 3–8.

Sexton, K., Needham, L., and Pirkle, J. 2004. "Human Biomonitoring of Environmental Chemicals: Measuring Chemicals in Human Tissues Is the 'Gold Standard' for Assessing Exposure to Pollution." *American Scientist* 92: 38–41.

Seydlitz, R., Spencer, J. W., and Lundskow, G. 1994. "Media Presentations of a Hazard Event and the Public's Response: An Empirical Examination." *International Journal of Mass Emergencies and Disasters* 12: 279–79.

Shalowitz, D. I., and Miller, F. G. 2005. "Disclosing Individual Results of Clinical Research: Implications of Respect for Participants." *Journal of the American Medical Association* 294 (6): 737–40.

Shapiro, M. 2007. *Exposed: The Toxic Chemistry of Everyday Products and What's at Stake for American Power.* White River Junction, VT: Chelsea Green.

Sharabi, Y., Danon, Y., Berkenstadt, H., Almog, S., Mimouni-Block, D. S., and Atsmon, J. 1991. "Survey of Symptoms following Intake of Pyridostigmine during the Persian Gulf War." *Israeli Journal of Medical Sciences* 27: 656–58.

Sharp, R. R., and Foster, M. 2002. "Community Involvement in the Ethical Review of Genetic Research: Lessons from American Indian and Alaska Native Populations." *Environmental Health Perspectives* 110 (Supp. 2): 145–48.

Sheehan, H. E., and Wedeen, R. P. 1993. *Toxic Circles: Environmental Hazards from the Workplace into the Community.* New Brunswick, NJ: Rutgers University Press.

Shendell, D., Barnett, C., and Boese, S. 2004. "Science-Based Recommendations to Prevent or Reduce Potential Exposure to Biological, Chemical, and Physical Agents in Schools." *Journal of School Health* 74 (10): 390–96.

Shenon, P. 1996a. "Advisers Condemn Pentagon Review of Gulf Ailments." *New York Times*, November 8.

———. 1996b. "Gulf War Panel Reviews Researcher's Ouster." *New York Times*, December 24.

———. 1997a. "Defense Secretary Vows Thorough Inquiry on Gulf War Illnesses." *New York Times*, March 6.

——— 1997b. "Half of Gulf-Illness Panel Now Calls Gas a Possible Factor." *New York Times*, August 19.

——. 1997c. "House Committee Assails Pentagon on Gulf War Ills." *New York Times,* October 26.

Shepard, P. M., Northridge, M. E., Prakash, S., and Stover, G. 2002. "Preface: Advancing Environmental Justice through Community-Based Participatory Research." Special issue of *Environmental Health Perspectives* 110 (Supp. 2): 139–40.

Shonkoff, S., Morello-Frosch, R., Pastor, M., and Sadd, J. 2009. "Minding the Climate Gap: Implications of Environmental Health Inequities for Mitigation Policies in California." *Environmental Justice* 2 (4): 173–78.

Shostak, S. 2004. "Environmental Justice and Genomics: Acting on the Futures of Environmental Health." *Science as Culture* 13 (4): 539–62.

——. 2005. "The Emergence of Toxicogenomics: A Case Study of Molecularization." *Social Studies of Science* 35 (3): 367–403.

Sightline Institute. 2004. "Flame Retardants in the Bodies of Pacific Northwest Residents: A Study of Toxic Body Burdens." www.sightline.org, accessed November 2, 2007.

Silent Spring Institute. 2007. *The Cape Cod Breast Cancer and Environment Study: Results of the First Three Years of Study.* Newton, MA: Silent Spring Institute.

——. 2009. *Breast Cancer and Environment Study.* Silent Spring Institute, www .silentspring.org/our-research/communities-high-breast-cancer-rates/cape-cod-breast-cancer-and-environment-study, accessed June 4, 2010.

Snow, D. A., and Benford, R. D. 1988. "Ideology, Frame Resonance, and Participant Mobilization." *International Social Movement Research* 1: 197–217.

Snow, D. A., Rochford, B., Worden, S. K., and Benford, R. D. 1986. "Frame Alignment Processes, Micromobilization, and Movement Participation." *American Sociological Review* 51: 464–81.

Spector, M., and Kitsuse, J. 1977. *Constructing Social Problems.* Menlo Park, CA: Cummings.

Spencer, J. W., and Triche, E. 1994. "Media Constructions of Risk and Safety: Differential Framings of Hazard Events." *Sociological Inquiry* 64 (2): 199–213.

Speth, J. G. 2004. *Red Sky at Morning: America and the Crisis of the Global Environment.* New Haven, CT: Yale University Press.

Srinivasan, S., O'Fallon, L., and Dearry, A. 2003. "Creating Healthy Communities, Health Homes, Healthy People: Initiating a Research Agenda on the Built Environment and Public Health." *American Journal of Public Health* 93: 1446–50.

SRP (Superfund Research Program). n.d. Description on home page. www.niehs.nih.gov/research/supported/srp, accessed January 4, 2008.

Staggenborg, S. 1986. "Coalition Work in the Pro-choice Movement: Organizational and Environmental Opportunities and Obstacles." *Social Problems* 33 (5): 374–90.

Stallings, R. 1990. "Media Discourse and the Social Construction of Risk." *Social Problems* 37: 80–95.

Star, S. L., and Greisemer, J. R. 1989. "Institutional Ecology, 'Translations,' and Boundary Objects: Amateurs and Professionals in Berkeley's Museum of Vertebrate Zoology, 1907–39." *Social Studies of Science* 19: 387–420.

Stokstad, E. 2004. "Pollution Gets Personal." *Science* 304: 1892–94.

Strand, K., Marullo, S., Cutforth, N., Stoecker, R., and Donohue, P. 2003. *Community-Based Research and Higher Education: Principles and Practices.* San Francisco: Jossey-Bass.

Strandman, T., Koistinen, J., and Vartiainen, T. 2000. "Polybrominated Diphenyl Ethers (PBDEs) in Placenta and Human Milk." *Organohalogen Compounds* 47: 61–64.

Suk, W. A., and Anderson, B. E. 1999. "A Holistic Approach to Environmental Health Research." *Environmental Health Perspectives* 107 (7): A338–39.

Sullivan, K., Krengel, M., Proctor, S., Devine, S., Heeren, T., and White, R. 2003. "Cognitive Functioning in Treatment-Seeking Gulf War Veterans: Pyridostigmine Bromide Use and PTSD." *Journal of Psychopathology and Behavioral Assessment* 25: 95–103.

Sullivan, M., Kone, A., Senturia, K. D., Chrisman, N. J., Ciske, S. J., and Krieger, J. W. 2001. "Researcher and Researched-Community Perspectives: Toward Bridging the Gap." *Health Education and Behavior* 28 (2): 130–49.

Szasz, A. 1994. *Ecopopulism: Toxic Waste and the Movement for Environmental Justice.* Minneapolis: University of Minnesota Press.

———. 2007. *Shopping Our Way to Safety: How We Changed from Protecting the Environment to Protecting Ourselves.* Minneapolis: University of Minnesota Press.

Sze, J. 2007. *Noxious New York: The Racial Politics of Urban Health and Environmental Justice.* Cambridge, MA: MIT Press.

Sze, J., and Prakash, S. 2004. "Human Genetics, Environment, and Communities of Color: Ethical and Social Implications." *Environmental Health Perspectives* 112: 740–45.

Taylor, D. 2003. "Building Networks to Assist in Community Research Protections." Conference on Dialogues for Improving Research Ethics in Environmental and Public Health, Providence, RI, May.

Thompson, H. J. 1992. "Effect of Amount and Type of Exercise on Experimentally Induced Breast Cancer." *Advances in Experimental Medicine and Biology (USA)* 322: 61–71.

Thornton, J. W., McCally, M., and Houlihan, J. 2002. "Biomonitoring of Industrial Pollutants: Health and Policy Implications of the Chemical Body Burden." *Public Health Reports* 117 (4): 315–23.

Tickner, J., and Hoppin, P. 2000. "Children's Environmental Health: A Case Study in Implementing the Precautionary Principle." *International Journal of Environmental Health* 6 (4): 281–88.

Tilly, C. 1978. *From Mobilization to Revolution.* Reading, MA: Addison-Wesley.

Timmermans, S., and Berg, M. 2003. "The Practice of Medical Technology." *Sociology of Health and Illness* 25 (3): 97–114.

Toxics Use Reduction Institute. 2003. *TURNing Partnerships into Progress in Massachusetts Communities: A Retrospective of the Toxics Use Reduction Networking (TURN) Grantmaking Program.* Lowell: University of Massachusetts, Lowell.

Tuite, J. J., III. 1997. Testimony to the Presidential Advisory Committee on Gulf War Veterans' Illnesses. Salt Lake City, UT. Cited in Committee on Government Reform and Oversight, *Gulf War Veterans' Illnesses: VA, DOD Continue to Resist Strong Evidence Linking Toxic Causes to Chronic Health Effects.* Second report. Washington, DC: House of Representatives.

US Army Environmental Health Agency. 1994. *Final Report: Kuwait Oil Fire Health Risk Assessment Report No. 39-26-L19291.* Brooks Air Force Base, TX: Department of the Air Force.

US Bureau of Labor Statistics. 2007. *Union Members in 2006.* Washington, DC: United States Department of Labor.

US Department of Health and Human Services, National Institutes of Health. Public Welfare: Protection of Human Subjects. Revised 2005. 45 CFR §46.103.

US Environmental Protection Agency. 1992. *Environmental Equity: Reducing Risk for All Communities.* Washington, DC: US Environmental Protection Agency.

———. 1998. *Cumulative Exposure Project.* US Environmental Protection Agency, www.epa.gov/CumulativeExposure, accessed June 21, 2003.

———. 2000. "EPA Orders Extensive Cleanup of Mass. Military Reservation on Cape Cod." Washington, DC: Environmental Protection Agency, www.epa.gov/region1/pr/2000/010700.html, accessed June 1, 2007.

US General Accounting Office. 1997. *Gulf War Illnesses: Improved Monitoring of Clinical Progress and Reexamination of Research Emphasis Are Needed.* Washington, DC: General Accounting Office.

———. 1999a. *Indoor Pollution: Status of Federal Research Activities* GAO/RCED-99-254. Washington, DC: US Government Printing Office.

———. 1999b. Pesticides: *Uses, Effects, and Alternatives to Pesticides in Schools.* Washington, DC: US General Accounting Office.

———. 2004. *Federal Gulf War Illnesses Research Strategy Needs Reassessment.* Report to the Chairman, Subcommittee on National Security, Emerging Threats, and International Relations, Committee on Government Reform, House of Representatives. Washington, DC: General Accounting Office.

US Preventive Services Task Force. 2009. "Screening for Breast Cancer: U.S. Preventive Services Task Force Recommendation Statement." *Annals of Internal Medicine* 151 (10): 716–26.

Usher, P. J., Baikie, M., Demmer, M., Nakashima, D., Stevenson, M. G., and Stiles, M. 1995. *Communicating about Contaminants in Country Food: The Experience of Aboriginal Communities.* Ottawa, ON: Inuit Tapiriit Kanatami.

Van Dyke, N. 2003. "Crossing Movement Boundaries: Factors That Facilitate Coalition Protest by American College Students, 1930–1990." *Social Problems* 50 (2): 226–50.

Van Vliet, P., Knape, M., de Hartog, J., Janseen, N., Harssema, H., and Brunekreef, B. 1997. "Motor Vehicle Exhaust and Chronic Respiratory Symptoms in Children Living near Freeways." *Environmental Research* 74 (2): 122–32.

Vasquez, V. B., Minkler, M., and Shepard, P. 2006. "Promoting Environmental Health Policy through Community Based Participatory Research: A Case Study from Harlem, New York." *Journal of Urban Health: Bulletin of the New York Academy of Medicine* 83 (1): 101–10.

Vastag, B. 2001. "CDC Unveils First Report on Toxins in People." *Journal of the American Medical Association* 285: 1827–28.

Vyner, H. 1988. *Invisible Trauma: The Psychosocial Effects of the Invisible Environmental Contaminants.* Lexington, MA: D. C. Heath.

Wagner, W. E. 1997. "Choosing Ignorance in the Manufacture of Toxic Products." *Cornell Law Review* 82: 773–855.

Wallerstein, N., and Duran, B. 2003. "The Conceptual, Historical, and Practice Roots of Community Based Participatory Research and Related Participatory Traditions." In *Community Based Participatory Research for Health*, ed. M. Minkler and N. Wallerstein, 27–52. San Francisco: Jossey-Bass.

Washburn, R. 2007a. "Human Biomonitoring and the Lived Experience of Body Burdens." Annual meeting of the Society for the Social Study of Science, Montreal, October.

———. 2007b. "In Pursuit of the Molecule: Making and Making Sense of Chemical Body Burdens in the United States." Conference on the New Chemical Bodies: Biomonitoring, Body Burden, and Endocrine Disruptors, Philadelphia, March.

Weijer, C. 1999. "Protecting Communities in Research: Philosophical and Pragmatic Challenges." *Cambridge Quarterly of Healthcare Ethics* 8: 501–13.

Weinberg, A. 1972. "Science and Transcience." *Minerva* 10 (2): 209–22.

Weisman, C. S. 2000. "Breast Cancer Policymaking." In *Breast Cancer: Society Shapes an Epidemic,* ed. A. Kasper and S. Ferguson, 213–34. New York: Palgrave.

Wesseley, S., and Freedman, L. 2006. "Reflections on Gulf War Illness." *Philosophical Transactions of the Royal Society, Biological Sciences* 361 (1468): 721–30.

West, D. W., Glaser, S., and Prehn, A. W. 1998. *Status of Breast Cancer Research in the San Francisco Bay Area.* Union City, CA: Northern California Cancer Center.

Whyatt, R. M., Rauh, V., Barr, D. B., Camann, D. E., Andrews, H. F., Garfinkel, R., Hoepner, L. A., et al. 2004. "Prenatal Insecticide Exposures and Birth Weight and Length among An Urban Minority Cohort." *Environmental Health Perspectives* 112: 1125–32.

Williams, D. R., Sternthal, M., and Wright, R. J. 2009. "Social Determinants: Taking the Social Context of Asthma Seriously." *Pediatrics* 123 (Supp. 3, 3): S174–S184.

Williams, G. 1984. "The Genesis of Chronic Illness: Narrative Reconstruction." *Sociology of Health and Illness* 6: 175–200.

Williams, P. R. 2004. "Health Risk Communication Using Comparative Risk Analyses." *Journal of Exposure Analysis and Environmental Epidemiology* 14: 498–515.

Williams, S. J., Birke, L., and Bendelow, G. A., eds. 2003. *Debating Biology: Sociological Reflections on Health, Medicine, and Society.* London: Routledge.

Wilson, M. P., and Schwarzman, M. R. 2009. "Toward a New U.S. Chemicals Policy: Rebuilding the Foundation to Advance New Science, Green Chemistry, and Environmental Health." *Environmental Health Perspectives* 117: 1202–9.

Winn, D. M. 2005. "Science and Society: The Long Island Breast Cancer Study Project." *Nature Reviews Cancer* 5 (12): 986–94.

Wolfe, J., Erickson, D. J., Sharkansky, E. J., King, D. W., and King, L. A. 1999. "Course and Predictors of Posttraumatic Stress Disorder among Gulf War Veterans: A Prospective Analysis." *Journal of Consulting and Clinical Psychology* 67 (4): 520–28.

Wolff, M. S., Toniolo, P. G., Lee, E. W., Rivera, M., and Dubin, N. 1993. "Blood Levels of Organochlorine Residues and Risk of Breast Cancer." *Journal of the National Cancer Institute* 85 (8): 648–52.

Wolfson, M. 2001. *The Fight against Big Tobacco: The Movement, the State, and the Public's Health.* New York: Aldine de Gruyter.

Woolcock, A. J., and Peat, J. K. 1997. "Evidence for the Increase in Asthma Worldwide." *Ciba Foundation Symposia* 206: 122–34.

World Wildlife Federation. 2004. "Bad Blood? A Survey of Chemicals in the Blood of European Ministers." www.wwf.fi/wwf/www/uploads/pdf/badblood.pdf, accessed May 10, 2011.

Wu, N., McClean, M. D., Brown, P., Ashengrau, A., and Webster, T. F. 2009. "Participant Experiences in Breastmilk Biomonitoring Study: A Qualitative Assessment." *Environmental Health* 8 (4).

Wynne, B. 1996. "May the Sheep Safely Graze? A Reflexive View of the Expert-Lay Knowledge Divide." In *Risk, Environment, and Modernity: Towards a New Ecology,* ed. S. Lash, B. Szerszynski, and B. Wynne, 4–83. Thousand Oaks, CA: Sage.

Zald, M. N., and Useem, B. 1987. "Movement and Countermovement Interaction: Mobilization, Tactics, and State Involvement." In *Social Movements in an Organizational Society,* ed. M. N. Zald and J. McCarthy, 247–72. New Brunswick, NJ: Transaction Publishers.

Zald et al. 2009 See ch 2, n1.

Zavestoski, S. 2009. "The Struggle for Justice in Bhopal: A New/Old Breed of Transnational Social Movement." *Global Social Policy* 9 (3): 383–407.

Zavestoski, S., and Brown, P., eds. 2005. *Social Movements in Health.* Oxford: Wiley-Blackwell.

Zavestoski, S., Morello-Frosch, R., Brown, P., Mayer, B., McCormick, S., and Altman, R. G. 2004. "Embodied Health Movements and Challenges to the Dominant Epidemiological Paradigm." *Research in Social Movements, Conflict and Change* 25: 253–78.

Zones, J. S. 2000. "Profits from Pain: The Political Economy of Breast Cancer." In *Breast Cancer: Society Shapes an Epidemic,* ed. A. S. Kasper and S. J. Ferguson, 119–52. New York: St. Martin's Press.

Zota, A. R., Rudel, R., Morello-Frosch, R., and Brody, J. G. 2008. "Elevated House Dust and Serum Concentrations of PBDEs in California: Unintended Consequences of Furniture Flammability Standards?" *Environmental Science and Technology* 42: 8158–64.

CONTRIBUTORS

CRYSTAL ADAMS, Department of Sociology, Brown University

REBECCA GASIOR ALTMAN, Community Health Program, Tufts University

MARA AVERICK, Science and Technology Studies Program, Brown University

JULIA GREEN BRODY, Silent Spring Institute, Newton, Massachusetts

PHIL BROWN, Department of Sociology and Center for Environmental Studies, Brown University

ALISON COHEN, School of Public Health, University of California, Berkeley

ALISSA CORDNER, Department of Sociology, Brown University

SARAH FORT, Harvard University Law School

ELIZABETH HOOVER, Center for the Study of Race and Ethnicity, Brown University

BENJAMIN HUDSON, Department of Geological Sciences, Institute of Arctic and Alpine Research, and Community Surface Dynamics Modeling System, University of Colorado

MEADOW LINDER, Department of Sociology, Brown University

THEO LUEBKE, Duke University Divinity School

MERCEDES LYSON, Department of Sociology, Brown University

JOSHUA MANDELBAUM, Lane and Waterman LLP, Davenport, Iowa

BRIAN MAYER, Department of Sociology, Criminology, and Law, University of Florida

SABRINA MCCORMICK, Department of Environmental and Occupational Health, School of Public Health and Health Services, George Washington University

RACHEL MORELLO-FROSCH, Department of Environmental Science, Policy, and Management and School of Public Health, University of California, Berkeley

MANUEL PASTOR, Department of American Studies and Program on Environmental and Regional Equity, University of Southern California

CARLA PÉREZ, Movement Generation Justice and Ecology Project, Oakland, California

RUTHANN A. RUDEL, Silent Spring Institute, Newton, Massachusetts

JAMES SADD, Department of Environmental Sciences, Occidental College

LAURA SENIER, Department of Community and Environmental Sociology and Department of Family Medicine, University of Wisconsin–Madison

RUTH SIMPSON, Department of Sociology, Bryn Mawr College

REBECCA TILLSON, Jackson Hole Conservation Alliance, Wyoming

STEPHEN ZAVESTOSKI, Department of Sociology and Environmental Studies Program, University of San Francisco

DEPs. *See* dominant epidemiological paradigms

developing countries, research opportunities in, 266

diesel exhaust, 115, 116

direct action, 196; in asthma activism, 115, 120; in the environmental breast cancer movement, 62, 157, 159

dominant epidemiological paradigms (DEPs), 12, 24, 25*fig.*, 84, 95–96; asthma, 108; breast cancer, 51–52, 55, 147, 149–50, 166, 167, 266; contestation and, 84–85, 96, 105, 106; EHMs as challenges to, 10, 18, 20, 24–27; field analysis and, 51–52; Gulf War–related illnesses, 82, 84–86, 95–98, 102–6; media interaction with, 85–86; politicized collective illness identity and, 23

Dotson, Ethel, 227

Downs, A., 86

EBCM. *See* environmental breast cancer movement

ECHO (Environmentally Compromised Home Ownership) loan program, 217–19, 220

economic arguments against health/environmental reforms, 170, 178, 190, 197, 204, 206

ecosocial histories, 127–28, 144; exposure responses and, 127–28, 139–40, 141–42

EDCs. *See* endocrine-disrupting compounds

Edelstein, Michael, 35, 39, 127

EHMs (embodied health movements), 10, 15, 16–32; as boundary movements, 24, 27–29; defining characteristics, 16, 18–21; as DEP challenges, 10, 18, 19, 24–27; embodied illness experience, 18–19; historical context analysis, 48–49, 62; interactions with wider social movements, 30–31; nonstate activist targets, 31; policy goals and opportunities, 26–27; political opportunities, 30–31; politicized collective illness identity, 15, 16, 18, 22–24; research and, 19–21; research background, 17

Ehrenreich, Barbara, 15

EJLRI (Environmental Justice League of Rhode Island), 272, 274

embodied exposure experience. *See* exposure experience *entries*

embodied health movements. *See* EHMs

embodied illness experience, 16, 18–19, 54. *See also specific illnesses*

empowerment, 28, 44, 109, 111–12, 116–17, 162, 167, 252

ENACT (Environmental Neighborhood Awareness Committee of Tiverton), 214, 217, 218*fig.*, 220, 263

endocrine-disrupting compounds (EDCs), 8, 144, 150, 247, 254

endocrine-disruptor hypothesis, 26, 43, 51

environmental breast cancer movement (EBCM), 12, 18, 27–28, 147–68; activist reflections, 164–66; anticorporate stance, 148, 150–51, 156, 157, 159, 160–61; as boundary movement, 27–29, 148–49, 153–54, 156, 164–65; breast cancer DEP challenges, 51–52, 55, 150, 166, 167; case study methodology, 151; citizen-science alliances in, 20–21, 148–49, 151, 154, 158, 159, 161–62, 164–66, 167; education initiatives, 156, 157, 158; effectiveness of, 163–64, 167; emergence of, 49, 147–48, 149–51; environmental groups/advocacy and, 153, 156, 158, 159–60; environmental justice activism, 157–58; feminism and, 163; field analysis, 47, 49–52, 50*fig.*; goals of, 148; health care access advocacy, 159; internal group interactions, 55, 56, 152; Long Island, 62, 148, 151, 152–54, 161, 162; mainstream movement and, 16, 17*fig.*, 150, 155–56, 159–60; Massachusetts, 148, 151, 154–57; media relations and coverage, 153; policy focus, 47, 161; policy goals and outcomes, 155–56, 156–57, 158–59, 262; political alliances and government relations, 153, 158; politicized illness experience, 162–64, 166; precautionary principle orientation, 148, 156, 158; radical groups and positions, 156, 159–61; San Francisco Bay Area, 148, 151, 157–61, 162; and the scientific community, 149, 152, 154, 158, 164–66; site differences, 62, 161–62. *See also* breast cancer *entries*; *specific organizations*

Environmental Cancer Prevention Center, 196

environmental causation, 26; medical treatments as environmental causes, 82–83, 106n3; research funding, 26. *See also specific conditions*

environmental health movement, 20–21

environmental justice: children's toxics exposure, 65; health inequalities and, 31–32; LAUSD toxics study implications, 71–72; policy goals, 64–65; precautionary principle and, 64, 74–75; research and, 3–4, 34, 260, 270; research needs and priorities, 71

environmental justice activism, 20–21, 23, 30, 272; ACE transit racism campaign, 115–16;

114; health tracking, 112, 121; San Francisco breast cancer efforts, 157–58. *See also* Green Cleaners Project

public participation, 4–5, 6, 19, 75; biomonitoring results communication, 234–35; contaminated community decision making, 211–12. *See also* CBPR; citizen-science alliances; community outreach

public policy. *See policy entries*

public transit, 115–16

Purcell, K., 212

pyridostigmine bromide (PB), 80, 83, 88, 90, 100–101

QSR NVivo, 194

qualitative research methods, 33–46, 264; access and trust issues, 36–37; funders and, 33, 45; history and legacy of, 35–36; hybrid quantitative-qualitative methods, 34; interviewing techniques, 38–39; objectivity, empathy, and researcher worldview, 38, 39–41; roles, reflexivity, and member validation, 41–44; sharing research data, 42, 44; study design, 37–39, 41; theoretical frameworks, 39. *See also* CBPR; field analysis; policy ethnography; research *entries*

Quandt, S. A., 235, 238

quantitative research methods, 41, 64, 264; hybrid quantitative-qualitative methods, 34; for risk assessment, 64, 71

RAC (Research Advisory Committee on Gulf War Veterans' Illnesses) report, 79, 82, 87–88, 98, 100, 101, 106–7n4, 107n5; reactions to, 102, 103, 104–5. *See also* Gulf War–related illnesses

race disparities: asthma incidence, 110–11, 114; breast cancer incidence, 158; in LAUSD toxics exposure study, 69, 69*fig.*, 70–71; lead exposure, 74. *See also* environmental justice *entries*

Race for the Cure, 160

racism, in the health care system, 30

RaDAR Committee, Massachusetts DPH, 253, 254, 257

RAND Corporation research, Gulf War–related illnesses, 87

Rapp, R., 54

Ray, Raka, 48

Reagan, Ronald, 195–96

The Real Disaster is Above Ground (Kroll-Smith and Couch), 35, 37–38

REEP (Roxbury Environmental Empowerment Project), 116

reflexivity, in research, 39–44

regulation: viewed as jobs threat, 190. *See also* air quality regulation; toxics regulation

regulatory agencies: contaminated community residents and, 211, 221. *See also specific agencies*

Reich, Michael, 35–36

research. *See* dominant epidemiological paradigms; research *entries* below; science; *specific illnesses*

Research Advisory Committee on Gulf War Veterans' Illnesses. *See* RAC

research collaborations, 7–10, 43–44, 211, 269–70, 271, 272–74; field analysis and, 52; IRB concerns, 248–51, 256–57; trust issues, 154, 211, 212, 219–20. *See also* CBPR; citizen-science alliances; coalition dynamics; interdisciplinarity; *specific projects*

research data reporting, 42, 44, 231, 246, 270–71; CBPR-IRB conflicts over, 247, 251–54, 257–58; ethical issues, 228, 243–44, 251–52; research opportunities, 259; right to know/access rights, 13, 126, 128–29; voluntary sharing of results, 237–38, 243, 252. *See also* biomonitoring results communication; community outreach; exposure information reporting and responses; research translation; right to know

research ethics: Belmont Report principles, 231, 245–46, 249, 252, 253, 254, 258; issues in qualitative methods, 38, 39–44; teaching, 265

research evaluation, 58, 61, 63, 265

research funding, 26, 264, 270, 273, 274; breast cancer, 149, 151–54, 156–57, 158; challenging funding decisions, 27; environmental causation, 26; interdisciplinary research teams and, 264; IRB requirements and protocols, 237–38, 239–40, 243; lobbying restrictions and, 161. *See also specific funders and projects*

research methods, 11; new approaches, 46–48; sharing, 271. *See also* CBPR; field analysis; policy ethnography; qualitative research methods

Research Priorities for Airborne Particulate Matter, 113